SOVEREIGN NECROPOLIS

SOVEREIGN NECROPOLIS

THE POLITICS OF DEATH IN SEMI-COLONIAL SIAM

TRAIS PEARSON

CORNELL UNIVERSITY PRESS
Ithaca and London

First published 2020 by Cornell University Press

Library of Congress Cataloging-in-Publication Data

Names: Pearson, Trais, 1979– author.
Title: Sovereign necropolis : the politics of death in semi-colonial Siam / Trais Pearson.
Description: Ithaca : Cornell University Press, 2020. | Includes bibliographical references and index.
Identifiers: LCCN 2019026365 (print) | LCCN 2019026366 (ebook) | ISBN 9781501740152 (cloth) | ISBN 9781501740176 (pdf) | ISBN 9781501740169 (ebook)
Subjects: LCSH: Death—Political aspects—Thailand—History. | Death—Proof and certification—Thailand—History. | Thanatology—Thailand—History. | Political culture—Thailand—History. | Thailand—Foreign Relations—1782–1945.
Classification: LCC HQ1073.5.T5 P33 2020 (print) | LCC HQ1073.5.T5 (ebook) | DDC 306.09593—dc23
LC record available at https://lccn.loc.gov/2019026365
LC ebook record available at https://lccn.loc.gov/2019026366

To Phi Pha and the Sukwong Family, who took in a twenty-one-year-old wanderer and helped him find his way.
To Su-Ping, Quinn, and Josephine—the life and light in my world.

Archives do not record experience so much as its absence; they mark the point where an experience is missing from its proper place, and what is returned to us in an archive may well be something we never possessed in the first place.
—Sven Spieker, *The Big Archive: Art from Bureaucracy*

The chronicler, who recounts events without distinguishing between the great and the small, thereby accounts for the truth, that nothing which has ever happened is to be given as lost to history.
—Walter Benjamin, *Selected Writings, Volume 4, 1938–1940*

CONTENTS

Illustrations

NOTE ON NAMING CONVENTIONS, SOURCES, TRANSCRIPTION, AND TRANSLATION

The nation-state of Thailand was known as the Kingdom of Siam until 1939. In the interest of historical accuracy, I refer to the polity and its population as Siam and Siamese, respectively, throughout most of this book. I have followed the Royal Thai General System of Transcription (1999) with some minor changes: I have transliterated "จ" as "*j*" when it appears in initial position (as in *jao phraya* or *jao phanak ngan*). Other exceptions have been made to conform to recognized spelling conventions in the case of proper names (e.g., Chulalongkorn).

I have chosen to retain Thai-language titles and honorifics more or less in accordance with their historical usages in the archival documents. These include markers of age, gender, (commoner) social status, and ethnicity such as *amdaeng* (Miss), *nai* (Mister), and *jin* (the ethnic marker for a male of Chinese birth or ancestry). Readers will also note three distinct titles used to signify medical expertise: (1) the English-language title Doctor (Dr.) was used to refer almost exclusively to Western-born and Western-educated physicians; (2) the Thai term *phaet* was also used in reference to these doctors, as well as Thai (or other non-Westerners) whose medical training was recognized as being in the Western tradition; (3) the term *mo* was typically used to refer to physicians trained in Siamese or local Asian medical traditions. Finally, the title *phra* was used in two contexts: when it appears before a Buddhist monk's personal name, the term is an honorific meaning "Venerable." When used before a civil servant's name, it signifies a bureaucratic rank, as in Phra Thep Phlu, with *phraya* and *jao phraya* signifying elevated ranks or offices. In the case of individuals who appear throughout the study but whose titles and ranks may have changed along with their office, I have elected to use a single, consistent honorific to aid in recognition; such is the case with Prince Naret Worarit, who occupied the office of Minister of the Capital during seminal years covered in this book.

The Siamese currency was in flux during the transitional period discussed in this book. Foreign-language sources most commonly used the Portuguese/Malay loanword *tical* when referring to the Siamese currency until 1897, when it was standardized using a decimal system whereby one hundred *satang* equaled one *baht*. The term *catty* (plural: catties; Thai: *chang*) referred to a larger denomination of the Siamese currency; it was based on a standardized Chinese measure of weight. One catty amounted to eighty baht (or *ticals*).

The empirical core of this book is a collection of documents from the National Archives of Thailand labeled "Death by various causes" (*tai duai het tang tang*; NA R5 N 23). The collection consists of the documentary records of inquests, or investigations into cases of unnatural or suspicious deaths in the Siamese capital city beginning in 1890. They are a diverse and uneven lot, containing voices ranging from illiterate subalterns to the king himself, often treading on every rung of the cosmopolitan social ladder in between. In making sense of and ultimately translating portions of these documents, I have benefited greatly from the help of Sirinan Bunsri and Ngampit Jagacinski. Any errors, of course, are my own.

In the only other work of published scholarship to make extensive use of the inquest files, Takashi Tomosugi has analyzed the documents as evidence of the changing nature of urban lives at that time; see his *Reminiscences of Old Bangkok: Memory and the Identification of a Changing Society* ([Tokyo]: The Institute of Oriental Culture, University of Tokyo, 1993), 131–50. These documents deserve much greater attention, and I urge scholars to pay them their due. Like the dead whose passings they recount, they have been hiding in plain sight for too long.

SOVEREIGN NECROPOLIS

Introduction

> The life of sovereign power is a life that is lived in
> the shadow of death—many deaths, nameless and
> innumerable, disavowed and forgotten.
>
> —Stuart J. Murray, "Thanatopolitics: On the Use
> of Death for Mobilizing Political Life"

On July 19, 1906, the queen consort of King Ch-
ulalongkorn of Siam was involved in a fatal car accident when the motorcar
she was traveling in struck and killed a pedestrian in central Bangkok. Although
the queen informed the king of the event the next morning, seven days passed
before news of the accident reached him through official channels in the Siamese bureaucracy. Chulalongkorn was incensed. He penned a letter to the responsible party, noting, "Since time immemorial, whenever a human being
died under unusual circumstances—such as being struck by lightning, burned
in a fire, drowning, or being stabbed or shot—whether by an act of the Gods
or not, if it happened in this city it was the duty of the Ministry of the Capital
to report it to the king without delay."[1]

Chulalongkorn's letter might be seen as in keeping with a paternalistic vein
in the Thai monarchical tradition. It harkens back to a pastoral kingdom where
the subjects did not want owing to the "fish in the water and rice in the fields,"
and where petitions could be voiced to the sovereign himself, who hung a bell
over the palace gate and "if any commoner in the land has a grievance which
sickens his belly and gripes his heart . . . he goes and strikes the bell which the
King has hung there; King Ramkhamhaeng, the ruler of the kingdom, hears
the call; he goes and questions the man, examines the case, and decides it justly
for him."[2] In this reading, Chulalongkorn's concern for the dead resounds as

a beneficent extension of the Siamese king's traditional mandate as "Lord of Life" (*jao chiwit*) to include jurisdiction over the dead as well. There is, however, an alternative reading, one that hints at darker realities of modern Thai history. In that view, the sovereign's concern for the dead is not a simple ethnographic anomaly, a testament to some ahistorical facet of Thai culture, but is rather a vision of Siamese political culture that intersected in crucial ways with the reality of the kingdom's semi-colonial status and the pragmatic actions being taken by the state to address those conditions.

By the turn of the twentieth century, the Siamese king's sovereign power over both the living and the dead had been dramatically curtailed. Since the mid-nineteenth century, unequal trade treaties had granted extraterritorial legal privileges to foreign residents. Consular courts administered justice to the growing contingent of foreigners residing in Siam, including immigrants from across Asia who likewise claimed privileged status as "protégés" (protected subjects) of the imperial powers. Bangkok, the Siamese royal capital, a cosmopolitan city of some half a million residents, thus became a plural legal arena, and death—especially death under unnatural, accidental, or suspicious circumstances, which might entail civil or criminal legal action—became a matter of transnational concern and expert intervention.[3] Barristers, physicians, police, consular officials, juries, and newspaper editors all disputed the Siamese monarch's claim to power over life and death, raising questions of evidence, liability, and jurisdiction. *Sovereign Necropolis* attends to these debates over the dead and injured and asks what they might reveal about the practice of sovereign politics in the (semi-)colonial world.

The social, cultural, and political lives of the dead have long been a topic of concern for anthropologists, who have endeavored to capture the symbolic, spectral, and affective presence and agency of the dead.[4] All of these forms of agency and concern for the dead are well attested to in the interdisciplinary field of Thai studies. Whether as victims of political violence or the looming spirits of those who suffered financial ruin or displacement by new urban lifeways, the dead figure prominently in much recent anthropological scholarship on Thai society.[5] The dead, however, are much more than just symbols and specters. They have a physical presence in the form of material remains that require diverse forms of care ranging from the custodial to the curatorial and can prompt forms of attention ranging from filial to forensic.[6] In their very physicality, the dead offer a carnal and charnel rejoinder to anthropological work fixated on the spectral and symbolic.[7] Yet these practical forms of engagement with the dead can themselves inspire a great deal of angst in the unaccustomed observer, as noted by Michael Taussig and by recent work in the field of death studies.[8]

In its early days, death studies scholarship tended to focus on longitudinal studies of deathways in homogeneous (largely European) cultural contexts.[9] By contrast, studies attuned to the ways in which cross-cultural encounters "challenged established Western deathways" or "the ways in which empire building and evangelization invested death with new significance for colonized communities" have been comparatively rare.[10] But the few notable exceptions, including Erik Seeman's *Death in the New World* and Vincent Brown's *The Reaper's Garden*, have helped to establish that historically death has been "one of the most important channels of communication between peoples of different cultures"—an insight that is borne out by modern Thai history.[11]

For foreign residents and visitors to Siam, indigenous deathways have historically been a topic of macabre fascination, ethnographic interest, and medical scrutiny. Travelogues attest to the fact that Wat Saket, a Buddhist temple located just outside of the city walls that was renowned for its role as a charnel ground, was an essential stop on the itinerary of any adventurous foreign visitor to the Siamese capital city in the late nineteenth century. "Oh! no I will not die here," vowed Ludovic Marquis de Beauvoir (1846–1929) after witnessing a corpse—seemingly resurrected—dance on top of a funeral pyre at Wat Saket, limbs flailing as the heat of the pyre scorched tendons and connective tissue.[12] One particularly graphic news item from the late nineteenth century chronicles the execution of a Siamese criminal who had been convicted of a brutal murder by bludgeoning while in the commission of a robbery.[13] Five foreign journalists attended the gruesome proceedings, along with an American physician named Dr. T. Heyward Hays. After the executioner's sword had severed the spinal column of the condemned man, Hays knelt down to take his pulse. Eyes fixed on the halting but rhythmic ticks of the seconds hand on his watch, Hays kept count as the pulse of the deceased grew fainter under the pressure of his pointer and middle fingers. The execution was very much a Siamese affair, but like so many other aspects of life and death in the colonial world at the end of the nineteenth century, Western science brought a new form of scrutiny to bear on it. The uninvited gaze of the foreign residents signaled the arrival of a new manner of concern for the dead and dying in the Siamese capital.

It is perhaps not surprising that such forms of disciplinary and charnel pageantry should have provoked the interest of foreign observers, but this study calls attention to quotidian and forgotten instances of death and injury in the city's streets, canals, gardens, and temples. Specifically, it explores the Siamese state's burgeoning interest in the fate of its dead and injured subjects and the increasingly systematic ways in which it investigated the circumstances of their passing and attempted to assert their rights in the plural legal arena of fin-de-siècle Bangkok. In contrast with the public spectacle of executions and the gruesome labors of undertakers, this study reveals the progressive sequestration of the dead as their bodies increasingly became the terrain of expert concern and intervention.

Sovereign Necropolis argues that the investigation of unnatural death was an early—and unlikely—site of direct interaction between the state and its subjects. By bringing agents of the state into direct relations of concern with its previously anonymous subjects, the inquest effectively sidestepped the hierarchical social relations that characterized the traditional sociopolitical order in Siam. It therefore stands in stark contrast to institutions like corvée labor and taxation, for example, whereby interactions between state and subject were mediated by the social relations of the feudal order and the tax-farming system, respectively.[14] Although these might appear *prima facie* to be liberalizing developments consistent with a growing recognition of subjects as rights-bearing citizens, I argue that in fact they were not. Although unnatural death became a new interface between the state and its subjects, it was not a trajectory that tended toward democratic politics or the formation of recognizable forms of civil society. Rather, the new legal and medicolegal channels of concern for the bodies of Siamese subjects maintained and even bolstered traditional forms of authority and authoritative political culture both within and outside of the state bureaucracy.

Moreover, I argue that the adoption of these forms of forensic expertise was part of a broader implementation of a conservative grammar of rule that spoke to conditions ranging from the nature of legal and political subjectivity to the metaphysical constitution of the social world. In short, *Sovereign Necropolis* makes the case that reforms in the arena of civil law and legal medicine were not intended to secure justice for the masses, but rather to meet the practical challenges faced by the Siamese elite in their ongoing engagement with imperial powers. The result was a form of necropolitics, in the general sense of discursive and practical actions oriented around dead bodies, which has important implications for our understanding of Thai history in the era of high imperialism and beyond.[15]

The Sovereign Exception (or, Exceptionally Sovereign?)

The emergence of a necropolitical regime at the turn of the twentieth century offers a troubling rebuke to the master narrative of modern Thai historiography: namely, the doctrine of Siamese/Thai exceptionalism. Thailand's status as the only nation-state in Southeast Asia to avoid direct control by European imperial power marks it as a singular state with an exceptional past. It is a narrative that has been touted by royal-nationalists and twentieth-century authoritarian advocates of development alike, who unanimously point to Siam's independence as evidence of its singular virtue. When confronting the question of how Siam remained independent, these scholars have looked first to the nation's leaders, specifically the monarchs of the reigning Chakri dynasty. In the view of Thai historians like Prince Damrong Rajanuphap, King Mongkut (Rama IV, r. 1851–1868) and his son and successor King Chulalongorn (Rama V, r. 1868–1910) were clear-eyed and farsighted leaders who ushered in reforms to anticipate and defuse the demands of the foreign powers for greater control over Siam.[16] Such historical narratives, which have been labeled the royal-nationalist mode of historiography, glorified the kings and purported to identify the true genius of the Thai people: the selective adaptation of the foreign.[17]

It is a narrative that has not gone unchallenged, however. By the mid-twentieth century, revisionist perspectives informed by Marxist theory began to seep in from the margins of Thai historiography, injecting a measure of skepticism. Pulling back the curtain on the drama of foreign aggression and the countervailing efforts of Thai monarchs to preserve the independence of the kingdom, these scholars saw evidence of both semi-coloniality and feudal social relations. With respect to the kingdom's semi-colonial status, scholars looked to unequal trade treaties that Siam had signed with European imperial powers beginning in 1855. The treaties transformed the Siamese economy by liberalizing the terms of foreign trade and enshrining extraterritorial legal privileges for foreign residents, which exempted them from Siamese judicial institutions.[18] Evidence of feudalism included a developed hierarchical system of social ranking that bestowed (royal) elites with the figurative power to control rice patties (*sakdina*) as well as the literal power to command human labor.[19] Thai scholars working in the Marxist tradition saw living remnants of these feudal traditions in mid-twentieth-century Thai society.[20]

More recently, scholars have revealed Siam's engagement with colonial modernity by charting the impact of technologies, institutions, and forms of expertise, including maps, laws, and medicine.[21] These works have advanced our understanding of how the Siamese state employed new forms of expertise to address the conditions of its constrained sovereignty in ways that often seemed to model the conditions of colonial states throughout the region. They decenter the monarchy by highlighting both the work of foreign advisers and the constrained conditions under which Thai modernity evolved.[22] Moreover, by revealing the transformative effects of foreign technologies and modes of expertise on Thai society, these works have gone a long way toward upending Whiggish historical narratives that explain the arrival of Western modernity through sanguine metaphors of adoption, adaptation, and transplantation. *Sovereign Necropolis* advances these efforts by revealing the ways in which new forms of technology, institutions, actors, and expertise helped to reconfigure Siamese political life with a view to the dead.

Outside of Thai studies, the notion of sovereignty itself has increasingly come under scrutiny. Scholars have come to see the idea of sovereign power as a notion profoundly "unsettled, inconsistent, fraught with contradictions"—troubled, for example, by an incessant need for outside recognition and by inherent inconsistencies surrounding the very nature of power over life.[23] These insights have gone a long way to upset classical conceptions of sovereignty as a stable attribute, a function of violence over territory.[24] They suggest that sovereignty is better understood as a precarious set of practices oriented around bodies, especially through the assemblages of law and medicine.[25] The bodies themselves, however, no longer bear any resemblance to those of the romantic subjects of normative political theory. In the colonial world, sovereign politics—like law itself—could have perverse outcomes when it attempted to humanize its subjects.[26] Achille Mbembe has extended these insights to the postcolonial state, demonstrating the ways in which sovereign power has engendered hybrid forms of political life that constitute a third zone between subjectivity and objecthood.[27] Together, these revisionist challenges to the nature of sovereign power reveal the state itself to be little more than a collection of contingent and heterogeneous modes of governing.[28] They have also brought to light the fetishization of life and the disavowal of death as the sine qua non of classical iterations of sovereign biopolitics.[29] In the process they have helped to spur a posthumanist turn in studies of political sovereignty, one that creates space for the agency of the dead—symbolic and otherwise. Armed with these insights, we can begin to see the outlines of the Siamese necropolitical state at the turn of the twentieth century and to grasp its significance both to Thai social and political life and to our understanding of sovereignty more broadly.

The sense of necropolitics employed in this study differs in important respects from the canonical understanding, which focuses on "the power and the capacity to dictate who may live and who must die."[30] For Mbembe and other theorists, necropolitics, along with the closely related idea of thanatopolitics, has been used to refer to the deployment of violence against lives that had been deemed expendable.[31] The term has also been invoked to theorize the ways in which human lives have been subsumed under differential regimes of value—whether imperialist, capitalist, or biocapitalist.[32] Such normative forms of necropolitics were also in evidence in late nineteenth-century Siam. One might cite, for example, the lives and labors of Chinese immigrants and

prostitutes, respectively, whose bodies were sacrificed for economic development. This connection is surprisingly literal in both cases: Chinese coolies
expended their labor building canals and other infrastructure—paying a triennial tax for the privilege to do so; they then patronized the state-granted
monopoly on the sale of opium in order to allay the physical pains of their
toil, as well as the emotional pains of migration.[33] At the same time, the state
similarly earmarked the tax proceeds from female sex work toward the construction and maintenance of the capital's roadways in the euphemistically
named "road maintenance tax."[34]

The necropolitical regime in turn-of-the-twentieth-century Siam was distinct from, though not unrelated to, these other historical formations. It too
was a product of practical efforts aimed at addressing changing historical circumstances, such as the decline of the feudal bonds that had long structured
the deployment of labor and the allotment of social status in Siamese society.
In their place were emerging more direct relations between state and subject—
the historical constitution of what David K. Wyatt described as "a compromise or amalgam between the old concept of the 'subject,' stripped of the
intermediaries that stood between the king and the peasant, and the modern
concept of the 'citizen.'"[35] What marked the new form of late nineteenth-
century necropolitics as distinct, however, was above all the fact that it
emerged out of the practical efforts taken by the royal elite to assert sovereignty in the face of particular constraints imposed by unequal trade treaties.
The treaties enshrined extraterritorial legal privileges for foreign residents, created a plural legal arena, and opened up the kingdom to the arrival of new
forms of social actors, including technology, expertise (legal and medical), and
interests—most notably foreign capital in all its nascent assemblages. It was
in this cauldron that modern Siamese necropolitics took shape: as the Thai
royal elite became more assertive about the rights of their subjects, these conditions conspired to place the emphasis on the dead and injured. The forms
of expert intervention—both legal and medicolegal—that state officials
adopted in turn created peculiar forms of legal and political subjectivity and
a distinctive polity whose crucial constituents were the dead.

Morbid Subjects and Anomalous Archives

This is a book about morbid subjects. In the first and literal sense, the book
concerns death and the ways in which we care for and assert the rights of the
dead. Accordingly, its pages are filled with lost lives and limbs—victims of misfortune, misadventure, and even malevolence. From pedestrians run down by

tramway cars to corpses found floating in Bangkok's waterways, quotidian tragedies and suspicious deaths prompted a range of legal and medicolegal interventions aimed variously at investigating the cause of death or injury and determining the appropriate form of compensation or restitution for the victim and their relatives. The documentary records of these seemingly disconnected deaths constitute an anomalous archive, a testament to anonymous historical actors whose lives were interrupted and whose fortunes were transformed by the confluence of foreign capital, expertise, technology, and institutions with indigenous forms of faith, custom, and absolutism. This is the second, figurative sense of morbid subjects, which refers to the kinds of legal and political subjectivity that were constituted when the Siamese state entered into new relations of concern with the bodies of its dead and injured subjects.

In spite of the anonymity of the morbid subjects of the Siamese state—the vast majority belonged to the ethnically diverse subaltern classes of the Siamese capital—their stories have been preserved in a peculiar collection of archival documents bearing the enigmatic label "Death by various causes" (*tai duai het tang tang*).[36] Compiled by the Siamese Ministry of the Capital beginning in 1890, the collection consists of the documentary records of inquests, or investigations into cases of unnatural or suspicious death in Bangkok. The documents attest to a forensic turn in Thai history and, in combination with the correspondence of Siamese state ministers and bureaucrats and reports in the local press, they make it possible to provide a social and institutional history of civil law and forensic medicine in turn-of-the-twentieth-century Siam in a way that is attentive to Siam's semi-colonial status.

The current investigation begins with an emic account of indigenous cultural forms of concern for "inauspicious" or "bad" death (*tai hong*). Attending to the Siamese state's archives of unnatural death, chapter 1, "Bad Death," identifies distinct registers of different semantic projects focused on the corpse. State interventions—including vernacular forms of forensic investigation and the "verdicts" rendered by the Ministry of the Capital—conflicted with subaltern forms of care and concern for the dead. Reading against the grain of the state archive, the chapter recovers fragments of subaltern lives and voices, as well as evidence of their efforts to resist the imposition of state-mandated forms of medicolegal concern as the forensic regime of "suspicious" death overcame sociocultural concerns for "inauspicious" death.

Chapters 2 and 3 analyze the ways in which urban passenger rail travel and its attendant tragedies helped to rewrite the rules governing loss and liability in Siam in ways that transcended both social conventions and codified sources of law. Chapter 2, "Indemnity and Identity," makes the case that compensatory arrangements made in the aftermath of injury and death effectively constituted a new and distinctive mode of legal subjectivity in the form of persons endowed with certain privileges and obligations, and in contradistinction to prior forms of rights and responsibility grounded in social relations. In nineteenth-century Siam, death required compensation, typically in the form of an ex gratia payment made to the relatives of the deceased without the intervention of courts or the admission of legal or moral responsibility. In the case of the Chinese man killed by the queen's motorcade, for example, the matter of compensation was handled through extrajudicial channels in the form of a monetary payment.[37] King Chulalongkorn found no fault in this arrangement—indeed his ministers had signed off on any number of such transactions, deeming them in each case an adequate and appropriate outcome, as the following chapters demonstrate. These compensatory arrangements, which were often reached outside of legal institutions and independent of judicial authority, were predicated not on a sense of universal rights and the dignity of human life but rather on customary modes of action and hierarchical social assumptions inherent in acts of *noblesse oblige*.[38] It was not just the Siamese elite, however, who enjoyed this privileged position of status and the entitlement to regard the lives of others with beneficence. These forms of privileged (extralegal) action were extended to foreign residents and limited liability corporations alike. Inspired by work in sociolegal studies, I examine these practices to consider not only the diverse forms of logic, interest, and authority that gave rise to them, but the manner of legal subjectivity that they might be said to have constituted. How did these practices determine what it meant to be a human being subject to law, and with what incumbent rights and responsibilities?

Since foreign lives and limbs were deemed more precious than those of subaltern Siamese subjects, chapter 3, "Treaty Port Tort," considers the kinds of legal and medicolegal disputes that arose when foreign residents sustained injuries on the tracks of the Bangkok Tramway Company. What kinds of expertise and institutions were responsible for adjudicating claims for compensation? And what of the rights of the Bangkok Tramway Company, its employees, managers, and shareholders? In answering these questions, the chapter analyzes "jurisdictional politics," "conflicts over the preservation, creation, nature, and extent of different legal forums and authorities," in the plural legal arena of treaty port Bangkok.[39] It deconstructs historical metanarratives about the "Westernization" or "modernization" of Thai law by revealing the fractious nature of Western law, including evidence of internecine squabbles between the representatives of legal and medical expertise—barristers and physicians—but also among the laypeople who advocated for particular brands of European legal tradition. It therefore complicates celebratory narratives of legal liberalism by demonstrating how nationalist sentiments (Dane versus Brit, for example) and professional self-interest (physicians and barristers) were the true impetus for legal change, not any grand imperial ambitions for bestowing law as a civilizing force.

Chapter 4, "Accidental Metaphysics," steps back to consider the more abstract side of these practical questions about law and liability for accidental death and injury. It analyzes the adoption and adaptation of tacit assumptions about human identity, agency, and responsibility that underlie legal liberalism, a notion that I call the metaphysics of civil law. Crucial to any effort to understand the boundaries of human agency and responsibility lies the notion of the accident. Although the accident masquerades as timeless and commonsensical, it is in fact a historical and cultural artifact: *ubatihet*, the Thai term, is a neologism dating to the late nineteenth century. Charting its introduction through etymological and historical linguistic evidence—as well as in practice as part of municipal governance—the chapter argues that the accident functioned as one axis of a metaphysical grid for representing social life and as a means of further codifying the identity of the Siamese legal subject. In both respects, the accident must be understood as part of a conservative grammar of rule: predicated on a secular-naturalistic vision of social life, it defined the legal subject in negative terms—through a constrained sense of agency rather than through the positive articulation of rights. Attending to the accident—and related terms such as negligence (*pramat loen loe*)—as a historical site of cultural production, the chapter destabilizes the naturalistic posture of legal reasoning and undermines celebratory narratives of law as a humanizing force.

Collectively, chapters 5 and 6 depict what might be called a forensic turn in Thai history, when in the final years of the nineteenth century the Siamese state suddenly began to invest in new forms of expertise to attend to the dead. That is not to suggest, however, that previously Siam was utterly devoid of medicolegal or forensic modes of concern for the dead. Even within this brief moment of awakening, one can discern a transition from long-standing forms of social and cultural interest in the dead to something resembling more modern scientific, medicolegal modes of concern. The transition encompasses a shift from vernacular forms of forensic interest in the dead to professional medical techniques that is best encapsulated by the change from *kan-chanasut phlik sop* (literally, "flipping the corpse over to inspect [for injuries]") to *kan-pha sop* (surgical forensic examination). But the transition is nevertheless stark when compared with the case of late imperial China, for example, which had a highly developed and standardized classical tradition of legal medicine.[40] The forensic turn in Thai history occurred in the context of severe constraints on Siamese sovereignty in the form of unequal treaties that established extraterritorial legal privilege for foreign residents in Siam and was part of the Siamese state's pragmatic efforts to address those conditions.[41] It also corresponded with a significant transitional moment for Siamese state and society, as direct relations between the state and its subjects gradually replaced hierarchical forms of feudal social organization that had previously mediated relations between the sovereign and his subjects.

Chapter 5, "Morbid Subjects," reveals how Siamese state officials came to see unnatural death as a specter of foreign violence against Siamese bodies and how they appealed to medicolegal science to address this problem. In stark contrast to other colonial legal jurisdictions, where medical jurisprudence helped to bolster (white) racial privilege, the chapter argues that medicolegal concern rendered the dead and injured bodies of Siamese subjects into potentially powerful pieces of leverage against foreign residents who enjoyed extraterritorial legal privileges and the consular officials and institutions who protected them.[42]

Chapter 6, "Incisions and Inscriptions," follows the dead body as it moved out of the public spaces of vernacular forensics and into the sequestered space of medicolegal science, the morgue. It attends to the efforts of the Siamese state to implement medicolegal science in the form of autopsies (incisions) capable of producing forms of documentary evidence (inscriptions) that foreign consular courts would recognize in the prosecution of foreign residents accused of having harmed Siamese subjects. Engaging with science studies scholarship on the work of mediation, the chapter focuses on the collaborative work of Dr. P. A. Nightingale, a British physician in the employ of the Siamese state, and Mo (Dr.) Meng Yim, his Sino-Thai assistant and translator. It discovers in the documentary fruits of their collaborative labor, the death certificate, a "boundary object" capable of entertaining discordant forms of knowledge, and a testament to the emergence of a new form of necropolitics in Siam.[43]

In the following pages, we will take King Chulalongkorn at his word and consider seriously the idea of the dead as a political constituency. What sorts of legal, medical, and bureaucratic practices and discursive acts allow the state to assert responsibility to and for its dead? And what manner of polity do such practices create? A historical analysis of medical and legal interventions in death reveals that constitutional decisions regarding the identity of the legal subject, the value of a human life, the nature and limits of human responsibility, as well as the political relations between the state and its subjects were forged in death, not life. *Sovereign Necropolis* thus exhumes the long-interred constitution of a necropolitical state and its morbid subjects.

CHAPTER 1

Bad Death

> Attitudes toward death often lie at the heart of social conflict, and the dead are frequently objects of contention and struggle.
>
> —Vincent Brown, *The Reaper's Garden*

In September 1890, unnatural death entered the archives of the Siamese state. What had previously been the preserve of cultural beliefs and social forms of action became a matter of state concern. The archival life of unnatural death in late nineteenth-century Siam speaks to what Ann Laura Stoler has identified as a crucial facet of state sovereignty, namely, "the power to designate arbitrary social facts of the world as . . . concerns of the state."[1] The very existence of a cache of inquest files, or documents related to the investigation of unnatural deaths, is a testament to the fact that unnatural death—a feature of social life—was becoming a matter of political concern for the Siamese state. The causes of this new facet of state concern for the dead are discussed in chapter 5, but here I am concerned primarily with the nature of this transition as documented in and through the archives. What did early state interventions into the realm of death look like, and how did they relate to traditional forms of concern for the dead? What do these new forms of forensic concern tell us about the nature of authority within the Siamese bureaucracy, and what implications, if any, did they have for Siamese political life?

Death Enters the Archives

On September 23, 1890, a Nai (Mr.) Mak hired three laborers to take down a ceremonial arch that had been constructed on the occasion of King Chulalong-korn's birthday celebration.[2] The arch, which was decorated with festive garlands, had been erected at the edge of the Chao Phraya River on the premises of a warehouse owned by a member of the Siamese elite. It was intended to serve as a backdrop for the king's ceremonial procession along the river. At just after four in the afternoon, one of the laborers, a Siam-born ethnic Chinese man named *Jin* (Chinaman) Pao cut one of the two wooden support beams holding up the arch. The arch immediately collapsed and all three laborers fell toward the river. One of the laborers, Jin Ma, was fortunate to fall in the vicinity of a passing boat, and was able to cling to the side of its hull. The second laborer, whose name is not known, fell straight down and caught hold of the riverbank. Jin Pao, however, disappeared into the brackish tidal river. Phraya Intharathibodi Siharatrongmueang, in his capacity as head of the police of the eastern districts of Bangkok, dispatched a single police officer to go and investigate the matter in the company of the district official (*nai amphoe*). The records of the case do not offer a detailed account of the methods of investigation employed by the police officer, but they do not appear to have been very detailed or scientific. Locating the body of Jin Pao was not the first priority in the investigation.

Three days later, on September 26, a man named Nai Chum spotted a corpse floating downriver near the mouth of the Toei Canal (*khlong toei*). The sighting was reported to police, who fished the body from the water. The police paid a visit to Jin Ma, one of the two surviving laborers, and asked him to come and identify the body. Jin Ma refused, claiming that he was still recovering from injuries sustained in the accident. The police then halted the investigation. The official documents do not make any mention of what happened to the body of Jin Pao. There is no indication, for instance, of whether the body was inspected for evidence of injuries that would suggest foul play, even though this had long been an established practice in cases of unnatural death.

The death of Jin Pao marks a significant change in the nature of state concern for cases of unnatural death in Siam. It is the first case that appears in the "Death by various causes" (*tai duai het tang tang*) files compiled by the Ministry of the Capital. The somewhat generic designation of these files speaks to the ambiguous nature of the archive in the early years of its existence. Insofar as the files contained within it are records of police investigations into cases of untimely or unnatural death, the logic of the archive corresponds to the British inquest, a medicolegal institution that Prince Naret Worarit (1855–1925), head of the Committee for Local Government (*khomitti krom phra nakhon ban*), may have learned about during his tenure at the Siamese legation in London in the 1880s.[3] Although there are no archival records that speak to the original decision to begin investigating such deaths in Bangkok, the fact of its creation suggests a juridical orientation that was quite opposed to Siamese traditional beliefs surrounding inauspicious death. In the early years of the inquest in Siam, however, these juridical inclinations remained unvoiced. It was not until March 1893 that we begin to see evidence of the explicit logic behind these investigations, when Prince Naret used the term "suspicious" (*na song sai*) to describe the conditions surrounding a double-suicide in the same household.[4] Similarly, in March 1897, Mo (Dr.) Meng Yim, a physician in the employ of the Siamese police, referred to an inquest investigation as pertaining to a "[Siamese] subject who died under suspicious circumstances."[5] Statements such as these reveal how the juridical logic of the "Death by various causes" files was slowly articulated, but in its early years the institution remained inherently ambiguous in both its conception and execution. This ambiguity is indicative of the faltering nature of the Siamese state's early regard for the dead: it appears to have adopted the trappings of European institutional forms of concern without articulating the intention or significance of the reforms.

As the case of Jin Pao demonstrates, the entrance of unnatural death into the archives was likewise an ambiguous development in terms of execution. First, the documents related to the case reveal the cursory and improvisational nature of police investigational techniques at the time. Second, the case of Jin Pao, and numerous others from the early era of record keeping, shows that the corpse was rarely the focus of police inquiries, which regarded the corpse only in passing and instead hinged on witness testimony. Finally, although the entrance of unnatural death into the archives marks a significant development in the state bureaucracy in terms of both oversight and documentation, it did not correspond to progress in the areas of forensic science or legal medicine. In spite of these limitations, the inquest was nevertheless an innovation that bore potentially important implications for political life in Siam from its very inception.

The inquest constituted a novel form of engagement between the state and its subaltern subjects in and around the capital city. In the case of Jin Pao, the arrival of police on the scene effectively brought the corpse of a previously anonymous laborer into a direct—though not reciprocal—relation with the state. There were, of course, other transactions and forms of obligation and imposition through which the Siamese state had traditionally interacted with subjects of little social standing, including the institution of corvée labor. Corvée obligations were twofold: on the one hand, every free individual was responsible to a patron to whom they rendered service a few days a year; on the other hand, they were also obligated to serve the state for a longer period each year, and that service was often defined according to the status of their patron within the state.[6] By the end of the nineteenth century, however, the system was in a state of dramatic decline. The peasant classes (*phrai*) and, more so, the patrons or lords who controlled their labor power through the feudal (*sakdina*) system of social ranks had increasingly opted to commute their corvée obligation through a cash payment.[7] Moreover, corvée could not really be considered a channel of direct interaction between the state and its subjects, since the conscription of manpower had always operated through the *sakdina* system. Corvée labor obligations to the state were therefore mediated by more personal forms of hierarchical patron-client relations.[8]

The peculiarly Thai institution of debt slavery was another form of social life that brought the subaltern to the attention of the state. Under the conditions of debt slavery in Siam, which was distinct from the chattel slavery practiced in much of the colonial world, the owner of the debt had complete mastery over the labor of the slave; debt slaves were therefore exempt from corvée labor obligations.[9] This exemption made debt slavery a challenge to the state's ability to muster manpower, and thus the institution was of some interest to the state.[10] But with the exception of military conscription, these forms of mediated state-subject relations were slowly waning as the Fifth Reign (1868–1910) witnessed the ascension of more absolute forms of monarchical rule.[11] Viewed in the context of these declining forms of mediated relations, police inquests into cases of unnatural death—much like the contemporaneous rise of civil legal interest in cases of accidental injury and death, discussed later in chapters 2 through 4—are remarkable. They are evidence of a new form of engagement between the state and its subaltern subjects, one that centered on states of death and injury and that would increasingly come to be dominated by novel modes of authority and forms of expertise. Before examining the emergence of these novel modes of state concern for the dead, however, one should first try to get a sense of the status of unnatural death in social life outside of state involvement.

Tai Hong (Inauspicious Death)

The Siamese notion of *kan-tai hong* ("inauspicious" or "bad" death) constitutes both a taxonomy of types of deaths and a repertoire of actions for dealing with and making sense of those types of deaths.[12] In the broadest terms, it is concerned with relations between the human social world and the realm of spirits, which were believed to be the spiritual remnants of human lives lost through sudden or unnatural means. Historically, the notion encompassed a broad range of causes of sudden or unnatural deaths, including murder, drowning, suicide, certain forms of particularly virulent illness (such as cholera and symptoms associated with opium withdrawal), death in childbirth, accidents (such as those due to a fall from a tree or a natural event), and animal attacks. The common denominator in these diverse forms of death was impaired consciousness; death took the deceased largely unawares—or, as in the case of suicide, the deceased's consciousness was exceedingly troubled at the moment of death. The impaired or disturbed consciousness of the deceased was unable to move on in the process of reincarnation and had the potential to become a malevolent spirit.[13] Such spirits tended to adhere to the location where the death occurred, and they were thought to be a threat to the living. The overwhelming logic of dealing with such death was a notion similar to contagion: because inauspicious deaths had the potential to leave behind malevolent spirits that might harm others, they were seen as a threat to the community. Inauspicious death therefore required social action aimed at protecting the community from further effects. This regard for the potentially malevolent spirit of the deceased also translated into a distinctive sense of locality; in the aftermath of an unnatural death, members of the local community had to be attuned to the potential abodes of the spirits left behind.

On a practical level, the sense of contagion surrounding unnatural death translated into a general unwillingness to interact with corpses that were left behind by what were deemed sudden or unnatural causes of death. According to Stanley Tambiah's ethnography of religious life in rural Northeast Thailand, burials for such corpses were "devoid of ritual."[14] A body left behind by unnatural death was quickly buried "so that the earth may contain its dangerous powers," and monks were called to officiate over rites intended "to invest the deceased with merit and grant protection to the living" from the potentially dangerous spiritual remnants of the deceased.[15] Tambiah emphatically notes that the special treatment given to the dead in such cases was not a matter of taboos related to the impurity of dead flesh but was predicated on the widespread fear of the malevolence of the spirit of the deceased, which "hovers dangerously" after death and "may attack the closely related living kinsmen because of its previous attachment to kin, property, and house."[16]

Apart from these ethnographic accounts, we can find contemporary references to customs associated with inauspicious death in anecdotal evidence offered by foreigners residing in Siam at the end of the nineteenth century. Aage Westenholz, the Danish manager of the Bangkok Tramway Company, for example, noted that when Siamese rivercraft capsized, bystanders tended to shy away from assisting for what he understood to be "reasons of religious superstition."[17] Understanding this belief in the threat posed by malignant spirits might help to explain morbid reports that appeared in the foreign press from time to time, such as the occasion whereupon seeing the corpse of a newborn baby floating in a basket in the canal next to a temple, a group of Siamese children hurled rocks trying to sink the basket.[18] The fact that the city's Chinese residents refused to allow dead bodies to enter their homes was another common observation by foreign observers, and it further suggests the cosmopolitan nature of beliefs surrounding bad death in the Siamese capital.[19] While foreign residents paid heed to this tendency to shun the bodies of those who had succumbed to a bad death and the potentially malevolent spirits they left behind, they were less inclined to notice more subtle forms of action taken in the aftermath of unnatural deaths.

The burden of placating the dispossessed spirit of the dead fell upon the bereaved family, which was expected to sponsor appropriate ritual actions to placate the spirit and protect the community. The logic of this arrangement might best be explained through an appeal to what Shigeharu Tanabe has called "community culture," the pervasive belief that individual physical injury "can damage the community as a whole."[20] The primary ethic of concern in cases of unnatural death was communal well-being rather than medicolegal certainty; when confronted with a corpse, Bangkok residents sought restorative action over forensic truth. But this logic was upset by the arrival of Siamese police tasked with investigating unnatural death in the capital.

Dealing with Death: The Police Inquest

It is fitting in many ways that the death of Jin Pao, the first case that would find its way into the archive of unnatural death in Siam, occurred in the river. In contrast with the tramway tracks that foreground the discussion of injury and death in the following chapters, the rivers and canals that crisscrossed the city were the quintessentially Siamese mode of mobility. And like the tramway, the city's waterways claimed their share of victims, whose corpses became the object of concern for both inauspicious death and the forensic investigations of police into suspicious death. Bodies floating in the river and canals were a common occurrence in fin de siècle Bangkok. They appeared as often as every other week in the "Local and General" news columns of the *Bangkok Times* as well as in the "Death by various causes" files of the Ministry of Local Government. In the case of the local government files, the bodies were most often observed by the police themselves and then retrieved; in the newspaper columns, however, reports of corpses drifting downstream seem to be based on local gossip and likely often went unreported to the police (only a small number of such reported drownings actually appear it the state inquest files). To conduct an inquest, police often had to retrieve corpses from these waterways. In seeking out—as opposed to shunning—the corpse, police inquests implied a radically different manner of concern for the dead body than the culture of inauspicious death. But beyond their willingness to engage with the corpse, the "Death by various causes" files reveal that the actual practice of forensic investigation in the early days of the inquest left much to be desired. Moreover, the state's archive of unnatural death also demonstrates that although the state bureaucracy was prepared to administer the paper trail of investigations into cases of unnatural death, the police were often unwilling to take up the burden of dealing with corpses.

A little over a year after the death of Jin Pao, in October 1891, while dismantling the ceremonial arch for the king's birthday, the body of an unidentified woman was found floating in the canal next to Wat Saket, a prominent temple located just outside the city walls that was well known for its functions in funerary rites.[21] Although it appears in the inquest files, this particular case is notable not as an inquest—the investigation of a case of unnatural death—but simply as a case of an errant corpse. The inquest file does not contain any information about an investigation into the cause of death or an examination of the body of the young woman. The central document in the file is a letter written by Phra Phrasit, a monk residing at Wat Bowoniwet, a prominent royal temple located some distance from Wat Saket and the floating corpse. On October 19 he wrote to the police ordering them to remove the body that very evening.[22] Phra Phrasit explained that monks from Wat Saket had reported the matter to police two days previously and that police had not taken any action to remove the corpse. He castigated the police, noting that the situation "was entirely unseemly" and warning them not to allow this to happen again in the future.[23] In the early days of police inquests, it was not at all uncommon for corpses to linger, as police were reticent to accept their new mandate over the dead.[24]

In cases where police did arrive in a timely manner and attempted to investigate the cause or circumstances of death, early records in the "Death by various causes" files convey a sense of the ad hoc nature of forensic investigations at the dawn of police inquests in Bangkok. To begin, the police and district officials charged with investigating the cases had no specialized knowledge or training in forensic investigational techniques or medicolegal expertise in matters of death.²⁵ When police arrived at the scene of an unnatural death, they would secure the corpse and conduct an on-site postmortem examination, a procedure known as *kan-chanasut phlik sop* (investigation [by means of] turning over the body). In the late nineteenth and early twentieth centuries, before the vocabulary and spelling conventions for these investigative techniques had stabilized, there was a great deal of variety in the spelling and terminology employed to describe police inquests.²⁶ As in the nomenclature, there seems to have been lack of uniformity in the actual conduct of forensic inspections of corpses. The colloquial sense of *phlik sop*, or "flipping the body over," seems to be an accurate description of the postmortem examinations conducted by police and district officials, which were often limited to inspecting the outside of the body for obvious signs of violence—or, in cases of suspected suicide or drug overdose, for signs of physical compulsion. Thus, the postmortem investigations conducted by police were quite accurately referred to as *phlik sop truat du bat phlae* (turning over the corpse to inspect for injuries).²⁷

Another indication of the ad hoc or vernacular nature of early police inquests was that postmortem examinations were limited to on-site viewings of the body, often in outdoor, public spaces. The police and district officials charged with the investigation often chose a nearby Buddhist temple (*wat*) to conduct the postmortem examination. In many cases, the temple was the original location where the corpse was discovered, making it the obvious choice for the examination. Buddhist temples attracted the desolate, destitute, and diseased. Open-air temple pavilions (*sala*), intended as a shady refuge for passing travelers, provided shelter for those without means or relatives to care for them. The Buddhist faithful furnished charity cases with food, care, and basic comforts, while allowing them to reside at the temple pavilions in their hour of need—or, very often, in their final hour. Charity and compassion made the temple *sala* an attractive destination for the terminally ill or suicidal, who were in effect entrusting their corpses to the care of the temple's benefactors, confident that their remains would be handled appropriately. In cases such as these, on-site postmortem examinations had to be performed in the open, accessible grounds of the local *wat*. Evidence from the "Death by various causes" files suggests that postmortem examinations were often well attended, to the point where police were not able to record the names of all the witnesses present.²⁸

In other cases, however, when the death did not occur within temple grounds, the *wat* was nevertheless chosen as the site for the postmortem examination. There were a number of reasons for this. First, temples were deemed public space, readily appropriated by police and local officials as a

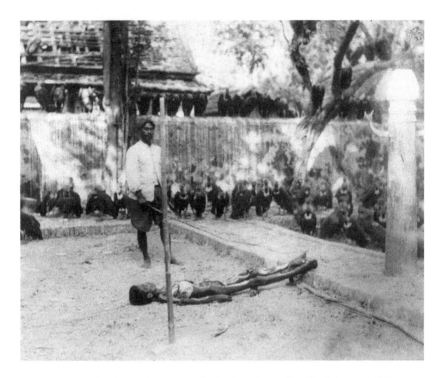

FIGURE 1.   An undertaker tends to a corpse in the charnel grounds at Wat Saket, ca. 1900. National Archives of Thailand, image # ภอ.ทต.2/33.

convenient landmark and gathering place. Many police stations were located next to temples from which they derive their names. This connection may simply reflect a long-standing mutual relationship that began with ad hoc local arrangements.[29] At a time when Bangkok was still known to foreigners as "the "Venice of the East" and waterborne transport remained a key mode of conveyance, temples often had frontage on rivers and canals. Beyond the matter of accessibility, open-air examinations at temples also had the added advantage of ventilation, which was crucial as corpses that had languished in the city's waterways for several days were likely well on their way to putrefaction. Yet another virtue of the temple as a locale for forensic investigations was that temples—especially those located outside of the city walls—were already associated with death.[30] Temples like Wat Saket administered a diverse (and hierarchical) array of funerary services, from charnel grounds where the bones of the destitute were picked clean by vultures (figure 1), to burial grounds where bones were temporarily interred in preparation for cremation rites at a later date, to elaborate funeral pyres and mausoleums prepared on the occasion of deaths among the social elite.[31]

Along with monks, who catered to the ritual needs of the deceased and their relatives, such temples employed in-house undertakers (*sapparoe*) who tended to the less ceremonious aspects of death in late nineteenth-century Bangkok. Among the responsibilities of the undertakers was the preparation of bodies before they were entrusted to carrion-eating birds in the charnel grounds. A late nineteenth-century travelogue penned by Lucien Fournereau offers a graphic account of the undertaker's activities, which included cutting "the flesh in long strips" and "launching" the pieces "as hard as he can to the dogs and the vultures which do not leave the temples." In cases of cremation, the undertaker had to "take the precaution" of severing the joints of the corpse; if he should fail to do so, once on the funeral pyre "the dead flesh appears to be born again and twitches; the electrified limbs stir, twist and relax; the dead, resurrected, grimaces and atrociously thrashes about on his bed of brands."[32] Beyond these macabre labors, undertakers played a pivotal role in early forensic investigations.

In an era when death remained a largely social and communal affair, the temple undertaker was often the last impediment to getting away with murder. Before the start of state intervention, when death occurred it fell to the relatives of the deceased to summon an undertaker and make arrangements for disposal of the body. In such cases, the undertaker was often the only figure with the opportunity and experience to note potential evidence of foul play before the body was either buried or dismembered for cremation. In October 1895, for example, an undertaker working at Wat Saket was called on to retrieve the body of a servant who had died in the home of her employers. By the time he arrived, the servant had been dead for some time; four Buddhist monks had earlier been called to perform ritual chanting over the corpse, and decomposition had already set in. The undertaker nevertheless took note of evidence of premortem bodily injury and he summoned the police.[33] Such cases were not exceptional, but it is important to note that undertakers were paid a fee for each body entrusted to them, so it is quite possible that their loyalties to the paying party might in some cases have outstripped their desire to see justice done. We see evidence of precisely this compromised position in the testimony of an undertaker named Khaek, given in response to an inquiry into a case of unnatural death in July 1896.[34] Khaek, a thirty-year-old man who had been working as an undertaker for five years and who had risen to a position of seniority within the ranks of undertakers at Wat Phrapiren (located just outside the gates on the southeastern edge of the city), admitted that he did not ask any questions of the people who had hired him to take away a body and he likewise did not remove the deceased's clothing to inspect for signs of injury.

In spite of the potential failings of undertakers as forensic experts, the temple was nevertheless the de facto site for postmortem examinations in cases of unnatural death in which the body was removed from the site of death. The most common cases of this nature were those of bodies found floating in the city's waterways. When floating bodies were observed by or reported to police, they were secured by police and taken to the nearest temple (unless they were spotted in the immediate vicinity of a police station, in which case they were sometimes taken to the station). Although the reports are not specific about the procedures for retrieving the bodies, archival evidence suggests that they were not removed from the water; instead, they were secured with ropes and towed to the boat launch of the nearest temple. Having reached the temple, the police would use the ropes to tether the body to the nearest tree on the temple grounds. It is not difficult to imagine these early postmortem examinations—those referred to as "turning the body over to inspect for wounds"—conducted with sticks as the body bobbed around at the end of a coarse hemp rope. The police then left the body—often unattended—in order to go off in search of witnesses or relatives of the deceased, who might be able to provide a narrative for the death and take charge of making funerary arrangements.

Given the limited and ad hoc nature of the postmortem examination, it is not surprising that police tended to rely on other means of gathering information in the investigation of cases of unnatural death, notably by collecting witness testimony. The new mandate of the police to investigate cases of unnatural death undercut local autonomy and interrupted the sociocultural habits of thought and practice associated with "inauspicious death." In effect, police intervention usurped the authority to forge meaning and take action in the wake of unnatural death from relatives, neighbors, and local authorities (such as village headmen or elite patrons). Yet the police nevertheless relied on the testimony of these same people to create their own narrative of the cause and meaning of cases of unnatural death. After securing and inspecting the body for evidence of injuries, the police would branch out in search of witnesses who could identify the deceased or help to clarify the circumstances surrounding the death. The crucial investigational tactic employed by police was the "search for local witnesses" (*kan-suep phayan rangwat*). In their search the police employed a sense of locality that was distinct from the culture of inauspicious death, with its concern for the topography of human-spirit interaction, yet in practice it seems to have retained some commonalities.

The fixation on proximity in the search for witnesses is perhaps best illustrated by police canvassing efforts in cases of bodies found floating in the city's waterways. After receiving reports about waterborne corpses—sometimes already secured by rope to a local pier or tree, but more often still adrift in the brackish waters of the city's rivers and canals—police would take custody of the body, check for injuries, and then set out in search of relatives or witnesses. Regardless of the degree of decomposition (*nao*) of the body—a recognized indicator of how long the body had been in the water—police concentrated their canvassing efforts on the immediate vicinity where the body was discovered. In cases of reported drownings police showed a clear understanding of the tidal influences of the river and they immediately connected corpses appearing downstream with such reports.[35] The "Death by various causes" files reveal, however, that police searching for local witnesses seem not to have applied this insight in their search for the original site of a drowning or the home village of the deceased. The idea of a "local witness" seems to have been somehow inextricably—and irreparably—linked to the discovery of the corpse and its final resting place.

At a time when forensic investigations into cases of unnatural death were limited to inspecting the corpse for external signs of injury and locating local witnesses, witness testimony was key to forging a meaningful narrative. The formal title for offering witness testimony in cases of unnatural death was "to offer legal testimony concerning the inspection of the corpse" (*hai thoi kham kotmai chanasut phlik sop*). The colloquial idea of "inspecting the corpse by turning it over" (*chanasut phlik sop*) was thus common to both lay witness testimony regarding cases of unnatural death and the forensic investigative practices of police and district officials. This suggests that there was no qualitative distinction made between forensic evidence offered by police or district officials and that offered by equally untrained laypeople who happened to be nearby at the time of the discovery of the body. Moreover, there is evidence to suggest that lay testimony at times went beyond cursory external examinations to touch on more specialized forensic evidence such as blood pattern analysis.[36]

Transcriptions of witness statements make up a significant portion of the documents archived in the "Death by various causes" files of the Ministry of the Capital. Even the comprehensive police reports that introduce the inquest files are often little more than paraphrased recitations of the original statements offered by witnesses, which are included in the files. The statements given by witnesses in cases of unnatural death reflect vernacular modes of thought and colloquial expressions of local cultures of death. But these statements were then collated by police into reports of the findings of the investigation, which were submitted to their superiors in the Ministry of the Capital. Witness testimonials in cases of unnatural death constitute a rare archive of the words, thoughts, and experiences of the subaltern masses in turn of the century

Siam. Burgeoning state interest in death effectively created a bureaucratic channel and an archival space for recording subaltern voices. In many cases, the statements were physically composed by clerks or local mediators and bear only the signature or mark of the unlettered witness. Such statements were likely shaped by a process of homogenization, as police coerced, cajoled, or simply directed witnesses, mediators, and translators to exact a particular kind of statement about the circumstances surrounding the death. Although the rough edges of colloquial speech and local concerns in cases of death were likely blunted by these interventions, the documents are nevertheless a significant archive of subaltern perceptions and concerns, as well as a record of the changing conditions of daily social and commercial life.

When they canvassed the local community in the wake of an unnatural death, the Siamese police encountered witnesses whose testimony brought assumptions and concerns to the experience of being near to death that were different from those of the police and officials in the state bureaucracy. Police officials, or their clerks, would compose a report offering an overview of the facts in the case, including the testimony—both forensic and otherwise—of local witnesses. As noted previously, their reports did not differentiate between forensic evidence offered by local witnesses and that of police and district officials. Adding to the social—even civic—nature of these early inquests was the fact that forensic investigations took place in the open air in public spaces in full view of the curious and concerned public. In spite of the intervention of the police and district officials, early police inquests in Bangkok seem to have been inextricably rooted in local meaning and practice. Police and local witnesses alike conducted forensic investigations and offered testimony on the cause of death. How then, was a single homogeneous sense of meaning distilled from the mélange of voices, habits, and cultures that constituted the early Siamese police inquest?

The Semantics of Death: Meaning by Executive Fiat

The institution of police inquests in cases of unnatural death in late nineteenth-century Bangkok did not imply a revolution in the actual investigation of such cases. Police records betray the improvisational nature of forensic methods. Although the state had usurped the authority from local officials and villagers to make sense of such cases of death, its agents continued to rely on vernacular forensic practices and colloquial witness testimony. From the start, district officials (*nai amphoe*) who were called on to inspect corpses alongside the police acknowledged that conducting forensic postmortem examinations was "beyond [our] capabilities" (*luea wikhro*).[37] Moreover, there appears to have been no fundamental sense of agreement at different levels within the state bureaucracy over the meaning of such deaths or the need for police investigation. Neglecting for the moment the question of how the cosmopolitan populace of the capital city responded to state intervention in the administration of unnatural death, one might well be skeptical that even the Committee for Local Government, the senior Siamese police officials, and district officials shared a common sense of the meaning and import of unnatural death in the early years of state involvement. When state authority first became involved in the investigation of unnatural deaths in the capital, it was left to the highest reaches of the Committee for Local Government and the office of the king himself to make sense of death. In the early era of police involvement, the semantics of death were decided by executive fiat.

Each of the early "Death by various causes" files crossed the desk of Prince Naret Worarit, a younger half-brother of King Chulalongkorn who presided over a recently reformed bureaucratic body charged with governing the capital city. The Committee for Local Government replaced the former governing body, known as the Capital Department (*krom mueang*), in 1886. Prince Naret, who had recently returned from serving as the head of the Siamese legation in London and an extended tour of the United States, was appointed to the committee.[38] When the committee was transformed into the Ministry of the Capital (*krasuang nakhonban*) as part of the sweeping government reforms of 1892, Naret was charged with heading up the new institution. From the start, the Ministry of the Capital was concerned with many of the same functions that had occupied its antecedents, including overseeing the administration of taxes, policing, and medicine.[39] In the coming years, sanitation and public works would become a crucial part of the ministry's mandate, accounting for nearly half of its expenditure by 1906.[40] When the ministry's work is viewed through the lens of financial expenditures, however, it is easy to overlook important shifts in the governmental work of the ministry. Alongside capital expenditure on public works projects, archival records reveal that the ministry was increasingly concerned with the well-being of its living residents and the material fate of the deceased. In the waning years of the nineteenth century, for example, the archives of the Ministry of the Capital show a dramatic increase in documents related to the oversight of the cattle industry and slaughterhouses as well as causes of death and burial practices.[41]

If expenditures are a potentially misleading metric of the work of the Ministry of the Capital, then sheer volume of documentation might offer a more reliable quantifier. The "Death by various causes" files compiled by the Ministry of the Capital, which occupy twenty-five boxes (or seven reels of microfilm) and are perhaps its single largest collection of documents, suggest that unnatural death was a topic of great concern to those responsible for governing the capital.[42] Throughout his tenure in the top office of the ministry, Prince Naret apparently spent a considerable amount of his time poring over inquest files compiled by the Siamese police as part of their investigation of cases of unnatural death in Bangkok. In the coming years, he would invest significant energy and political capital in reforming the procedures involved in investigating such cases (these developments are chronicled in chapters 5 and 6). In the early years of the 1890s, however, Prince Naret exercised near-complete authority over the cases, scribbling judgments at the end of each file that would either corroborate police findings or offer an alternative interpretation of the causes and significance of the death in question. Prince Naret's judgments in cases of unnatural death, which I refer to as "verdicts," are brief comments appended near the final page of many of the "Death by various causes" files of the Ministry of the Capital. They are sometimes titled "decision" (*kham tat sin*) but more often appear as telegraphic remarks without any introduction, though usually bearing his signature. After rendering a "verdict," Prince Naret would submit the files to the private secretary of King Chulalongkorn for royal endorsement.

Documents concerning the death of a thirty-three-year old monk named Phra Mongkhon by apparent self-immolation in January 1892 reveal an early iteration of the role of executive authority in metropolitan police inquests.[43] According to his sister, Amdaeng Daeng (who was a debt slave working as a household servant), Phra Mongkhon had been ordained as a monk for at least nine years, having taken up his most recent residence at Wat Khruawan some four years before. Amdaeng Daeng noted, however, that her brother had not been well mentally for some time, long before the fateful morning of January 4, 1892, when she was summoned to the temple to find him lying scorched and lifeless beneath a papaya tree under the window of his monastic chamber. Police were summoned and a postmortem examination took place on site, attended by the district official, police officers, monks from the temple, Phra Mongkhon's sister, and several other unnamed male and female bystanders. Witnesses noted that the corpse was covered in burns that penetrated to the bone on all parts of the body save for the left foot, which was not burned. Nearby, they found a square metal canister, which was empty but smelled distinctly of oil.

The following day, police submitted documents concerning the case to the Committee for Local Government. On reviewing the documents, the committee immediately found them to be lacking, and so a committee member (Phra Anatinarakon) drafted a letter to the senior police officer, Phra Thep

Phlu, complaining that the police report was not sufficiently clear.[44] He therefore summoned Phra Thep Phlu, along with the district official who had helped to collect the witness testimony in the case, to come before the committee in order to give a more complete account of the causes of this "strange event."[45] He instructed the two officials to arrive at the appointed time and place—11 a.m. the following morning, January 6, at the Police Court—on time, and not to waste official government time. The meeting amounted to an official state inquest into the death of Phra Mongkhon, which was conducted at the highest levels of the newly formed metropolitan government administration. The inquest proceedings, however, were sequestered in the halls of state government—in marked contrast to the postmortem examination and on-site investigations conducted by police.

Once the details of the case had reached the desks of the officials who comprised the Committee for Local Government, it became a matter of executive authority, with the district official submitting to an interrogation by the members of the committee.[46] Following the inquest proceedings at the Police Court, Prince Naret ordered a new copy of the police report to be compiled, reflecting the revised testimony as recorded in the minutes of the inquest proceedings.[47] Finally, the redacted report of the inquest into the death of Phra Mongkhon was submitted to the office of the secretary of the king on January 20. The final report relies on the testimony of Phra Mongkhon's sister and his fellow monks, and it constructs a narrative whereby Phra Mongkhon "had succumbed to madness, and had never recovered."[48] His death, the report concludes, was a confirmed suicide, with no one else having done him any harm. The case of Phra Mongkhon reveals the authoritative role of the Committee for Local Government in cases of unnatural death, which involved the compilation of a definitive narrative stating the cause of death.

Although the governing body and procedures behind the exercise of this authority would change during the early years of police inquests, the nature of this mode of executive authority over cases of unnatural death in the capital city would not. When Prince Naret was appointed minister of the newly founded Ministry of the Capital in April 1892, he found himself invested with the full authority formerly wielded by the committee. In some cases, Naret's verdicts did not extend beyond his role as the head of the metropolitan police: for instance, those that pointed out shortcomings in the police reports and demanded further investigation. In other cases, however, Naret's role was not unlike the office of the coroner in Anglo-American legal medicine: after reviewing evidence collected by police, Naret constructed plausible narratives explaining the causes of death and submitted those judgments to the highest authority in the land, the king.[49]

Documents recording the accidental drowning of an elderly monk named Phra Jong at Wat Suthat in central Bangkok similarly reveal Naret's role in collating the evidence gathered by police.[50] Phra Jong was reported missing before dawn on the morning of April 24, 1892, by junior monks who had come to his quarters to rouse him for the morning observances. The same monks then went in search of Phra Jong, eventually finding his lamp at the edge of the well where they later recovered his body. On being informed of the death, Phraya Intharathibodi, of the metropolitan police, dispatched two district officials to the temple in order to conduct a postmortem examination. The officials inspected the body for signs of injury, and, not finding any, they presumed that Phra Jong had gone to fetch water during the night, had become faint, tripped, and fell into the well, where he drowned. After reviewing the evidence, Prince Naret entered his "verdict" in the case; he sent a letter to King Chulalongkorn on May 2, 1892, informing him that he agreed with the police report, citing the lack of marks on the monk's body and Phra Jong's reported habit of fetching water late at night.

When two members of the same household died under unusual circumstances in March 1893, Prince Naret took a more active role in creating a narrative that would explain the deaths. In the early hours of March 2, 1893, police were informed that Amdaeng Mon, aged 46, had used a white cloth to asphyxiate herself in the home of her husband.[51] Some hours after her death, Jin To Than, her nephew by marriage, consumed a lethal combination of alcohol and opium in his uncle's home. Police were informed and Phraya Intharathibodi dispatched officials to the home, where they found the bodies of Amdaeng Mon and Jin To Than—the latter having died while police were en route that morning. After examining the bodies, officials found no evidence of injury to Amdaeng Mon, and likewise no evidence of compulsion or foul play in the death of Jin To Than. They therefore concluded that the former had hung herself and the latter had taken an overdose of alcohol and opium in apparently unrelated events.

When the documents pertaining to the case reached Prince Naret, however, he viewed the circumstances from afar, with a different sense of causation. In Naret's verdict, which is undated, he observed that the coincidence of the two deaths was "suspicious" (*na song sai yu*). Given the unlikely concurrence of the two deaths in the same household on the same day, Naret speculated that there must have been a link between them: "Perhaps they were illicit lovers together, since after Amdaeng Muan [*sic*: Mon] hung herself, Jin To Than consumed poisonous drugs and was dead before the following dawn."[52] Naret instructed the police to continue the investigation and to inquire among those in the household whether they could offer any explanation for the simultaneous deaths. He specifically ordered Phraya Intharathibodi to canvass the neighbors and ask whether they had ever observed any "coarse behavior" (*kiriya yaep*) between the two that would confirm his suspicion that they were surreptitious lovers. Whatever the outcome of this particular case—the documents end with Naret's instructions to the police to continue the investigation— it clearly shows that as Minister of the Capital, Prince Naret acted as arbiter over cases of unnatural death within the Siamese capital, and his dominion went beyond the oversight of the police under his command. In his efforts to uncover the reasons behind cases of unnatural death, Naret at times passed over the physical evidence and witness accounts and looked instead for other patterns of causation that escaped the notice of the police and bystanders.[53]

Other records of Prince Naret's interventions into police inquests show an awareness of the lack of medical expertise possessed by state officials investigating cases of unnatural death. In the case of Amdaeng Lap, who died of suspected poisoning in June 1892, for example, Naret reviewed the conflicting witness accounts and the conclusions reached by the police. Although Naret concurred with the police that it appeared to be a case of poisoning, he added that it was an unusual case of death, which required a complete investigation.[54] He then ordered police to reinterview all of the witnesses and to speak with the two physicians who were called in to tend to all of the victims who were poisoned along with Amdaeng Lap, paying special attention to the symptoms that the physicians observed when they arrived at the scene. Naret's verdict in the case of Amdaeng Lap was the first instance where the police were directed to seek the input of medical practitioners in the investigation of an unnatural death by the metropolitan police. Although the physicians in this case were consulted not because of their expertise per se but simply because of their proximity to the case as witnesses, the role of medical expertise would nevertheless increase in the coming months.

Prince Naret later interceded when a corpse found floating in a canal led to a disagreement between police and physicians working for the Hospital Department. When a male corpse was found floating in the Mahanak Canal in central Bangkok, police canvassed the area and soon learned that the man, Nai Jui, had been a long-term resident of the hospital at Wat Thepsirin where he was being treated for cancer (*rok mareng rai*).[55] Neighbors told police that Nai Jui often left the hospital grounds to bathe at the canal's edge, where he may have slipped, fallen in, and drowned. The physician in charge of the hospital, a minor royal named Momratchawong Wong, told police that Nai Jui had indeed been a patient of the hospital, but that he was released after his cancer had been cured. The police, skeptical of the doctor's account, conducted a postmortem examination, claiming to have seen evidence of cancerous legions on the man's face, body, and feet. They faulted Momratchawong Wong and the hospital administration for allowing patients to leave the hospital grounds. Naret's verdict in the case, dated September 19, 1893, rejects the testimony of the police officers, noting that they were not used to performing such medical diagnoses. He advised the police that there is no use arguing with physicians over such matters and ordered an end to the investigation.

In sum, Naret's verdicts reveal a great deal about the nature of forensic investigations in the early years of the police inquest and the status of authority within the Siamese bureaucracy. To begin, they go a long way toward concealing the messy reality of early police inquests into cases of unnatural death in Bangkok. Naret's executive authority over the meaning of death allowed him to disregard the forensic findings of the rudimentary—and communal—postmortem examinations conducted at the river's edge or on the grounds of the local *wat*. His verdicts likewise eliminated the dissonant voices of witness statements, with their lay judgments concerning forensic evidence. In short, Naret articulated a new semantics of death, substituting executive authority for the rough edges of vernacular inquests.

Naret's role as the final arbiter over the semantics of unnatural death in state inquests also provides important insight into the nature of authority within the Siamese bureaucracy during a time of dramatic transformation. In the final years of the nineteenth century, the administrative structure of the Siamese state underwent a thorough reformation intended to "rationalize" the bureaucracy by organizing distinct ministries according to function rather than geography.[56] But in spite of these sweeping changes in the structure and function of the bureaucracy, William J. Siffin has argued that in many respects the deeper organizational characteristics of the traditional bureaucracy persisted, particularly the hierarchical nature of social relations within the bureaucracy. "As the Reformation [of the bureaucracy] proceeded," according to Siffin, "continued reliance upon the hierarchical principle as the prime basis for defining and ordering relationships was unquestioned."[57] Naret's verdicts, which often supplanted the work of police officers and silenced the voices and concerns of subaltern witnesses, demonstrate how elite social status implied a unique form of authority. Thus it can be said that the new form of state concern for the dead and its attendant procedures was consistent with long-standing patterns of authority.

This would not be true in the coming years, however, when the social and political conditions of extraterritorial law in Siam combined to elevate forensic medical expertise. The executive authority of Siamese officials would then yield to new forms of expertise as described in chapters 5 and 6. For the time being, however, Naret's executive authority would continue to hold sway—at least in the context of the state. Naret's verdicts, scribbled as marginalia on police reports, belie the ambiguous findings of the police and testify to the power of executive authority, but they ultimately fail to repress dissenting voices in the "Death by various causes" files.

Registers and Resistance

State intervention into cases of unnatural death in the Siamese capital at the end of the nineteenth century did not go unchallenged. The transition from the local, vernacular mode of concern for "inauspicious" death to the new forensic logic of "suspicious" death administered by police and state officials required uprooting and supplanting long-standing habits of mind and custom.[58] Reading against the logic of "suspicious" death, the inquest records compiled by the Ministry of the Capital contain archival traces of the persistence of local sociocultural ideas pertaining to death. In spite of the arrival of police and state officials who spoke a more bureaucratic language inflected by the forensic concerns of "suspicious" death, local residents continued to make sense of unnatural death on their own terms. Careful reading of the colloquial register of witness testimonial statements compiled by the police reveals the persistent logic of "inauspicious" death. Moreover, when it came to dealing with corpses—the cultural object of local, vernacular forms of forensic interest—local residents and witnesses resisted the new forms of state intervention.

For witnesses who were party to a case of unnatural death, locality was a preeminent concern. In their statements to police, witnesses focused on the place where the death had occurred, often noting the position of the body with respect to a tree. Recall, for instance, the case of Phra Mongkhon, whose sister's testimony stated that the body was found "under a papaya tree" outside the window of his monastic chamber.[59] Witnesses noted the type of tree and its proximity to the body because they understood that unnatural death had the potential to leave behind a malevolent spirit, and that the spirit might take up residence in the nearest tree. In cases of suicide by hanging, for example, witness statements show a tendency to identify the type of tree from which the deceased was found hanging and to repeat this identification in their statements. When a commoner named Nai Won committed suicide by hanging in an orchard near his home, his wife learned of the death from relatives and went to see for herself. In her testimony given to police, she reported having found her husband "hanging dead from the branch of a mango tree in the orchard of Nai Nak."[60] Similarly, when Amdaeng Im committed suicide by hanging, her husband's statement given to police shows a marked fixation with the fact that she was found hanging from the branch of a durian tree.[61]

It is worth noting once again that the extant witness statements in the inquest archives compiled by police were shaped by the conditions of their composition. In most cases, the statements were transcribed by clerks (*samian*) who accompanied the police during such investigations—since many of the people providing statements were undoubtedly illiterate—or were recorded in translation, having been mediated by a translator. The clerks, for their part, likely did not have the same fixation on place and may have scrubbed witness statements of some of these repetitive elements. Witnesses would perhaps also have engaged in a degree of self-censorship as well, suppressing elements of their testimony in accordance with the perceived interests of police.[62] Still, when taken collectively, the traces that do survive provide evidence of subaltern modes of concern for the dead, marked by a fixation on the specific location of the corpse—as evidenced by the recurring identification of tree types in witness testimony.

Witness testimonies referring to bodies hanging from mango (*mamuang*), durian (*thurian*), persimmon (*tako*), guava (*farang*), ashoka (*sok*), mulberry (*khoi*), and bulletwood (*phikun*) trees, among others, are more than a naturalistic catalog of fruit-bearing trees in turn-of-the-twentieth-century Bangkok.[63] They constitute a tacit testament to the persistence of long-standing sociocultural habits of mind associated with the Siamese culture of unnatural death. Insofar as the culture of inauspicious death focused on potential interactions between humans and spirits, the location of spirits in the human world was of great concern for those who were party to a case of unnatural death. Trees, which were thought to serve as abodes for spirits—malevolent and otherwise— were therefore an important feature of the topographical map of the intersection of the realm of spirits and that of humans.[64] Such is the force of the testimony, for example, when a debt slave found her compatriot, a runaway named Ai Am, dead after apparently committing suicide by hanging, and she identified a persimmon tree in an orchard belonging to their shared owner as the location; or a distraught husband, on finding his wife hanging dead from a tree behind their home, who lingers over the fact that it was a guava tree that he had cut her down from and under which he had tried to resuscitate her.[65] These passages suggest that for bystanders the shock of an untimely and unnatural death was perhaps mitigated by the sense of fear and dread that they associated with a haunting spirit.[66] For local residents who bore witness to unnatural death in late nineteenth-century Bangkok, trees marked the potential abode of such spirits, and the fixation on these trees is a testament to their distinctive forms of concern for unnatural death.

In addition to the surviving traces of the culture of unnatural death in the statements given by witnesses, and the ways in which these local concerns were at odds with those of the state when it came to administering unnatural death, there is evidence of more direct resistance to new forms of state intervention in death. The new mandate of the Siamese police to investigate cases of unnatural death, which amounted to a novel forensic concern with corpses, provoked forms of outright resistance from those invested in a culture of inauspicious death. In one particularly striking case, local Siamese residents cut the same corpse loose from its temporary moorings on at least two separate occasions after it had been retrieved from the river.[67] This particular corpse belonged to a foreign resident named J. J. Grant who had only recently arrived in Siam by way of Rangoon in British Burma. Upon arrival in Siam, he had taken a job working for the holders of the opium tax farm in Bangkok. (*Tax farming* was a system whereby the Siamese state auctioned off monopoly rights to collect a tax on the distribution, consumption, or use of certain goods in a specified area for a period of time.) His disappearance prompted rumors of foul play related to his line of work. In that case, the *Bangkok Times* explained, "The fact of the body having been twice cut adrift was . . . due to the customs and superstitions of the Siamese, who[,] believing that the deceased's spirit might somehow affect them if left near their houses, naturally objected to the presence of the corpse."[68] Indeed, evidence suggests that these traditional beliefs concerning the potential danger of spirits associated with corpses typically held sway when the city's residents observed bodies floating in the river, and local residents permanently entrusted the corpses to the river. The "Local and General" news column of the *Bangkok Times* is rife with reports of waterborne corpses during the last decade of the nineteenth century.[69] In most cases, the reports were based on "rumors" and there is no indication of what became of the corpse. Cases of voluntary intervention, however, were rare, and worthy of special note in the local press. In December 1901 the *Bangkok Times* ran a story noting, "The dead body of a Chinaman floated down Klong [*sic*: Khlong] Kut Mai yesterday afternoon. It was, however, brought ashore by some kindly disposed person for cremation. There were no marks of violence."[70]

Apart from police intervention in cases of unnatural death, there is also evidence of local resistance to early instances of medicolegal inquiries conducted by physicians. In December 1889, when physicians at the Bangrak Hospital conducted a postmortem examination on the body of an ethnic Chinese man named Ah Heng, a crowd of "about 300 or more Chinese were congregated outside waiting for the verdict of the doctors."[71] In August 1898 the body of a suspected murder victim went missing from the police morgue before the physician arrived to conduct a postmortem examination.[72] The editors of the *Bangkok Times* surmised, "the relative of the murdered man had carried the body home," perhaps in protest of the interruption of traditional funerary practices or the prospect of postmortem medical procedures.

Resistance to the state's intervention, however, was not limited to non-state actors. Siamese police were likewise reluctant to take up their new burden as overseers of unnatural death. Dereliction of duties and jurisdictional disputes over the dead provide evidence of police reticence to fulfill their new mandate. Two cases in June 1900 help to demonstrate the ways in which police could eschew their new responsibilities to the dead. On June 5, 1900, the *Bangkok Times* noted, "The body of a dead Chinaman was lying by the tramline near Wat Rajabophit this morning. There was a small crowd around it, evidently waiting till a policeman should happen to come along from some quarter to remove the body."[73] Later that month, the corpse of an ethnic Chinese man was observed "lying by the side of the road near the Sam Yek [*sic*: Yaek] police station," where it had been left to fester for over twenty-four hours.[74] Although the body was evidently in sight of the central police station in Bangrak, police overlooked it, ignoring even "the relations of the dead," who "for some time before [its] removal . . . were burying gold paper etc. by the side of the body."[75]

Finally, the question of responsibility for dead bodies prompted a number of disputes—jurisdictional and otherwise—between police and quasi-state officials as well as private residents in the capital. In August 1895 the *Bangkok Times* noted a spate of corpses found dead in rickshaws around the city.[76] The brief notice concerned a recent case where "a Chinaman in a collapsed condition was found in a rick'sha [*sic*] yesterday morning, and taken by a constable to the Bangrak Police Station, where, after having been seen by a doctor, he died. On the remains being conveyed to their late home they were, in accordance with the Chinese custom of refusing the entrance of a dead body, denied admittance."[77] While the editors of the paper evidently understood the refusal to accept the body as part of a Chinese taboo, they nevertheless posed the rhetorical question of "whether this practice of putting dying men into rick'shas is also a Chinese method of preventing deaths taking place inside lodging houses."[78]

It was not only owners of boarding houses who were reluctant to take responsibility for those who might perish while residing in their premises; the tax farmers who ran gambling parlors likewise wanted to avoid the added expense and trouble of dealing with the dead. In spite of their ostensibly official standing as representatives of the Siamese state, Chinese tax farmers fought the police when corpses appeared in the areas surrounding their businesses.[79]

Early state intervention in the administration of unnatural death was thus marked by both outright and tacit forms of resistance to a new mode of concern for the dead and its associated responsibilities.

From Inauspicious to Suspicious Death

When unnatural death entered the purview of the Siamese state, it marked a break with traditional forms of concern for the dead. Siamese and ethnic Chinese residents of the city tended to view such deaths as "inauspicious": the body of the deceased was viewed as a threat to the community and was therefore shunned, while its spirit was placated in order to quell its potentially malevolent powers. Siamese officials, however, were beginning to view unnatural death from a more juridical perspective, as a matter of suspicion that merited police investigation and documentation. With the institution of police inquests into cases of unnatural death in 1890, the municipal authorities of the Siamese capital instituted a new archive for records of such investigations. The "Death by various causes" files of the Ministry of the Capital contain evidence of the improvisational nature of early police investigations, including indifferent attention to the corpse, vernacular postmortem examinations, and a reliance on witness testimony.

These early proceedings, entirely lacking in medical or forensic expertise, were documented by police and submitted to the officials responsible for the administration of the capital. The elite Siamese officials who wielded executive power over police inquests helped to collate police evidence and witness testimony in order to create a single authoritative narrative for each case of unnatural death. These narratives, recorded in the judgments of the officials of the Ministry of the Capital, suggest a new sense of meaning surrounding cases of unnatural death—that of "suspicion." But this new mode of concern did not go unchallenged. The state archives of unnatural death also provide a record of diversity and dissent among the cosmopolitan populace of Bangkok and the police officials charged with the administration of death in the capital.

Beyond providing a record of a new facet of state concern for the dead and the resulting forms of subaltern dissent, however, the "Death by various causes" files also suggest an important development in Thai political culture. When Siamese police were dispatched to investigate reports of an unnatural death in the capital city, they in effect instituted a new means of engagement between the state and its subaltern subjects. It was not, however, a reciprocal encounter, but rather one through which the state interrupted sociocultural forms of concern for the dead and obstructed local forms of sovereign agency.

By seizing the corpse and imposing a new regime of juridical concern for un-natural death, the state barred the culture of "inauspicious" death and asserted its own preeminence over the semantics of death. This transition in forms of authority over death has been documented in other geographical and histori-cal contexts: whether as an interaction between the state and its emissaries as they asserted sovereignty over the realm of unnatural death, or as an interac-tion between the practitioners of modern medical science who were intent on advancing their own agendas with respect to the dead, in each case these were inevitably asymmetrical encounters.[80] State and expert interventions in death had the effect of interrupting pathways of social thought and action as-sociated with bad death in ways that might be likened to a surgical extraction: they removed the body from its social, communal, and even spiritual relations in order to render it as an object of forensic concern. In this transaction, ex-ecutive authority won out, effectively displacing the hierarchical patron-client relations that had formerly served to mediate between the state and its sub-jects and foreclosing other possibilities of civic organization and interaction with the state. In the coming years, however, these new forms of state con-cern for the dead would become embroiled in transnational forms of legal and political contestation. These developments would invite new forms of expert knowledge to intervene in and mediate the relationships between the state and its subjects.

In much the same way that the new juridical culture of concern for the dead—and the new interest of the Siamese state in unnatural death—interrupted the Siamese culture of inauspicious death, the coming years would witness a challenge to the executive authority of Siamese officials over the semantics of death in the capital city. Imperial politics and the plural legal arena in Bangkok would provoke a new, medicolegal regime of concern for death, characterized by the rise of forensic medicine as an authoritative mode of knowledge. Executive authority over the semantics of death would thus be-come untenable, as increasingly specialized forms of expert knowledge were brought to bear on corpses. Amid these changes, and within the context of the plural legal arena created by extraterritoriality, the dead would rise to oc-cupy a position of prominence in transnational politics, a development that would mark the formation of the sovereign necropolis. Forensic medicine, however, was not the only form of interest and intervention into the domin-ion of unnatural death. In the realm of civil law, juridical concerns with re-sponsibility often yielded to questions concerning the appropriate ways to make restitution for a lost life. These negotiations likewise took place across cultural divides, where the dead were invoked for disparate means and ends.

CHAPTER 2

Indemnity and Identity

> Rather than regarding person as a legal concept to
> be studied in abstraction from history and material
> practices, it is more illuminating to regard person as
> a forensic fact that is not self-evident but that must
> be ascertained by accepted social practices.
>
> —William Pietz, "Person"

On August 10, 1889, a concise report appeared in the "Local and General" news column of the *Bangkok Times* concerning a serious injury sustained by a passenger on the Bangkok Tramway line:

> On Monday last a Siamese girl, named E. Nak, in stepping from a tram-car near the Royal Barracks missed her footing and fell, the wheels of the car passing over the calf of one leg and breaking the bone. The unfortunate woman was immediately placed in a carriage and taken to the Bangkok Hospital by Mr. [Aage] Westenholz [manager of the Bangkok Tramway Co.,] and it was there found necessary to amputate the limb.[1]

Apart, of course, from the fact of permanent disability, readers were assured that "the operation was successfully performed on Tuesday morning last and we understand that the patient is doing fairly well." The young woman would not be the first or last person to be permanently maimed or killed by the tramcars that had begun plying the narrow, crowded, and pitted streets of the city in 1888.[2]

The metal rails, ponies, and especially the electrical-powered motors of the tramway delivered to the Bangkok streets what Marc Bloch has described as "one feature, the most distinctive of all" that distinguishes "contemporary civilization" from its predecessors: *speed*.[3] Paul Virilio, standing on Bloch's shoulders and gazing back at the wreckage of the twentieth century, suggested a second distinctive feature of modern society, which is corollary to speed: *the accident*.[4] According to Virilio, the "innovation of a motor or of some other substantial material" that makes rapid mobility possible is "equally the invention of the 'accident.'"[5] But accidents are only known to us through "a process of fortuitous discovery" that Virilio calls "archeotechnological invention": "To invent the sailing ship or steamer is *to invent the shipwreck*. To invent the train is *to invent the rail accident* of derailment."[6] For Virilio, every form of technological innovation is accompanied by its own "specific negativity," its own accident, and this co-origination spawns further technological progress and ever more accidents.[7] But is it possible to think of the accident as a creative force outside of Virilio's closed system of technological progress? What might the accident itself be said to *invent*?

This chapter is an inquiry into the sociocultural implications of tramway accidents in late nineteenth-century Siam. It interrogates the legal and extrajudicial consequences of the intersection of bodies, rails, wheels, and law. This marks a dramatic departure from the familiar terrain of the historiography of modernizing legal change in Siam, which has typically been fixated on the process of codification—the translation and promulgation of positive law—as the path to restoring Siamese jurisdictional sovereignty.[8] Recent scholarship has revealed how the process of translation was crucial to forging a sense of Siamese legal modernity that codified elite forms of privilege.[9] These scholars have also helped to decenter the royal elite as the sole agents of change by highlighting the work of transnational legal advisers.[10] To date, however, there has been little effort to attend to law outside of the corridors of royal power and expressions of codified law.

Bangkok was a cosmopolitan port city long before serious efforts were under way to revise Siam's legal codes, and its residents had to negotiate fundamental questions concerning social and commercial life across a dizzying array of cultural practices and beliefs. These negotiations inevitably included questions of liability and responsibility for loss, injury, and death. The narrative of codification is unable to account for these pragmatic interactions and the kinds of cross-cultural negotiations that they implied. Forms of extrajudicial action that evolved out of these practical deliberations constitute a particularly glaring blind spot for scholars interested in the social and cultural history of law in Siam. We also lack a clear sense of the indigenous precedents that correspond to civil legal process and action and the ways in which practical forms of legal action were shaped in accordance with the logic of these Siamese antecedents.[11]

In an effort to address this lacuna, this chapter explores the creation of the Siamese legal subject *by accident*. That is, it examines the ways in which subaltern Siamese subjects came to be defined in legal terms through fatal encounters with tramcars. These encounters offer a resolutely empirical and materialist vision of the sociohistorical conditions for the constitution of legal subjects by moving out of the elite halls of justice and into the streets of the capital, where Siamese bodies felt the impact of new modes of mobility, finance, and legality. Like recent theoretical inquiries into law and society in the colonial and postcolonial world, which reveal the ambiguous outcomes of efforts to tether human life to legal regimes, this chapter charts the emergence of an impoverished form of legalistic life.[12] Through these quotidian tragedies—events that brought Siamese subjects into no less traumatic forms of engagement with foreign capital (in the form of limited liability corporations) and alien forms of legal reasoning—the ghosts of Siamese cosmology were summoned and commanded to life.

The inquiry will proceed in four parts, beginning with an introduction to the Bangkok Tramway Company, its legal and physical existence, its agents and investors, its acceleration and its accidents. Next, it considers the legal and extralegal fate of the victims of tramway mobility by attending to modes of remediation for the loss of human life. How did these arrangements come about, and what was their legal standing? Third, it considers how these practical arrangements for compensation related to modes of thought and action in traditional Siamese sociolegal life. Finally, the last section of the chapter situates these encounters within what was an important transitional and transformational moment in Thai history. It presents accidents and acts of remediation as evidence of a distinct legal regime, on the one hand, and as a marker and maker of novel forms of legal subjectivity, on the other.

"The Slow and the Dead": Urban Rail Travel Comes to Bangkok

Four bells jangle on the harness of an approaching horse. The brassy tone of an infantry bugle pierces the air, signaling the approach of a southbound tramcar on the New Road line.[13] Drivers coax their horses and ponies into motion, and a sea of pedestrians bearing fruit, vegetables, and dried fish and trailed by children parts around the iron tracks laid into the pitted road. The horse-carts, rickshaws, and any number of other improvised vehicles traveling the New Road tended to avoid the iron tracks installed by the Bangkok Tramway Company, preferring the wider and relatively unmarked road surface. The absence of street traffic quickly made the tramway tracks the de facto pedestrian thoroughfare along the heavily trafficked New Road, so long as pedestrians remained wary of the warning sounds of an approaching tramcar.[14]

The Bangkok Tramway Company was founded in 1887, when the government of the kingdom of Siam granted a concession to build a tramway system to two foreign entrepreneurs who were longtime residents of the city. The concessionaires, a British subject, Alfred John Loftus, and a Dane, Andre du Plessis de Richelieu, were granted "sole and exclusive right to construct and maintain . . . the Tramways hereinafter described . . . and to work and use the same for 50 years from the date hereof."[15] The concession allowed for the eventual construction of seven tramway lines and fixed standard passenger rates of six *at* (1/64 of a *baht*) per three-mile interval (or twelve *at* for "superior" seats at the front of the car).[16] Tramway line number one, which would run for a distance of six miles roughly parallel to the Chao Phraya River from the commercial district of *Bang Kho Laem* in the south of the city to *Tha Thian* pier near the southern walls of the Grand Palace in the north, would be constructed first (figure 2). The concessionaires were only allowed to construct a single rail track for each of the proposed tramway lines, meaning that tramcars travelling in opposite directions would pass one another at designated sidings along the route.[17]

The concession stipulated that the New Road line (line number one) would have to be built within three years to meet the growing demand for passenger transit in the congested central part of the city, but the city's residents would not have to wait nearly that long. Loftus and Richelieu hired an ambitious young Dane named Aage Westenholz to serve as manager of the company and by 1888 tramcars were already plying the number one line, each car being towed by a team of ponies. By Westenholz's own admission, the "first two months," when the tramcars were first unleashed on the city streets being towed behind untrained ponies, "were full of mishaps and accidents."[18] In October 1890, after a spate of injuries along a particular stretch of the New Road line, police officers were posted to prevent passersby from stopping on the tracks, where they could peer into a newly established theater. In a letter to the district police chief at Sam Yaek station, Westenholz expressed his gratitude for the work of the police and enclosed a reward of eight *ticals* [baht] to be distributed among the officers.[19] In spite of these mishaps, the company, which was a public limited liability corporation, rewarded shareholders with a healthy semiannual dividend, and within two years of its opening Westenholz was already laying out an ambitious scheme to introduce electric power along the New Road line.

King Chulalongkorn (King Rama V, r. 1868–1910) was also a major shareholder in the Bangkok Tramway Company, so when early plans for electrifi-

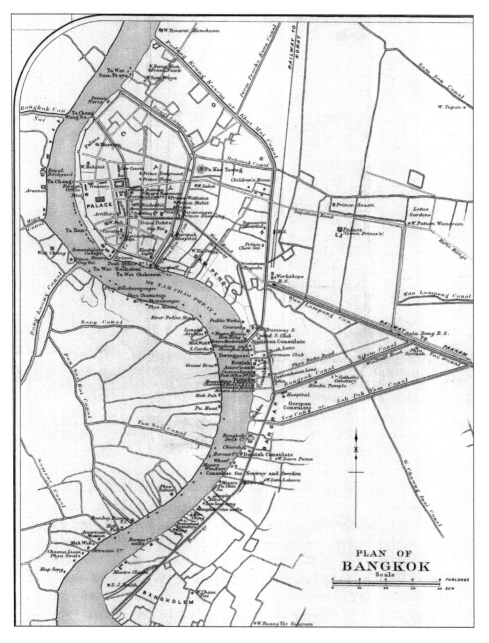

FIGURE 2. Map of central Bangkok, ca. 1900. The New Road tramway line is highlighted, running roughly north to south parallel to the Chao Phraya River. *Map of the Kingdom of Siam and Its Dependencies* (Edinburgh: W. & A. K. Johnston, [1900?]). Photo courtesy of Olin Library Maps Collection, Cornell University.

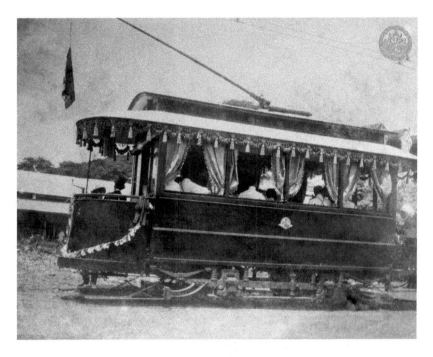

FIGURE 3. A tramcar photographed at the inaugural ceremony following conversion to electric power in 1893; King Chulalongkorn (Rama V, r. 1868–1910), in top hat, boarding an electrified tramcar at the opening ceremony following conversion to electric power in 1893. Prince Damrong Rajanuphap Library, Bangkok, Thailand (image # R105–091).

cation were announced the venture was regarded as a sure thing to gain the approval of the Siamese state (see figure 3). Unfortunately, as an American trade publication noted, the company was viewed as such a sure bet to succeed that "stock [was] not to be had at any price."[20] Westenholz traveled to Europe and the United States to study the operations of electrical tramcar systems and to visit the manufacturers of the required equipment, which included "dynamos, motors, line appliances, and trucks."[21] He would eventually place an order with the Short Electric Railway Company in Cleveland, Ohio, for all the necessary equipment needed to electrify the New Road line with the exception of the posts for hanging the overhead lines—for those, local teakwood was used.[22] The first tramcars under electric power travelled the number one line on February 20, 1893; a full contingent of six cars was in operation under electric power only a month later.[23]

Despite the commercial success of the company, hazards abounded along the New Road tramway line. Over its six-mile course, the line passed over a total of fourteen canal bridges, each of which acted as a choke point for traffic, including pedestrians.[24] The speed and weight of the tramcars were another hazard. Initially, drivers of the horse-drawn tramcars relied on a handbrake and likely shouted commands such as *"cha noi"* (slow down) to rein in the ponies at designated stops and intersections. In 1891, Westenholz engineered a footbrake that allowed the driver to exert more stopping pressure, which was presumably more efficient at slowing the tramcars.[25] After 1893 and the transition to overhead electric power along the length of the New Road line, the driver would ease back on the throttle, slowing but not stopping the cars for passengers to disembark and board. Surveying the scene, Westenholz remarked, "it is a pleasure to see how well even old women with babies or trays of glassware in their arms jump on or off the" moving tramcars, whose "pace is slackened down to a walk" only "if the [disembarking] passenger desire[s] it."[26] In 1895, Westenholz was praised for speeding up transit times along the tramway line by ordering tramcar drivers to roll through all intersections and passenger boarding areas without coming to a stop. He thereby accelerated transit times along the length of the line by nine minutes (reducing the time required to travel the entire six-mile length of the line from fifty-five to forty-six minutes). "The acceleration," the *Bangkok Times* noted, "is not obtained by actually running the cars more quickly, but by avoiding stoppages at the terminal and crossings, and also by putting a stop to the dawdling which has hitherto been so annoying."[27]

These operating conditions render it unsurprising that in the early years of the Bangkok Tramway Company, death and injury along the tramway tracks were so commonplace that they gave birth to their own mythology. As early as November 1889, little more than a year after the tramway had commenced operations, the *Bangkok Times* reported on the growing suspicions of the company's Siamese employees concerning the ill-fated cars under their direction. Following three fatal accidents involving tramcar number five, employees of the company had come to a consensus that the number five was a particularly inauspicious number.[28] Interestingly, the article faults not the novelty of the technology, which clearly posed a danger to unaccustomed residents, but rather the fact that Bangkok's denizens had already become inured to the warning calls of approaching tramcars and had become heedless. Under questioning at the police court, the man driving tramcar number five at the time of the most recent accident "claimed that the bugle notice of the coming of the tramcar was sounded as usual, but," the newspaper notes, "it is notorious that familiarity with the tramcars has the usual effect of making people careless about keeping out of their way."[29]

In two separate incidents on the same ominous Saturday in February 1892, a Chinese man was injured while disembarking from a tramcar and an old Siamese man was run over and killed. The sardonic news item in the *Bangkok*

Times—titled "The slow and the dead"—reported that in the latter case, "The driver blew his bugle, but the old fellow was blind, and deaf, and lame, and several other things, and he never knew what hit him. Mr. Westenholz, the tramway manager, gave his family a catty [80 Baht], however, to soothe their grief."[30] In the former case, the American Dr. T. Heyward Hays, chief physician at Bangrak Hospital, attended to the Chinese man, who "jumped gracefully off a tramcar on Saturday, without waiting for it to slow down. He alighted on his pigtail, and had to be galvanised into consciousness by Dr. Hays." The press coverage of these cases of death and injury suggests an important distinction in respect to the victims of the tramcars: for the Siamese and ethnic Chinese who did not enjoy the extraterritorial legal protections enshrined by Siam's trade treaties with the European powers, civil litigation against the Bangkok Tramway Company in the case of death or injury was not a viable option. The family of the old Siamese man killed by the train was awarded a single *catty* (eighty baht)—apparently at the sole discretion of the company and its management—and the injured Chinese party likely received little more than free medical care from Dr. Hays, himself a major shareholder in the Bangkok Tramway Company.[31]

These anecdotes concerning the loss of life and limb on the tramway tracks help to situate the Bangkok Tramway Company within the indeterminate civil legal system in Siam at the turn of the twentieth century. Those who fell victim to the erratic jolts of the ponies pulling the cars, the errant traffic patterns on the city streets surrounding the tramway tracks, the negligence of the drivers, or simply their lost footing on the ill-maintained roadways all became subject to the brutal and unpredictable calculus of loss and liability in late nineteenth-century Bangkok.[32] When the tramcars crushed and severed limbs and ended lives, the Bangkok Tramway Company and its managers understood the nature of their liability in terms of Western legal traditions, but the plural legal environment created by extraterritorial law provided the opportunity to appeal to local customs and institutions in order to define their liability in more advantageous terms. Accidental death and injury along the tracks of the Bangkok Tramway Company therefore demonstrates the malleable nature of civil law in the context of a cosmopolitan colonial treaty port.

Kan-tham khwan: Restoring the Spirit of the Deceased

In February 1892, a sixty-two-year-old Siamese man named Nai Ao, who worked as an undertaker, was struck and killed by tramway car number seven.[33]

The incident occurred near a shrine erected by the Guangdong Chinese community in Bangkok, at the Sam Yaek intersection on New Road. Nai Ao was likely killed immediately by the impact, as the documents concerning the death at the Siamese Ministry of the Capital do not contain any discussion of the administration of medical care in the case. The managers of the Bangkok Tramway Company sought out Amdaeng Jan, a female relative of the deceased, and offered her a lump sum payment of eighty baht as compensation for the loss. Amdaeng Jan accepted the payment and had the body of Nai Ao taken to Wat Sam Jin for burial.[34]

As the death of Nai Ao demonstrates, in the immediate aftermath of an accidental death or dismemberment on the tramway tracks, the question of compensation was the predominant concern, and it was addressed according to Siamese customary practices. Amdaeng Jan had accepted the payment offered by the company and Nai Ao's corpse was already in the ground by the time Prince Naret, head of the Ministry of the Capital, learned of the incident in a handwritten letter received on February 16. The letter states that "the Bangkok Tramway Company requests [permission] to make a 'funerary payment' (*ngoen tham khwan*) to Amdaeng Jan, a relative of Nai Ao [the deceased]."[35] The memo therefore presents the payment as a proposed solution to compensate relatives for the loss of Nai Ao's life; it implies that such compensatory actions required some degree of approval by the Ministry of the Capital, which had geographical if not formal legal jurisdiction over such events. In actuality, however—and as the report later notes—the payment had already been offered and accepted; the evidence of the death, Nai Ao's corpse, had already been interred in the cemetery at the temple. In spite of the seeming finality of these arrangements, they were in fact made outside of the purview of the Siamese officials who were responsible for the civil governance of the capital city. With respect to the monetary compensation, Prince Naret noted with approval, "In this case, the company has paid a sum [amounting to] the funeral expenses (*bia pluk tua*) of the deceased to his relatives, which is appropriate."[36]

The payment made to Amdaeng Jan in the wake of Nai Ao's death is notable for three reasons. First, there is the manner in which the payment corresponded with traditional Siamese practices of remediation in cases of accidental injury and death. The report submitted to the Ministry of the Capital uses the language of traditional Siamese civil remediation, describing the proposed payment as "*ngoen tham khwan*" (money to restore the spirit [of the injured party]). This description of the payment helps to situate the actions of the Bangkok Tramway Company in the wake of the accident within the cultural milieu of traditional Siamese ideas on injury, loss, and remediation.

As discussed in the preceding chapter, the Siamese concept of unnatural death (*tai hong*) was a wide-ranging system of beliefs and practices for dealing with the aftermath of sudden or unforeseen losses of human life.[37] The relevant concerns and actions taken in the aftermath of unnatural deaths were dictated by the circumstances of the death and the perceived repercussions that it would have for the community. Generally, the occurrence of an unnatural death by violent or sudden means necessitated some action to placate and pacify the disembodied spirit of the deceased for the good of the community.

When death was caused by the neglect or default of another person, interested parties tended to invoke the metaphysical principle of the *khwan* as the subject of remediation and compensatory action.[38] Actions taken in the aftermath of such tragedies were characterized not by retribution or vengeance for the departed and their kin, but rather, in accordance with a restorative sense of justice, they were aimed at placating the harmed spirit and protecting the community from further loss. The notion of social differentiation is implied in such actions as an essential part of the broader cultural context of the practice: the cost of restoring the *khwan* was related to the social standing of the individuals involved. According to M. B. Hooker, traditional Siamese civil law was emphatically "status" based (as opposed to "contract" based), and did not assume the equal status of all legal parties.[39] In such a legal tradition, "one's obligations were ascribed upon the basis of one's rank in society."[40] Therefore, one's liability in the accidental death of another—as expressed through the amount of expected remediation—was likewise calculated according to the relative social standing of the parties.[41] There can be no doubt that in depicting the compensatory payment as a "funerary payment" (*ngoen tham khwan*), the Bangkok Tramway Company sought to participate in precisely these extrajudicial compensatory practices that were rooted in Siamese tradition and based on the assumptions of Siamese metaphysics.

The second notable feature of the payment made by the company is that it received the explicit endorsement of officials in the Siamese state. Prince Naret, for his part, helped to legitimize this mode of remediation when he referred to the compensatory payment as a "fee paid to cover the funeral expenses of the deceased" (*pia pluk tua phu tai*), another description of compensation actions used in traditional Siamese remediation practice, which was apparently used interchangeably with the idea of *ngoen tham khwan*. Just as important was Naret's verdict that the company had acted appropriately in the matter. Indeed, in response to another report on the same case, Naret reiterates that "the company had already paid [a fee] to restore the spirit of the deceased (*tham khwan*) to his relatives, and there is no need for further action."[42]

Naret's verdict highlights the third and final noteworthy aspect of the payment offered to Amdaeng Jan after the death of Nai Ao: it ostensibly put an end to the civil liabilities arising from the death. With the question of compensation settled, Prince Naret ordered an inquiry into whether the actions of the tramcar driver had played a role in the death of Nai Ao. He ordered police to determine the cause of the deceased's being struck by the car and whether it had been the fault of the driver.[43] Some two weeks later, on March 1, a police official named Luang Wisut informed Naret that the driver was, in fact, "at fault by means of [his] carelessness."[44] Although police concluded that the actions of the driver played a contributing role in the death of Nai Ao, the repercussions of such a judgment of culpability were anything but clear. Legal historians of Thailand have suggested that there was no formal distinction between penal and civil litigation in traditional Siamese law, so a finding of negligence would not necessarily result in any form of criminal or civil litigation—whether against the driver or his employer, the Bangkok Tramway Company.[45] Documents from the Ministry of the Capital, however, suggest that the question of the driver's liability in the death of Nai Ao was handled in an extrajudicial manner. Despite the finding of culpability by negligence, the police investigation into the death concluded with the note that Aage Westenholz, the Danish manager of the company, had dismissed the driver from service.[46] Thus, culpability in the death of Nai Ao never extended beyond the driver of the tramcar and did not result in any civil or criminal legal action.

In sum, documents concerning the death of Nai Ao indicate the manner in which a foreign corporation was able to make use of local practices and expectations to help define the limits of its liability in cases of accidental death and dismemberment. The payment offered to the relatives of Nai Ao amounted to an ex gratia payment according to Western legal ideas: a payment made out of a certain sense of moral obligation without an acknowledgment of legal culpability.[47] Siamese officials were complicit in this arrangement in three ways: first, by recognizing the proposed payments made by the managers of the Bangkok Tramway Company as commensurate with traditional compensatory practices; second, by approving the payments as a sufficient and appropriate outcome in cases of death and dismemberment caused by the tramway cars; and third, by applying (or acquiescing to) a constrained sense of liability in such cases. The case of Nai Ao is emblematic of a transitional period in Siamese legal history, when reforms had only recently been put in place to rationalize the structure and function of the judicial system and clear a backlog of cases.[48] It is possible that in the midst of this transition the managers of the Bangkok Tramway Company had no other recourse than to attempt to conform to the tacit rules of compensation according to Siamese customs. But there is reason to suspect that the decision was also a strategic one, aimed at limiting the liability of the company for civil damages. These actions in turn helped to constitute a distinctive sphere of customary law in Siam.

Traditional Siamese ideas and practices concerning remediation were not the only context for the actions of the managers of the Bangkok Tramway Company and the Siamese government officials in the aftermath of the death of Nai Ao. The logic and vocabulary of such practices conformed in large part to the preeminent source of traditional Siamese law: the so-called Law of the Three Seals. The Law of the Three Seals (1805) was the product of a formal recension of a diverse array of extant law codes undertaken by King Rama I soon after the founding of Bangkok.[49] At the end of the nineteenth century, before modern law codes had been promulgated as part of the effort to construct a national justice system, the Law of the Three Seals was the only codified source of Siamese law.[50] The codified form of the Law of the Three Seals, however, belies the ambiguous nature of its use and application in Siamese jurisprudence. The early historian of Southeast Asian law Robert Lingat asserted that "Siamese traditional laws came to us embodied in a single code, compiled in the early years of this century [the nineteenth century]. . . . Its provisions were really law [as opposed to custom], and were applied as such by Courts of Justice till the codes used to-day [modern legal codes] were promulgated [in the first quarter of the twentieth century]."[51] In actuality, historians do not have a definitive sense of how the Law of the Three Seals was implemented and what sort of demographic or geographical reach it might have had in application.[52] Moreover, as Tamara Loos has argued, "Implementation of the letter of the law, a foreign concept in any event, was also nearly impossible in practice. That is not to say that Siam was lawless, but that the regime of law did not operate primarily as an institution of codes emanating from Bangkok."[53]

For much of the nineteenth century, only three copies of the codes existed, and they were sequestered in places of royal power and not released to the public. David Streckfuss has noted that King Rama I, who ordered the codification of the codes, "might have wanted his dominions to follow the [Law of the] *Three Seals*, but part of its power was its limited accessibility."[54] Another Siamese sovereign, King Rama III, allowed the codes to be printed by an American missionary in 1849 but quickly changed his mind and had all the copies gathered up and destroyed.[55] Eventually his successor, King Mongkut (Rama IV), would allow the codes to be printed and disseminated to the public beginning in 1863, but according to Loos, this wider dissemination transformed the Law of the Three Seals, which were thenceforth "no longer a source of legitimacy and sacred power that had to be secluded."[56] The codes became instead "a source of applicable and practical law," albeit one that would soon be rendered obsolete by the propagation of modern law codes beginning in 1908.[57]

The cases of injury and death on the tracks of the Bangkok Tramway Company under consideration in this chapter fell within this transitional period, after the Law of the Three Seals had become part of the public domain but before the codification of modern legal codes and the constitution of national institutions of justice. For foreign residents seeking an understanding of Siamese civil law during this era, the Law of the Three Seals remained the preeminent source. Consular officials posted at the foreign legations of the imperial powers approached the Law of the Three Seals as part of an ethnography of law in Siam. William J. Archer, the British consul in Bangkok, published annotated translations of the laws related to physical assault and debt as part of this effort.[58]

It is no surprise, then, that when the Bangkok Tramway Company became embroiled in civil matters with Siamese legal subjects—who did not have the legal rights to file civil claims against it in the city's foreign consular courts—it turned to the same laws to determine the appropriate mode of civil remediation. By doing so, the managers of the Bangkok Tramway Company helped to institutionalize traditional forms of sociolegal action as part of a system of customary law under the plural legal system established by extraterritoriality in Siam. Other cases of accidental death and dismemberment in late nineteenth-century Siam involving the Bangkok Tramway Company reveal a similar engagement with traditional Siamese civil law as customary law. The company's managers, however, were privileged participants in the traditional Siamese practices, and they brought with them distinctive legalistic concerns, including a desire for documentation and indemnification that was inimical to Siamese customs.

The death of Jin Kim Hok (also known as Jin Jai) in May 1895 demonstrates the distinctive and exceptional nature of the ways in which transnational social actors interacted with Siamese customary law in late nineteenth-century Bangkok.[59] On the afternoon of May 20, Kim Hok went out on an errand to buy betel nut at the fresh market near Sam Yot Gate (figure 4). To reach the market, he had to cross over an iron bridge; but the bridge, as usual, was crowded with the traffic of horse-drawn carts and rickshaws. He decided to take a short cut by crossing over the section of the bridge reserved for the passage of tramway cars. As soon as he entered the bridge, however, he saw tramway car number two approaching from the opposite direction. Realizing his error, Kim Hok jumped to the side of the passageway and pressed himself against the wall to make way for the approaching tramcar. The passage was

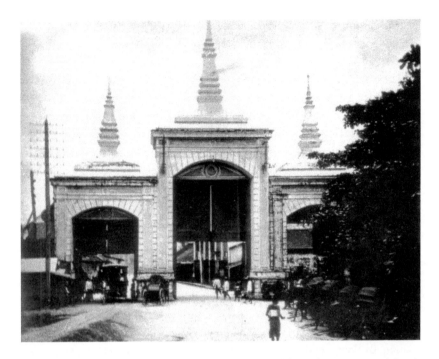

Figure 4. *Pratu Sam Yot* (Sam Yot Gate), ca. 1892. Pictured with horse-drawn tramcar at left and rickshaws awaiting fares at right. National Archives of Thailand, image # ภ.002 หวญ.52–31.

too narrow, however, and the tramcar crushed him against the wall, seriously injuring his head, shoulders, flank, legs, and toes.[60] Kim Hok's wife immediately had him placed in the tramcar and he was rushed to the care of Dr. Hays at Bangrak Hospital, where he died the next morning of injuries sustained in the accident.

In the aftermath of the accident, the managers of the Bangkok Tramway Company sought out Kim Hok's widow, a Siamese woman named Amdaeng Phring, and two of his male relatives, Jin Pin Thao and Jin Hok Huai, who had also emigrated from China. As representative of the tramway company, Aage Westenholz offered the relatively extravagant sum of three *chang* (240 baht) to cover the funerary costs of Kim Hok; the payment offered by the company was described as a *"kha phao phi,"* or a "fee for the cremation of the spirit [of the deceased]."[61] The very fact that Westenholz offered 240 baht at a time when most awards given out by the company were in the amount of 80 baht suggests that perhaps the company understood its liability to be somehow greater in this case than in others. In exchange for the compensation, Westenholz insisted on obtaining documentation that would both verify the payment and indemnify the Bangkok Tramway Company against future claims for damages related to the death.

On May 24, presumably at the appointed time for receiving the payment, Amdaeng Phring and Kim Hok's two male relatives arrived at the offices of the Bangkok Tramway Company, where they were greeted by a clerk named Nai Khian. Following the instructions of Westenholz, Khian accompanied them to the local police station, where he informed the district inspector, Inspector Sathonmorakha, of the events and asked him to draft up an "official contract" (*sanya pracham*) reflecting the agreement of the parties concerning the death and to stamp it with an official (state) seal. It is interesting to note that Inspector Sathonmorakha uses an elevated register to describe the actions of Aage Westenholz, referring to him as *"than mistoe"* (respected "Mister") and describing the manner in which he dispatched Nai Khian as *"chai . . . hai,"* which signifies the type of hierarchical social relations that would obtain between a social superior and their client in the Siamese feudal social order. Despite the deferential language, however, Inspector Sathonmorakha refused to draft the requested document, explaining, "in cases of death such as these I am unable to write up a contract out of fear that there would be some mistake."[62]

Nai Khian, the company's clerk, apparently understood that the notion of an "official contract" was the sticking point for Inspector Sathonmorakha. According to Sathonmorakha's account, Khian accepted his refusal without argument and proposed instead that the inspector "depose" the interested parties.[63] Sathonmorakha evidently deemed this a much more appropriate sort of intervention for a police inspector in what amounted to a matter of civil law, and he agreed to draft up a statement of the essentials of the case and to record the names of the interested parties and witnesses. He submitted a copy of the resulting document, which the parties called a "letter of agreement" (*nangsue sanya*), to his superior officer at the police station and requested that it be forwarded to the director and deputy director of police.

The letter of agreement that Nai Khian, on behalf of the Bangkok Tramway Company, extracted from Amdaeng Phring and Kim Hok's Chinese relatives clearly reflects the legalistic concerns of the company and its shareholders in cases of accidental injury and death. It demonstrates the Janus-faced nature of the company's interactions with Siamese subjects in matters of civil law: the company spoke the vernacular language of customary forms of compensation while demanding a legalistic explanation of the events and indemnification in ways that were in stark contrast to the former practices and discourses. In describing the actions of Chinaman Kim Hok on that fateful day, the letter says that after being unable to find a way across the public (*luang*) section of

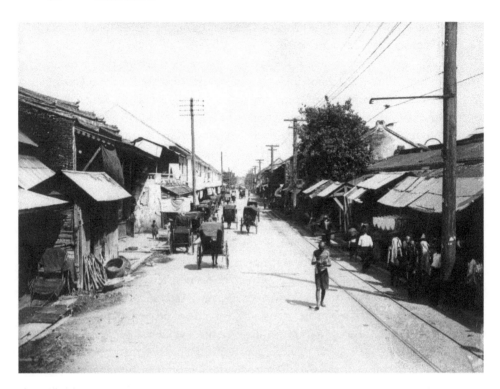

FIGURE 5. *Thanon jaroen krung*, also known as the New Road, ca. 1900. The tramway tracks are visible at right; electrical power lines run overhead. National Archives of Thailand, image # ก.002 หวญ.52/12.

the bridge (or finding it too crowded with traffic to permit easy passage), "Jin Kim Hok took an illegal shortcut by crossing over the narrow channel of the steam-powered train bridge."[64] The signatories to the letter—Amdaeng Phring, Jin Pin Thao, and Jin Hok Huai—were made to explicitly acknowledge that "they all agreed that" Kim Hok was at "fault [in the accident] for walking on the pathway of the steam-powered train," which had been granted to the tramway company.[65] Amdaeng Phring further stated that she did not bear ill will toward or have intentions of taking legal action against the tramway company.[66] Finally, the letter states that if any of the three concerned parties, Amdaeng Phring, Jin Pin Thao, or Jin Hok Huai, should attempt to file charges against the company in the future, the company could produce this letter and the parties in question would be subject to a fine and other punishment.

Concerning the monetary compensation offered by the company to the relatives of Jin Kim Hok, the letter of agreement gracefully utilizes the discourse of customary Siamese compensation practice while taking care not to admit fault. The agreement states, "the employees [managers] of the company

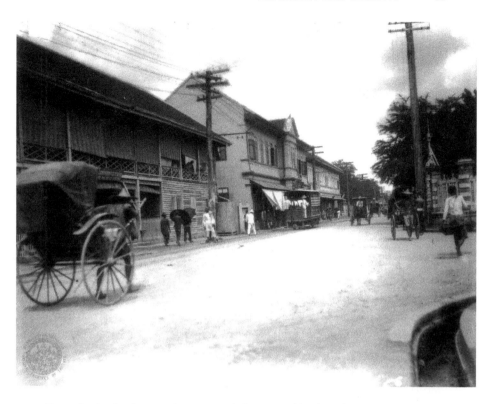

FIGURE 6. An electric-powered tramcar travels the New Road line (center) alongside other types of vehicles. National Archives of Thailand, image # 49M.00024 (หจช) 686–2409.

had compassion towards Jin Kim Hok, the deceased" and had "paid money in the amount of three *chang* [240 baht] as a funerary payment to Jin Kim Hok, the deceased."[67] The letter explicitly—and repeatedly—describes the money as a payment made to the deceased, not his relatives. This is in conformity with customary laws of remediation, where the focus was on the spirit of the harmed or deceased party, not the well-being or rights of surviving family.[68] Also, the letter describes the payment as a *"kha phao phi"* (a "fee [to pay for the cost of] cremating the spirit"), which is something of a departure from the standard vocabulary of compensatory actions—or, at the very least, an instance of the most colloquial of the terms used for compensatory actions. Finally, returning to the legalistic concerns that motivated the company's desire for documentation, the letter states that Amdaeng Phring and Kim Hok's two male relatives "willingly and gladly accepted the payment of three *chang* from the managers of the tramway company."[69]

The letter of agreement concerning the death of Jin Kim Hok is a crucial document for what it reveals about civil law in Siam in the last decade of the nineteenth century. In cosmopolitan Bangkok, social actors possessed radically different expectations and operated on divergent understandings of the implications of accidental injury and death. The managers of the Bangkok Tramway Company sought to participate in the customary practices of the Siamese by offering a funerary payment while at the same time attempting to obtain legal documentation that would serve to indemnify the company against possible litigation in the future. When the company first started operations, Siam had not yet taken concrete steps to establish the national legal institutions that had been part of King Chulalongkorn's public vision of reform since 1888, so it is quite possible that the managers of the Bangkok Tramway Company simply did not know where to file official notices of their compensatory payments to victims and their relatives in the case of accidents.[70] But in the wake of the sweeping administrative reforms of 1892, a new Ministry of Justice had been established along with lower courts responsible for criminal and civil adjudication, respectively.[71] There is reason to suspect, however, that despite their new luster, these institutions remained as opaque as courts under the former system—at least until a set of provisional rules governing civil procedure was promulgated in 1896.[72]

Rather than appeal to the newly formed Ministry of Justice, then, Aage Westenholz continued to deal with the Siamese police force in Bangkok, which was an administrative unit under the Ministry of the Capital. This in itself might be an indication of a strategic decision: Westenholz and the foreign managers of the company may well have appealed directly to the police for the express purpose of avoiding entanglements with new legal institutions and bureaucrats who were less familiar to them. Individual police inspectors, however, were understandably reluctant to engage in legalistic documentary practices that did not fall under their mandate. The letter of agreement that resulted from this engagement demonstrates the willingness of Siamese subjects to engage with transnational social actors (including corporate entities) so long as they fulfilled their cultural expectations—spoke their language—and likewise the desire of transnational actors to accommodate local practices, so long as the outcome was advantageous.

The manner in which the Bangkok Tramway Company accommodated local cultural expectations in dealing with matters of civil law concerning Siamese subjects suggests something of the liminal position of the company in Siamese society. The company appealed to traditional Siamese compensatory practices as an exceptional participant, able to indulge in culturally appropriate modes of extrajudicial action while appealing to Western legal practices and institutions for indemnification. This dual mode of action demonstrates that the company and its managers acted to secure their own best interests in such transactions without paying heed to the social institutions that enforced cultural expectations about compensatory practices in Siamese society. This peculiar form of agency, namely, the ability to engage with customary practices while remaining independent of the forms of sociocultural authority that made them obligatory, was characteristic of another segment of Bangkok's population as well: the Siamese elite.

"Merry Natives" and Noblesse Oblige: Liability and Privilege in Customary Law

The sense of privilege that informs the perspective of the Bangkok Tramway Company's management in cases of accidental injury is revealed by the cavalier manner in which Aage Westenholz treated the payment of compensation for injured Siamese and Chinese passengers. Writing in a Western trade publication, Westenholz observed of indigenous use of the tramway: "While all the Siamese are extremely alert, some of the Chinese are clumsy and too pig[-]headed to listen to the conductor's directions, and, in consequence, you sometimes see them turn head over heels, to the great delight of the other passengers."[73] Regarding compensation for injuries in such cases, Westenholz joked that the right to laugh at others unlucky enough to fall while exiting the tramcars was compensation enough. "On the whole," he flippantly remarked, "I am disposed to believe that the amusement in seeing thirteen other men fall more than compensates the inconvenience of one fall himself to one of these merry natives."[74]

In cases of more serious injury, however, and of accidents resulting in death, Westenholz was forced to find a more culturally appropriate idiom for responding to the loss experienced by the victims, as evidenced by the discussions of the cases of Nai Ao and Jin Kim Hok. That is not to suggest, however, that Westenholz and the shareholders of the Bangkok Tramway Company were forced to bow to local attitudes and expectations. Rather, the actions of the company and its management in conforming to local customs are more accurately viewed as strategic behavior aimed at limiting the liability of the company in cases of accidental injury and death. The assumptions about liability and the practice of compensation that the Bangkok Tramway Company adopted in cases of injuries sustained by Siamese legal subjects articulated with a distinctive strand of Siamese cultural practices in cases of injury and death. In many ways, they mirrored the practices of elite Siamese, which reflected a privileged sense of liability and the prerogative to dictate the terms of their own exposure and the amount of compensation due to injured parties.

One salient case in demonstrating the nature of this privilege is that of a traffic accident involving a high-ranking royal official named Prince Phichit Prichakon, a half-brother of King Chulalongkorn, in February 1896. An open horse-drawn cart (*rot keng*) was traveling along a main thoroughfare in the city when a sedan drawn by a pair of horses abruptly pulled out in front of it at a busy intersection at *Ban Mo*—an area of the central city known for, and named after, its pottery industry. The horse-drawn cart violently crashed into the back of the sedan. In the impact, the driver of the cart, named Nai Pao, was thrown clear of the scene, injuring his left elbow and temple when he landed on the road. Jin Kuai, the sixteen-year-old Chinese laborer who was with Nai Pao in the cart at the time of the accident, however, remained seated on the cart. The horse drawing Nai Pao's cart evidently veered away from the sedan, but the impact of the cart broke the real axle under the sedan and the weight of the rear of the sedan crashed down on Jin Kuai's chest.[75]

Nai Koet, the police officer who had been assigned to watch over the intersection, rushed to the scene of the accident and immediately apprehended the horses attached to the sedan so that the driver could not flee. The driver alighted from the sedan and approached the police officer, informing him that the sedan belonged to Prince Phichit and that the dignitary himself was seated in the sedan at the time of the accident. Prince Phichit then identified himself and ordered the police officer to release his sedan.[76] The police officer recognized the prince and followed his command, allowing him to go on his way. He then turned his attention to Nai Pao, ordering that he, his cart, and the young Chinese man be led to the local police station.

At the police station, Nai Koet assessed the injuries sustained by the two men. He first noted Nai Pao's bruised and scraped temple and elbow and then continued with the injuries of Jin Kuai, which were considerably more serious. Jin Kuai's chest was bruised and bleeding and blood was running from his mouth and nose.[77] Nai Koet realized the possibility that the young man had sustained injuries "inside his chest" that were beyond his ability to discern; he therefore decided to send Jin Kuai to the police Hospital, where he was attended to by the head physician, Jin Meng Yim.[78] (Jin Meng Yim, a physician of Chinese ancestry, was more commonly referred to as Mo [Dr.] Meng Yim in the state's archives. He had been the head physician at the police hospital in central Bangkok from its inauguration in August 1892 and would go on to play an important role in the introduction of forensic medicine in Siam, as discussed in chapter 6.)[79] Meng Yim's report on the physical condition of Jin Kuai attests to the presence of what he called "bad blood" (*lueat rai*) in his lungs.[80] Jin Meng Yim despaired at his chances of recovery, acknowledging that he was unable to purge the bad blood.

Prince Naret, head of the Ministry of the Capital, was informed of the situation by police in the wake of their investigation. He wrote a private letter to Prince Phichit concerning the events. In the letter, Naret addressed the injuries sustained by Nai Pao and Jin Kuai, and the inability of the doctors to purge the blood from the latter's lungs. Naret noted the possibility that the injuries could prove fatal.[81] In a telling passage, Prince Naret then suggested in deferential terms that Prince Phichit should show "kindness" (*khwam metta*) to the injured parties, and either "present a compensatory payment or make arrangements to take care of [the cost of] medical treatment."[82] He added that such were the appropriate measures given the circumstances, and according to Naret's view of the situation, if the prince showed "kindness and benevolence towards those common people who are suffering in the appropriate manner," then "[Your Highness] would be free from any fault that might lead others to criticize Your Highness."[83] Naret appended a copy of the police report and the opinion of the attending physician to his letter to Prince Phichit, so that there could be no doubt as to the gravity of the injuries sustained by the other parties.

The supreme irony of this case—and what elevates it above the status of mere historical anecdote—is that Prince Phichit was at the time the minister of the newly created Siamese Ministry of Justice.[84] A high-ranking prince, Phichit had been singled out at a young age from among King Chulalongkorn's many siblings as having a legal mind and served as an apprentice (to Prince Thewawong) during a formative era in the creation of the country's nascent national justice system. Unlike many of his siblings and royal contemporaries, however, Phichit was never sent abroad for his education; "for this reason," according to legal scholar David Engel, "his ideas of justice were more strongly rooted in the traditional than was true in the case of his brothers and nephews."[85] During his long and distinguished legal career, Prince Phichit had already served as the head of the Supreme Court (*san dika*) and the central civil court (*san phaeng klang*) in Bangkok. During his tenure as special commissioner (*kha luang phiset*) to Chiangmai in 1884, Phichit had been instrumental in establishing the International Court, which was invested with limited power to adjudicate commercial matters between Siamese and foreign (British) subjects in the northern capital.[86]

Apart from the hypocrisy of a sitting minister of justice eschewing the halls of justice for the adjudication of his own legal affairs, the accident involving Prince Phichit is important for what it reveals about the logic and agency behind compensatory gift giving in cases of injury and death involving elite Siamese parties. When the party at fault in a civil matter (the tortfeasor) was a member of the Siamese elite, that party's social and economic status mitigated the effectiveness of traditional modes of compensatory reasoning and practice. Both the appeals to communal well-being—the "restorative" logic—and the hierarchical social channels by which these expectations were enacted and enforced were largely inapplicable when the tortfeasor was a member of the elite royal classes. In such cases the tortfeasor therefore had a great deal of latitude in deciding the appropriate outcome. And in this era of rapid legal change, recourse to the formal institutions of justice was evidently seen as an optional or voluntary course of action at best, even for an official whose entire career had been devoted to establishing such institutions.

When tortfeasors were members of the Siamese elite, they were essentially free to unilaterally assess their own liability and the value of the loss incurred by the victim—up to and including the value of the victim's life—offering whatever compensation they deemed appropriate. Yet, despite the fact that they enjoyed greater license in these transactions than average Siamese subjects, the Siamese elite nevertheless couched their compensatory actions in the terminology of traditional forms of remediation aimed at repairing the social fabric in the wake of accidental loss in the community. That is to say, the compensatory gift giving of the Siamese elite ostensibly fell within the range of culturally expected behavior in cases of accidental injury and death, and payments were described accordingly.

Insulated by extraterritorial treaty protections, the Bangkok Tramway Company, its managers, and its legal representatives enjoyed a similar degree of license in their dealings with Siamese subjects and Chinese immigrants who experienced loss on the tramway tracks. Their compensatory gift giving conformed to the ethos of the traditional Siamese practices involved in communal mediation, yet they exercised a similar degree of autonomy in deciding the terms and conditions of their payments and the extent of their participation. Incidents in October and November 1898 reveal that up until the final years of the nineteenth century, the subject of compensation and liability in cases of injury remained a matter left largely to the discretion of the Bangkok Tramway Company. On October 17, 1898, the *Bangkok Times* announced, "The child who was run over recently by a tramway car has had its leg amputated, and is progressing favourably." "As to the matter of compensation," the article continued definitively, "everything is in the hands of the Company's lawyers."[87]

A few weeks later, a train was bearing down on an errant child playing on the tramway tracks when the child's grandmother rushed over to the rescue. She was too slow, however, and the tramcar ran over both her chest and the child's leg. The grandmother was killed instantly, while the child was not expected to survive the grave injuries. After registering their surprise that such "accidents in Bangkok are not more frequent," the editors of the *Bangkok*

Times concluded, "In the present case the occurrence has all the appearance of being a sheer accident, and the officials of the Company have shown every kindness towards the relatives of the deceased."[88] The language employed by the *Bangkok Times* in describing these instances of death and injury and the subsequent calculation of compensation suggests a peculiar legal subjectivity in traditional Siamese society. The Bangkok Tramway Company, like elite Siamese subjects, enjoyed substantial exemptions from the social mechanisms that enforced obligatory forms of action in lieu of civil litigation.

At the same time, there is evidence to suggest that in rare cases the Bangkok Tramway Company was able to capitalize on tacit forms of social allegiance akin to the patron-client social relations enjoyed by Siamese elites in order to mitigate its losses. Such appears to be the case when an employee of the company lost his own daughter on the tracks of the Bangkok Tramway Company. On a Sunday afternoon in the middle of the hot season, in April 1894, "while No. 3 car was traveling at a good speed along the middle section of the electric system, the driver suddenly noticed a Siamese infant of about 12 months old creeping across" the tracks in front of the approaching car.[89] The driver applied the brakes "and did everything possible to stop the car, and then jumped on the cow-catcher [a device intended to redirect would-be victims away from the wheels of the tramcar] in front, with the purpose of picking up the child, [however,] just as he bent forward to grasp the infant, a sudden jerk overwhelmed him, and he narrowly escaped being run over himself." The cow-catcher failed to save the child and the car passed over her, causing instant death. "The father of the child," the story notes in conclusion, "is employed by the Tramway Co. as a clerk." This particular case does not appear in the inquest files compiled by the Ministry of the Capital; the police evidently did not conduct an investigation into the death of the young girl, and no mention is made of compensation paid by the company to the girl's father.

Subject to Custom

When the Bangkok Tramway Company introduced passenger rail travel to the crowded streets of the Siamese capital in the final years of the nineteenth century, the alluring promise of urban transit was mired by the tragic loss of life and limb. The majority of those killed and injured were individuals who fell under the de facto category of Siamese legal subjects. In dealing with these socially and legally marginal victims, the foreign managers of the company worked through extrajudicial channels and offered forms of compensation that corresponded to traditional expectations arising out of Siamese social practices and cultural repertoires. The company's managers, who occupied a liminal but privileged status in the broader sociocultural world inhabited by the majority of Bangkok's residents, appealed to these practices in order to limit their financial liability. For tortfeasors who were protected by extraterritoriality—including foreign residents and business ventures—the ability to partake in traditional extrajudicial modes of remediation for loss provided a considerable amount of leeway in acknowledging liability and determining appropriate compensation. With the explicit approval of officials in the Siamese Ministry of the Capital, these instances of loss did not amount to a challenge to the Siamese legal system, such as it was. Instead, the valorization of the practices by Siamese officials and the Siamese subjects who were the victims of accidental loss helped to create a new form of legal life—a realm of customary law—within the plural legal arena of treaty port Bangkok.

Customary law was a product of middle to late nineteenth-century attempts to reimagine the colonial enterprise. It was a product of what Karuna Mantena has identified as a "broad transition from a *universalist* to a *culturalist* stance in nineteenth-century imperial ideology," which was institutionalized in the ideology and institutions of indirect rule.[90] Of course, as Martin Chanock and other scholars have long understood, customary law "was essentially a product of the impact of capitalism and colonialism; not the expression of some authentic communal tradition, as indirect rule theorists believed, but rather an instrument forged by local hierarchies to defend their interests."[91] Siamese customary law effectively extended the privileges enjoyed by elite Siamese social actors to foreign residents and their corporate endeavors; it also married these forms of privileged action with what were—in the Siamese context—unprecedented forms of documentation and indemnification. The forms of legal life that grew out of these practical encounters in what was an interstitial era in Siamese legal history are an overlooked aspect of modernizing legal change in Siam. In contrast to scholarship fixated on codification, these practical arrangements provide a window into the realities of social life under extraterritoriality. They impart a sense of contingency to the processes of legal change while attending to indigenous precedents. In short, they allow us to see Bangkok as a distinctive site of legal evolution in its own right—and one that can no longer be regarded as a fallow field waiting to receive the transplanted codes and institutions of foreign legal systems.[92]

Each case of the loss of life or limb on the tracks of the Bangkok Tramway Company was a discrete social entanglement that required practical cross-cultural labor to unwind. The individual outcomes—extrajudicial payments that suited the strategic interests of the company while appealing to the cultural sensibilities of Siamese subjects—were part of a broader pattern of cross-cultural engagements that were beginning to redefine social and political life in late nineteenth-century Siam. Although these encounters fall outside the purview of narratives of modernizing legal change, they are nevertheless a crucial part of the story of the formation of a modern legal system in Siam. The assemblage of customary law is a neglected part of the patrimony of elite efforts to achieve sovereignty through legal reform in the early twentieth century, "to purchase," as Sally Engle Merry has remarked of indigenous efforts to adopt Western law in Hawai'i, "independence with the coin of civilization."[93]

Yet beyond the institutional history of legal reform, the contingent compensatory arrangements discussed in this chapter have a broader referent. As "both a system of meaning and an institutional structure backed by the political power of the state," Merry argues, "[l]aws define persons and relationships, which create, if they do not already reflect, popular consciousness."[94] By attending to these tragic events and their aftermath, we apprehend the inchoate Siamese legal subject at a unique historical moment, as it was simultaneously constituted as the object of different but in many ways articulated cultural and social logics. The power of law in these historical encounters is more modest than the "humanizing" power claimed by colonial legal regimes, where positive law declared the ability to transform the subhuman into the human by virtue of bringing pre-colonial subjects into (colonial) liberal modernity.[95] Instead, I understand these extrajudicial compensatory arrangements as capable of codifying traditional metaphysical ideas of the human-in-death into a viable facet of the human as legal subject.[96]

The accidents, injuries, and compensatory arrangements discussed in this chapter reveal how the Siamese legal subject was identified in practice—through pragmatic encounters—at a historical moment long before its rights and obligations were codified and articulated in theory in the form of modern legal codes. The ahistorical constituents of a timeless Siamese feudal world were made historical by accident, through collisions with new modes of mobility, finance, and legality. The constitution of this distinctive form of legal subjecthood paralleled elite Siamese efforts to construct a modern legal regime that perpetuated aspects of the feudal social order in Siam. Unlike the discursive efforts of Siamese elites to capture the emancipating prospects of legal reform through the act of translating ideas like "rights" and "liberty," however, the forms of historically contingent subjecthood discussed here offer the possibility—perhaps uniquely—of bridging the chasm between historical iterations of subjecthood on the one hand, and subjectivity, on the other.[97]

From the perspective of Michel Foucault's notion of "the historical ontology of ourselves," invoking the *khwan* as a facet of the subaltern Siamese legal subject was not simply an act of power-knowledge in the objectifying sense.[98] The *khwan* was a metaphysical idea with long standing in the Siamese cultural world. It was undoubtedly one of the constitutive elements by which many Siamese understood human identity. In that sense, invoking the *khwan* also had ethical implications for the subaltern Siamese who were being constituted as—and likewise beginning to understand themselves as—legal subjects. The same could not be said of foreign residents who encountered loss on the tramway tracks, however. Foreign residents possessed a radically different sense of legal subjectivity, and, endowed with extralegal privileges, their traumas entailed very different forms of legal action. Their fortunes—as well as those of other privileged legal entities like the Bangkok Tramway Company—are the subject of the next chapter.

CHAPTER 3

Treaty Port Tort

> A tort system is a cultural artifact. Like "nature" and
> law more generally, tort is both an artifact and a tool
> for crafting other artifacts such as "liability." It is a tool
> of a particular sort, a tool for making a particular sort
> of sense. It is a tool for putting broken things back
> together. Tort is also a device for ordering relationships
> among strangers, for distributing risks and burdens,
> incentives and disincentives. It is a tool for doing justice.
> It is, more specifically, a tool for projecting and
> enforcing conceptions of reasonableness.
>
> —David Delaney, *Law and Nature*

In late 1891, the five-member juries of the British consular court in Bangkok took notice of the spate of injuries on the tramway tracks and began to award sizeable damages to plaintiffs who filed civil charges against the Bangkok Tramway Company. According to the *Bangkok Times*, the case of a British lawyer who had his foot run over by a tramcar helped set the precedent.[1] In that case, a British jury awarded the lawyer the princely sum of six thousand dollars in damages in addition to his legal expenses.[2] For Siamese subjects, suffering loss on the tramway tracks meant being placed at the mercy of the company's managers for compensation as discussed in chapter 2. For foreign residents, however—including the growing number of Asian immigrants who had registered as the legal subjects or protégés of foreign nations at their legations in Bangkok—even falling from a tramcar could result in a windfall.

Leaving behind the plight of subaltern Siamese subjects who met with tragedy on the tracks of the Bangkok Tramway Company, this chapter considers the fate of injured parties with legal standing in the city's foreign consular courts. Their efforts to seek legal damages against the company attest to the universal problem of the relationship between sociotechnical innovation and legal change. The tramway might be taken as a case study in the "unpredictable ways in which scientific and technological developments slice into settled social relationships and compel a redefinition, through law, of established rights and duties."[3] This is the first and most abstract of three scales for analyzing sociolegal life in this chapter, each of which speaks in turn to the fraught nature of sovereignty in a colonial treaty port, where jurisdiction was always in doubt.

The second scale is revealed by the cast of characters: the plaintiffs, defendants, jurors, and even corporate shareholders and journalists who people the pages mark this as a work of sociolegal history. It is fundamentally a story about ordinary people coming to terms with technological and social change through debates over loss, liability, and compensation. In Siam—just as in many Anglo-American metropolitan jurisdictions—common citizens were conscripted as jurors and empowered to adjudicate such matters in consular courts. Of course, the work of reconciling sociotechnical change and legal order is more often a matter of specialized knowledge, and medical and legal expertise played a fundamental role in discussions over law and liability in late nineteenth-century Bangkok, affirming Sheila Jasanoff's axiom that "law and science are involved in constructing each other."[4] I approach these forms of expert knowledge through their professional incarnations, barristers and physicians, and demonstrate the opaque interactions of the two in mediating the new social realities created by social and technological change. The foreign-language press was a surprisingly critical voice, helping to untangle and articulate the vested interests of these experts, while constantly alluding to the broader global—and imperial—stakes of debates over law and liability in Bangkok.

Finally, the global implications of these local debates are best apprehended through the lens of "jurisdictional politics," which refers to "conflicts over the preservation, creation, nature, and extent of different legal forums and authorities."[5] In plural legal arenas like Siam, jurisdictional disputes provided a forum for the assertion of cultural boundaries and were expressly manipulated by social actors for that reason, as the following discussion demonstrates. Although this chapter repeatedly invokes the plurality of the legal world in treaty port Bangkok, a crucial caveat is that none of the competing jurisdictions should be regarded as monolithic legal systems. Even the British consular court, which dominated the competition among the plural jurisdictions of the day, cannot be uncritically regarded as merely a local iteration of British metropolitan law in Siam; crucial developments in British common law in the nineteenth century were left on the docks of London, and pivotal debates over loss and liability had to be played out anew in the British consular court in Bangkok. The legal conflicts and discourses discussed here thus confirm Lauren Benton's maxim that "no legal sphere (whether defined by jurisdiction, municipal law, religious affiliation, or legal cultures) constituted a closed world;

in practice and in political imagination, legal relations always reached outside."[6] It is fitting then, that this inquiry into sociolegal change at the margins of the nineteenth-century imperial world should begin with a case study drawn from the very center.

"Moving to the Death": Railways and Legal Change in British History

Steam power revolutionized the production and movement of commodities in the early nineteenth-century world. By mid-century, as steamships and railways transitioned into a second phase of existence as modes of passenger transport, they increasingly became a threat to the public well-being. In metropolitan Europe and America, news of boiler explosions and the spectacular carnage that they wrought prompted public discussion of liability due to negligence in the context of industrial business ventures and public transportation. Passenger rail travel likewise produced highly visible cases of injury and death, inciting demands for greater legal oversight of industrial ventures, a more defined sense of liability, and a mandate for the compensation of victims. In mid-nineteenth-century Britain, the public nature of injury and deaths wrought by industrial steam power—and especially passenger rail travel—galvanized public opinion and had a direct role in the transformation of traditional British legal ideas and practices concerning accidental death.

The deodand was a legal instrument of British common law that could be applied by a jury that was convened by a coroner as part of an inquest into a case of sudden or unnatural death. It stipulated that in cases where "an animal or inanimate object caused or occasioned the accidental death of a human being," the object in question had to be forfeited by its owner.[7] The deodand evolved within common law as a way to deal with certain kinds of human deaths that were regarded as events whose effects "transcended mundane considerations, and entailed expiation in one form or another."[8] According to Jacob Finkelstein, the deodand is evidence of the British Crown assuming the responsibility of "vicar of transcendent concerns and values"—even over and above the church; foremost among those values was the "transcendent value of human life," the loss of which required an act of expiation.[9] In theory, the deodand, the surrendered object that had "moved to the death" of another person, was sold and the proceeds were used by the royal almoner to sponsor a religious rite (hence the Latinate name *deodand*, meaning "God-gifts").[10] In actual practice, the value of the forfeited item was often assessed and the owner was given the opportunity to pay a fine equal to the assessed value, which was often (though not invariably) given to the relatives of the deceased by the local authorities.[11] Although the deodand underwent significant change over time and showed considerable variance in its application across different jurisdictions, one crucial feature remained true: there was never a systematic relation between the deodand and the notion of fault. As a legal instrument intended to deal with "transcendent" aspects of loss and as a relic of "a more superstitious age," the deodand resisted explicit articulations of causality and fault.[12] The fortunes of the deodand as a legal instrument waxed and waned over the centuries, culminating in the mid-nineteenth century, when it made a brief but spectacular revival before being finally abolished by parliamentary act in 1846.[13]

The mid-nineteenth-century revival of the deodand was inextricably linked to railway disasters, which briefly transformed the deodand into a punitive instrument for assessing fault. In a single year, 1840, deodands awarded by coroners' juries in cases involving railway operators increased exponentially, rising from nominal amounts to thousands of pounds sterling based on the value of the railway engines that had contributed to injury and death.[14] A catastrophic train wreck at Sonning on Christmas Eve in 1841, which claimed the lives of nine passengers, proved to be the deciding event that transformed the deodand into a de facto legal instrument for assessing fault and awarding compensation to victims.[15] In a decisive break from the tradition of deodand common law, the coroner's jury summoned to hear the inquest called the Sonning wreck "willful murder" and awarded a deodand on the railway engine, which was owned by the Great Western Railway, in the amount of one thousand pounds sterling.[16]

The development of a new and potentially maiming technology such as industrial rail travel was not alone sufficient to transform the British legal apparatus surrounding accidental death; social interests and actors also played a crucial role. For politicians and industrialists alike, the Sonning railway disaster revealed the incongruity of traditional legal practices in the age of industry. Railway deaths were so pervasive and railroads so capital-intensive that the notion of deodand became "irrational" when applied to such deaths—at least from the perspective of the railway owners and investors.[17] While debating the merits of legal change, members of the British Parliament described the deodand as "extremely absurd and inconvenient."[18] In the wake of these developments, and with pressure from industrialists, Parliament abolished the common law of deodand in 1846 through the Deodand Abolition Act.[19] That same year, Parliament also passed the Fatal Accidents Compensation Act, a comprehensive measure aimed at indemnifying the railways in the event of fatal injuries. The Fatal Accidents Act also closed a vast loophole in British civil law, which stipulated that there could be no civil charges filed if the victim of a tort were deceased. The act made provisions whereby the family of the deceased could be awarded damages in the case of an accidental death.

The legal change surrounding the deodand reflects nothing less than a reordering of the sociocultural habits of thought associated with accidental death in the wake of the introduction of a new technology: passenger rail travel. With the death of the deodand came the possibility for a radical new ordering of responsibility for wrongful death. In theory, the owners of railroads, tramways systems, or other industrial ventures might be held liable for any and all accidents and deaths that occurred in association with standard operations. Judges and jurists recognized, however, that such a regime of strict liability was likely to place an overwhelming burden on new industrial ventures, which would ultimately stifle economic development. Instead of strict liability—or indeed, its antithesis, absolute immunity—they turned to the notion of negligence as an intermediate space for legal judgment. Negligence, the question of whether or not an accidental death occurred due to carelessness, or failing to uphold "the vague, subtle standard of the 'reasonable man,'" became the new metric of fault.[20] Thus, the abolition of the deodand helped to usher in a new era in civil law, the law of torts, whereby accidental death became a mundane violation of human civil law and culpability was transformed into a matter subject to measurement by degree through the principle of negligence. Similar developments occurred in other metropolitan jurisdictions as well.[21]

The implications of this specific negotiation between technological change and socio-cultural life, however, were apparently not modular. Although parliamentary law had helped achieve stasis in matters of liability and compensation in British common law in Great Britain, juries in the British consular court in Bangkok asserted their own—often antagonistic—views of liability for death and injury when adjudicating cases involving the Bangkok Tramway Company.

The Third Rail: Accidents, Compensation, and Tort Law in the British Consular Court

Despite the incredible carnage on the tracks of the Bangkok Tramway Company in its early years of operation, there was a decided shift in the coverage of the company and its legal fortunes in the local press some four years after tramcars began plying the streets in 1888. By early 1892, the solemn reportage of accidental deaths and injuries had given way to scathing editorials about the abuse of civil litigation at the British consular court in Bangkok. Foreign residents filing suit against the Bangkok Tramway Company had become so commonplace that it was a matter of farce.

In an article titled "The Law and the Profits," the editor of the *Bangkok Times* opined, "Considering the size of the European community in Bangkok there is just about as much litigation going on now as is to be found to the square mile anywhere [in the world]."[22] The article comments on the recent upsurge in cases of civil litigation for injury and libel in the British consular court. After the court—and more specifically its rotating juries of five British subjects—had proven charitable in awarding lavish damages to plaintiffs in civil cases involving injury and defamation, the caseload had only increased. The Bangkok Tramway Company had become the prime target for Bangkok residents with the financial means and legal rights to file a civil suit in the British consular court. The *Bangkok Times* satirically noted that since the city's "pathetic" fleet of horse-drawn carts and wagons could not muster sufficient power to cause injury to pedestrians, would-be plaintiffs were limited to filing suit against the Bangkok Tramway Company, "so the inoffensive tram-car has had to stand the judicial racket since the epidemic set in, last year [late 1891]."[23]

It is worth noting that in what appears to be a departure from the institutions and procedures of justice in British colonial jurisdictions, civil cases before the British consular court in Bangkok were decided not by a judge but by five-member juries composed of British-born residents.[24] It is possible that civil trials by jury were an overlooked part of other British legal regimes that were established outside of the confines of formal colonial control; there were at least twelve such regimes around the globe over the course of the nineteenth century if one includes the Ottoman Empire as a single jurisdiction.[25] In a study of one of these regimes in Qing China, Robert Bickers has highlighted the fundamentally ad hoc nature of the system, which was driven not by policy decisions emanating from London but rather from the practical guidance of the system's first chief justice, which in turn was informed by his "own assessment of how the British presence in China should be shaped."[26] Bickers has also noted the reality of diverse modes of orientation and operation across the courts in each of the distinct treaty ports in China.[27] These characteristics of British justice in Chinese treaty ports might help to explain the seemingly anomalous institutional reality of civil trials by jury at the British consular court in Bangkok.

Not long after damages had been awarded to an unnamed British attorney who suffered injury to his foot in 1891, a Chinese man injured his collarbone in January 1892, apparently as a result of falling from a tramcar. The Chinese man in question appears to have been registered as a British subject, which allowed him to file a claim against the Bangkok Tramway Company in the British consular court in Siam—with its sympathetic juries—in the amount of two thousand ticals (baht). (This seems to be a rather extravagant claim for what sounds like a broken collarbone—but it pales in comparison to the six thousand baht awarded to the British attorney only a few months before.)[28] When the charges were filed with the British consular court, the *Bangkok Times* noted sardonically that the tramcar in question had had the misfortune of injuring an "expensive Chinaman," meaning, presumably, a Chinese immigrant registered as a subject with the British Consulate who thereby gained the legal right to file a claim in front of the sympathetic juries of the British court. The management of the Bangkok Tramway Company erred on the side of experience in the case, hiring the same British lawyer with the injured foot who—as a plaintiff—had cost them six thousand ticals in damages only months before. The brazen lawyer balked at the Chinese man's request for damages and told the jury that "fifteen ticals was ample compensation" for the injury to the plaintiff's collarbone. The jury, however, "curled its lip scornfully and gave the Celestial [Chinese man] what he wanted, on the basis [precedent] created by the jury in the [British lawyer's] Feet *cause célèbre.*"[29]

The *Bangkok Times*'s editors lamented what they saw as widespread abuse of all manner of tort litigation in Bangkok's foreign consular courts, including the torts of libel and defamation. They remarked that "if this sort of thing goes on there will soon be but two classes of society here, the wealthy individuals with the soiled reputations or deteriorated feet, and the bankrupt parties who once expressed indiscreet opinions, and the insolvent tramway proprietors. And the Grand Panjandrum will be the lawyer man."[30] And still—flouting the calls for tort reform in the Bangkok press—the tramway cars continued to maim and kill. In September 1892, when a Mr. Maclachlan was thrown from his horse onto the tramway tracks and barely escaped being crushed by an approaching streetcar, the editors wryly noted that in this way he had "escaped being made wealthy."[31]

The discourse on the subject of civil litigation appearing in the English-language press shows an overwhelming commitment to the tenets of nineteenth-century British liberalism. The verdicts awarded by British juries against the Bangkok Tramway Company were viewed as a misappropriation of the rule of law and a threat to private property. The editor of the *Bangkok Times* lamented the evolution of a new regime of civil law in the British consular court that he viewed as a contradiction to the natural (that is, British liberal) order of society. Whether or not the growing number of civil claims against the company was indeed indicative of a wave of tort abuse as the editor suggests, it is notable that the timing coincided with what scholars of American legal history have recognized to be a broadly based and "dramatic transformation in in the attitude toward accidents and the assessment of responsibility between the 1870s when accident rates were still low and the 1880s and 1890s when accidents rates and lawsuits skyrocketed."[32]

Despite the objections posed in the English-language press, it can be said with some certainty that the British juries in Bangkok had accomplished a rather incredible feat: they had managed to turn back the clock on half a century of legal change under parliamentary rule in Britain, a period which had resulted in the eradication of an important element of British common law, the deodand. Through findings of liability and awards of punitive damages, juries in the British consular court in Bangkok had become a threat to the profitability of the Bangkok Tramway Company and a drag on the dividends paid to its shareholders. But, as a registered limited liability corporation under British law, the Bangkok Tramway Company was not without rights.

Locating Liability (I): Jurisdiction

In Bangkok, as in Europe, steam power transformed commerce and transport. Industrial boilers burning rice husks, bagasse, and other biofuels powered the mills that dotted the river's edge, where sugarcane and rice were threshed and milled. Massive boilers on ships and railcars also fueled the steam-powered engines that moved people and goods around the globe in the late nineteenth century. Boiler explosions, the underside of this narrative of progress, were horrific, killing stokers and leaving engineers and others permanently scarred and disfigured by burns.[33] News of high-profile industrial accidents in Europe reached Bangkok and prompted serious discussion of the regulation of risks associated with steam power in both industry and passenger transport.[34] In the final years of the nineteenth century, legislation governing negligence and liability had come to be seen as a requisite feature of the law codes of any country that aspired to the status of a "civilized" nation. Although corporate negligence and liability were discussed extensively in the Bangkok press at the time, the subject was never broached in relation to the proverbial elephant in the room: the Bangkok Tramway Company.

The omission of the Bangkok Tramway Company from contemporary debates about negligence and liability remains something of a mystery. In many ways, the company was a natural target for legal actions aimed at defining (or expanding) the limits of liability in late nineteenth-century Siam. Railways played a central role in the modern transformation of tort law in Anglo-American jurisdictions (as described earlier). The peculiar exceptionality of the Bangkok Tramway Company from discussions of tort reform in Siam seems to have roots in the original contract granting the tramway concession, which was drafted and signed in 1887 between agents of the Siamese government acting on behalf of the king and two foreign entrepreneurs residing in Bangkok (a British subject, Alfred John Loftus, and a Dane, Andre du Plessis de Richelieu).[35] That is not to say, however, that the granting of the concession was somehow exempt from legal reasoning. Far from it: the original tramway concession included extensive provisions governing the process of mediation over eminent domain land purchases, the value of property owned by the tramway concessionaires (in the event that the concession reverted to the state), and even the subject of reparations in cases where the tramway company damaged state-owned buildings. The question of liability in cases of injury, however, was left in a state of utter uncertainty that can only be explained with reference to the complicated matter of jurisdiction in a colonial treaty port subject to extraterritorial law.

The original contract governing the tramway concession broaches the topic of liability for accidents and injuries in the third clause, concerning the use of roads and land where the tramway lines were laid. According to the contract, the "free right of way over all roads" and other places used to construct tramway lines is granted

> provided always that such rights will be exercised with a due regard to the convenience of all other vehicles or persons using the same roads or places, and that in case of any collisions or accidents occurring through the default or negligence of the Concessionaires or their workmen, or servants, the Concessionaires shall be [held] liable in damages to be paid by the Tribunals having cognizance of such collisions or accidents in the same manner as if the said collisions or accidents had occurred through the default or negligence of a person not entitled to the benefit of this concession.[36]

The ambiguities of this clause are a direct reflection of the uncertain state of legal affairs in the Siamese capital at the time. Under extraterritorial law, jurisdiction was defined not by territory but by legal subject status. Injuries sustained by the residents of the Siamese capital could result in very different forms of legal (or often extrajudicial) action, which might likewise result in very different forms of remediation depending on their subject status.

In addition to the question of plural jurisdictions in the Siamese capital, the commonsensical reference to a normalized sense of "the default or negligence of a person" belies the fact that there was no agreement over these notions in cosmopolitan fin de siècle Bangkok. Notions of fault, negligence, and liability remained inextricably tied to distinct sociocultural worlds and, in a few instances, the legal institutions that were established to represent those worlds in accordance with extraterritorial legal privileges.[37] But the lack of specificity concerning liability for damages in cases of accidental injury or death was not limited to Bangkok. Modern legal understandings of negligence and liability were still being worked out in European and American metropolitan jurisdictions alike, where railroads and streetcars likewise played a pivotal role in fostering legal change.[38] The ambiguities surrounding notions of fault and liability in these metropolitan jurisdictions were imported along with the consular courts established by foreign powers in Siam.

In an article on the topic of "Liability for Criminal Negligence," the *Bangkok Times* observed that British law made provisions for such cases, while French law did not.[39] This meant that in cases of injury where a British subject was either harmed by or caused harm through negligence, the injured parties would have recourse to the British consular court. In cases such as a boiler explosion at a rice mill owned by a French protégé in May 1895, however, the victims (who were Siamese subjects by default of not being registered as foreign subjects) had no apparent legal recourse. According to the *Bangkok Times*, "judging from the absence of inquests upon fatal accidents, and of prosecution where criminal negligence is apparent," "French law makes no provision for such cases any more than does the Siamese"—a damning slight in the era of high imperialism, when law was regarded as an index of civilization.[40]

In the end, because the Bangkok Tramway Company was a limited liability corporation registered under British law, adjudication of civil cases against the company fell under the jurisdiction of the British consular court in Bangkok. Urban rail travel had altered the realm of social possibilities in the Siamese capital, and law was called on to mediate these changes through the "redefinition . . . of established rights and duties."[41] The British consular court was the stage for this contest, and the principal actors were the expatriate British jurors who were called on to use their legal power to mediate the effects of technological change in Bangkok. The managers and shareholders of the Bangkok Tramway Company, however, had other plans.

Locating Liability (II): Transnational Corporate Law

Before the abstract notions of negligence, liability, and fault could be debated in the aftermath of the arrival of passenger rail travel in Bangkok, the ramifications of corporate law would have to play out across the competing jurisdictions of the foreign consular courts. As British juries awarded generous verdicts to plaintiffs, the management and shareholders of the Bangkok Tramway Company looked to the privileges of extraterritorial law for shelter. In an article published in a Western trade publication, Aage Westenholz, the Danish manager of the company, acknowledged that in the wake of the "unreasonable verdict" of six thousand baht in the case of the British attorney who "got his foot squeezed [by a tramcar] . . . desperate efforts have been made to get under some other [nation's legal] protection."[42] It was very likely Westenholz himself who hatched the plot to disband the Bangkok Tramway Company, a registered corporation under British law, and reincorporate as a Danish limited liability corporation in order to escape the punishing verdicts awarded to plaintiffs by British juries.

The move came during an "extraordinary" meeting of the management and shareholders at the home of the company's director, Admiral Andre du Plessis de Richelieu, on March 5, 1892.[43] Those in attendance were likely focused on the first proposals mooted at the meeting, which concerned ambitious and expensive plans to introduce electric power on the New Road tramway line. The shareholders authorized the sale of 50,000 ticals' worth of bonds to pay for the improvements, which included the construction of a generating station and the hanging of electrical lines along six miles of a heavily trafficked central artery. The agenda then turned to the question of the company's legal status as a limited liability corporation under British legal protection. Three specific proposals were submitted, including (1) liquidating the assets of the Bangkok Tramway Company as currently constructed, (2) transferring and selling "this Company's business and property to another Company under Danish law with the same name and objects as this Company" with outstanding shares being converted as well, and (3) conducting the transfer under the stipulations of section 204 of the (British) Straits Settlements Companies Ordinance 1889.[44]

While the resolution to introduce electric power seems to have passed without discussion, the dissolution and reincorporation of the company provoked some challenges. Perhaps wary of leaving the well-established jurisdiction of the British consular court in Bangkok, shareholders questioned the wisdom of the move. Those responsible for the plot (likely the two Danes, Westenholz and de Richelieu) allayed their fears by appealing to fundamental cultural differences between British and Danish law: "it was unprecedented, for a man, through an accident, being made rich in Danish courts."[45] (While the article does not attribute this phrase to anyone specifically, it seems to hint at a nonnative command of English, and so might very well have been uttered by one of the Danes. Moreover, Westenholz's acquaintances report that he was "hesitant in his speech because he wanted to choose exactly the right words to express his thoughts."[46]) The plotters then appealed to standards of precedent in Danish tort law, asserting that "the highest damages heard of were a few thousand kroner; and that man [the plaintiff in that case] was killed on the railway."[47] By way of conclusion, the proponents of reincorporation cited the losses already incurred by the company due to the generous verdicts awarded by British juries. The resolutions were then put to a vote. They passed almost unanimously. The sole dissenting vote was cast by a Mr. J. Maclachlan, a British subject, "who said he was too patriotic" to vote in favor of abandoning British legal protection.[48] In retrospect, Maclachlan's dissent has an ominous quality, as the change in jurisdictions would soon become a matter of great personal concern to him, as discussed in the following section.

The matter of the Bangkok Tramway Company's incorporation underscores the contentious and nationalistic nature of debates over liberal forms of governance in a cosmopolitan port city. Efforts to shield the company and its shareholders from the costs of civil litigation gave rise to debates over the respective merits of political culture and business climate under particular national jurisdictions. The cold exigencies of personal financial interests intersected with the patriotic sentiments and longings of the expatriate entrepreneur. In the end, despite Maclachlan's protest, the move to reincorporate under Danish legal protection was largely celebrated by those connected with the Bangkok Tramway Company. According to a visiting foreign correspondent from Singapore, a "native associated with the Company" cheered the move to change jurisdictions, observing that "[while] the—[British] Consul deals out justice with a heavy hand, the Dane is different."[49] The anonymous native employee thereby registered a vote in favor of the business climate fostered by Danish corporate and civil liability law. Meanwhile, the manager, directors, and shareholders in the Bangkok Tramway Company all considered the scourge of punitive judgments awarded by British juries solved—until another accident occurred.

Expertise (I): "The Law and the Profits"

On the evening of October 24, 1893, "a child of about five years was run over by an electric tramcar . . . and sustained frightful injury."[50] The little boy was rushed to nearby Bangrak Hospital and into the expert care of the American physician, Dr. T. Heyward Hays, who assessed the injuries and promptly took action. Dr. Hays "found it necessary to amputate both arms and one leg, unfortunately without avail, death supervening a few hours after the accident."[51] Some two weeks after the boy passed away, Edward Blair Michell, an Oxford-educated barrister practicing law in Bangkok, filed a civil suit in British consular court on behalf of the father of the victim, claiming two thousand baht in damages. The claim, however, was not filed against the Bangkok Tramway Company or even the attending physician who had amputated three of his child's limbs. Instead, the suit was filed against Mr. J. Maclachlan.[52]

Maclachlan, a British subject working as a superintendent engineer at a rice mill in Bangkok, was not a manager, director, or even a driver in the employ of the Bangkok Tramway Company—nor was he present at the time of the accident or the ill-fated operation at Bangrak Hospital.[53] He was, however, a shareholder in the company. In filing suit against Maclachlan, Michell mounted a challenge to the received ideas of liability in the British consular court. Specifically, his suit called into question the corporate status of the Bangkok Tramway Company and the limited liability enjoyed by its shareholders. As the *Bangkok Times* astutely observed, "the action against Mr. Maclachlan, a British subject, may be considered in the light of a test case."[54]

While assessing his clients' legal options after the death of his son, Michell had likely initially explained that any claims against the newly reincorporated Bangkok Tramway Company would have to be argued in the Danish Courts in Copenhagen, where juries were reputedly more conservative in awarding damages. There was no Danish consular court in Bangkok at the time, so a registered Danish limited liability corporation would have had the right to insist that all civil claims against it be adjudicated in Denmark. The managers of the Bangkok Tramway Company likely considered this as another form of deterrence in limiting their liabilities when they hatched the plan to reincorporate. At some point, however, Michell had seized on the idea that although the Bangkok Tramway Company "was formerly a registered public Company [under British corporate law] . . . [it] had since been wound up [dissolved] and had then become an unlimited partnership" in terms of its de facto legal status vis-à-vis British law.[55] Under British corporate law, in an unlimited partnership—unlike in a limited liability corporation—individual shareholders were liable for damages in excess of the value of their shares in the company. Michell decided to test his theory by filing a claim for damages against a British shareholder in the company in British consular court. In the coal mine of civil liability in turn-of-the-twentieth-century Bangkok, Maclachlan was chosen as the ill-fated canary.

Bangkok's lawyers could smell blood in the water, and shareholders in the Bangkok Tramway Company held their collective breath as Michell's brief went before the officials of the British Consul in Bangkok. Then, strangely—

in spite of his own confidence in his legal argument and a general public consensus that the corporate charter and limited liability of the Bangkok
Tramway Company had indeed lapsed—Michell abandoned his claims for
damages against Maclachlan.[56] The proceedings, however, had already received
too much attention in the Bangkok press and had peaked the curiosity of the
tiny and incestuous community of barristers. Before long, W. A. G. (William
Alfred Goone) Tilleke, an ambitious Sinhalese barrister practicing law in Bangkok, took up the cause. Tilleke filed charges in British consular court on behalf of a Chinese man whose daughter had received permanent injuries when
she was struck by one of the Bangkok Tramway Company's horse-drawn cars.
Ironically, Tilleke used Michell's own strategy of pursuing the individual British shareholders in the company against him: He named Edward Blair Michell,
Esq., himself a shareholder in the Bangkok Tramway Company, as the defendant in his suit.[57]

Several months later, Edward Henry French, the British consul in Bangkok,
ruled in favor of Michell's claim that the Bangkok Tramway Company was
no longer a limited liability corporation under British corporate law. French
explicitly based his ruling on "the failure to produce proof that the Company
had been properly [re]constituted a Danish one."[58] The ruling had grave implications for the shareholders in the Bangkok Tramway Company, particularly those who were British subjects. According to French's ruling, when the
company was dissolved, it lost its legal status as a limited liability corporation
and therefore also the protections provided by British corporate law.[59] This
would not have been an issue had the company been properly reincorporated
under Danish corporate law, but French ruled that there was not sufficient evidence to prove that it had in fact done so. In the absence of the legal protections provided by limited liability law under any foreign jurisdiction, French
ruled that British shareholders in the Bangkok Tramway Company "were in-
dividually liable for damages" in the case of accidental death or injury. While
all the shareholders in the company were potentially at risk of civil litigation,
British shareholders were in a particularly precarious position, lacking the protections of limited liability and vulnerable to the punitive awards of British
juries at the consular court in Bangkok.

In the wake of French's ruling—and with the specter of the looming civil
suits over recent deaths and injuries—the management of the Bangkok Tramway Company convened an emergency meeting "for the purpose of considering the position of the British shareholders."[60] Aage Westenholz took the
lead in trying to secure evidence of the legal reincorporation of the company
under Danish law. He soon acknowledged, however, that his efforts to get the
Danish government to recognize the incorporation retroactively were not

likely to succeed.[61] Public debate on the controversy focused on the procedural merits of corporate registration under Danish law. Danes in Bangkok claimed that the company did not need to be physically registered in Copenhagen in order to be considered a Danish company.[62] But the squabbles over the process of incorporation and changing flags of multinational business ventures amounted to more than just a matter of immoderate British juries versus austere Danish ones. The public legal struggles over corporate law and registration masked a larger issue: the ambiguous and evolving sense of liability in Western jurisprudence during the nineteenth century. The debates being played out across the competing jurisdictions of foreign consular courts in Bangkok struck at the very core of the emerging assumptions of legal liberalism in modern Western juridical traditions, including fundamental questions about the legal rights of individuals and their obligations to one another. In late nineteenth-century Bangkok, foreign barristers and physicians—not legislators—dictated the terms of the debate.

Not long after he had abandoned the civil claims against Maclachlan on behalf of his client, the British attorney Edward Blair Michell mounted yet another legal challenge to the received notions of liability in the Siamese treaty port. This time the incident was a fatal stabbing on the grounds of the Borneo Company's holdings in Bang Kho Laem near the southern terminus of the New Road tramway line. Michell claimed damages against the Borneo Company in the death of a laborer named Maidin Picha, who died after being stabbed by another employee. While making his case for damages to be awarded to Picha's widow, Michell argued for a more expansive definition of liability in cases of injury or death. "Speaking of the question of legal responsibility," the *Bangkok Times* paraphrased Michell's argument, "in all cases where death or injuries occurred, they had, in considering who was responsible, not only to look [at] who actually caused the death, but to all persons concerned."[63] Michell's brief explicitly appealed to precedents set in cases against railway operators, noting, "In railway accidents caused by the negligence or improper conduct of servants, railway companies had, in hundreds and thousands of cases, had to pay compensation for deaths and injuries, and the same law applied in this case."

Michell's argument should be understood as an attempt to introduce the English common law doctrine of vicarious liability into the plural legal arena of Bangkok. The doctrine of vicarious liability holds that an employer might be found legally responsible for actions committed by an employee under certain circumstances.[64] The scope of the application of vicarious liability in Anglo-American law was not at all settled at the time of Michell's test case; the second half of the nineteenth century saw courts and jurists in both

British and American jurisdictions wrestling with the limits of its application, perhaps especially when it came to the matter of assault.[65] This ambiguity, however, did not stop Michell from effectively attempting to redefine local law through an appeal to metropolitan precedents. In the end, the jury disagreed with Michell, returning a verdict of no fault against the Borneo Company in the death of Maidin Picha. In this instance as in others, Bangkok proved to be an independent jurisdiction where questions of fault and liability played out anew according to distinctive local traditions and transnational dynamics, and largely irrespective of settled patterns and emerging trends in metropolitan jurisdictions. This was true even in the confines of the British consular court, where British judges and juries held sway.

While attorneys used their legal expertise to poke and prod at received definitions of liability and fault—as well as each other—they were lampooned in the English-language press. The *Bangkok Times* was particularly fond of criticizing the tiny cohort of legal professionals who dominated legal proceedings in Bangkok.[66] The newspaper held the attorneys responsible for the unrestrained growth of civil litigation in the British consular court in the final decade of the nineteenth century. In fact, there is reason to believe that the press was justified in its low opinion of the legal profession in Bangkok at the time, particularly the barristers practicing law at the British consular court.

In 1894, reports surfaced about how British barristers in Bangkok had conspired to keep their numbers small and to restrict the right to bring cases before British consular courts to lawyers who were British subjects.[67] W. A. G. Tilleke (the Sinhalese lawyer who had sued E. B. Michell), who arrived in Siam in 1890, was particularly jealous of the legal privilege to try cases in the British consular court. For a time, in 1892, Tilleke was "Bangkok's only lawyer"—meaning, in fact, the city's only credentialed British barrister. He seems to have been held in rather high regard at the time, and The *Bangkok Times* ran a report on his heritage, confirming rumors that he was, in fact, from an auspicious Ceylonese (Sri Lankan) lineage—"a real Kandyan chief," as the paper put it.[68] Tilleke was a vehement defender of the proprietary rules that prohibited non-British barristers from trying cases before the British consular court in Bangkok. When an American attorney named Kellet arrived in Bangkok intending to start a private practice, Tilleke objected vociferously at the prospect of encroachment on his terrain.[69] Tilleke himself, however, was regarded as something of an impostor by members of the foreign community, who deemed that a British barrister should not be a "product of local [Asian] manufacture" (and should presumably possess a whiter shade of skin tone).[70]

In time, Tilleke would nevertheless rise in esteem along with the growth of Siamese state legal institutions. He would eventually take the title of "Acting Attorney General" in association with his duties at the Siamese Criminal Court.[71] His rise within the legal apparatus of the Siamese administration was paralleled by his growing profile in the public sphere when he acquired ownership of the *Siam Observer*, the English-language competitor to the *Bangkok Times*. Tilleke was accused of using his editorial powers to advance his legal interests, which made him a target for challenges from foreign legal professionals and his competitors in the press. When he was found to be in contempt of court for publishing editorial comments on a pending case in which he was involved, the *Bangkok Times* cheered the penalty against him, commenting, "here we have once more emphasized the incongruity of a person engaged in running a newspaper being employed as 'Acting Attorney-General.'"[72]

On the occasion of another dispute over Tilleke's penchant for using his newspaper—"his organ" as the *Bangkok Times* would have it—as a forum for legal arguments, the *Bangkok Times* facetiously noted, "It is becoming more and more uncertain where Mr. Tilleke will go when he dies."[73] Tilleke's commercial endeavors were by no means limited to the legal profession and the press: in time he would also take an ownership stake in a shipping concern and would own and manage the famed Oriental Hotel. The *Bangkok Times* helpfully indicated his "multifarious businesses" and "other concerns of a speculative nature in which he busies himself" when Tilleke's health failed him in December 1899.[74] While Tilleke's karmic fate might have seemed in doubt to his contemporaries at the *Bangkok Times*, his imprint on the practice of law in Southeast Asia endures to this day: a prominent law firm, Tilleke & Gibbins, still bears his name.[75] Such instances of critical journalism cannot simply be attributed to—and dismissed as—commercial rivalry. In these and other cases, the foreign-language press proved itself to be a surprisingly astute observer and critic of the problematic wedding of expert knowledge and personal interests, a phenomenon that extended to the ostensibly altruistic field of medicine.

Expertise (II): Medicine and the Muddled Legality of Liability

Those who fell victim to the tramway along New Road had the good fortune to be hurt in the vicinity of Bangrak Hospital, by all accounts the premier medical institution in Siam at the time. The casualties of the tramway were either taken to the offices of the Bangkok Tramway Company at the end of the line or rushed directly to the hospital to be treated by the American physician Dr. T. Heyward Hays (figure 7). Hays, who arrived in Bangkok in October 1886

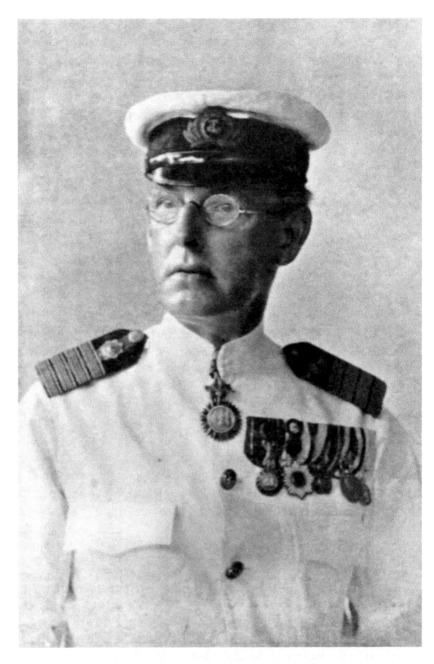

FIGURE 7. Dr. T. Heyward Hays. Archives of the Ministry of Public Health, Nonthaburi, Thailand. Photograph is reproduced in *Twentieth Century Impressions of Siam: Its History, People, Commerce, Industries, and Resources*, ed. Arnold Wright and Oliver T. Breakspear (London: Lloyd's, 1908), 134.

after having secured his medical credentials at the University of Maryland in the United States, had taken charge of Bangrak Hospital, where he held the title of Superintending Physician.[76] When the victims of tramcar injuries arrived at the hospital, Hays amputated limbs, dressed wounds, and performed emergency procedures. But complicating the issues of loss and liability in treaty port Bangkok was the fact that Dr. Hays was also a major shareholder in the Bangkok Tramway Company and a constant presence at shareholder meetings.[77] An American trade publication referred to "an energetic American, Dr. T. H. Hays," as the "president of the board of directors" of the Bangkok Tramway Company.[78] Hays is in many ways emblematic of the situation of medical expertise in the impossibly tangled web of law and loss in late nineteenth-century Bangkok.

For Siamese subjects who were injured on the tramway tracks, the medical expertise of Dy. Hays was often their only consolation. For British subjects and protégés who were injured and who filed suit against the Bangkok Tramway Company, however, Hays was not only a physician but also an expert medical witness, who was called on to present evidence concerning the extent of injuries sustained by victims of accidents under his care. His testimony often proved decisive for establishing the extent of liability faced by the Bangkok Tramway Company in cases of accidental injury. In spite of his very active and public involvement as an investor in the company, however, Hays's status as an impartial expert medical witness in cases of injury involving the Bangkok Tramway Company seems to have gone entirely unchallenged in the British consular court in Bangkok. In all of the cases where Hays was called to give testimony, the question of his impartiality as an expert medical witness seems to have come to light only once, when the case moved outside of Bangkok on appeal.

On Wednesday, June 29, 1892, an appeal in the case of Teo Ah Paeng versus the Bangkok Tramway Company was heard before the British Court of Appeal of the Straits Settlement in Singapore. In the original case, Teo Ah Paeng claimed that he had sustained serious injury on December 4, 1891, when a passing tramcar rode up an embankment and overturned onto him as he waited to board. The plaintiff claimed that the accident had "render[ed] him insensible, and inflict[ed] serious injuries which prevented him following his employment and had [thereby] caused him considerable expense."[79] To the outrage of the Bangkok Tramway Company, the jury that heard the case in the British consular court in Bangkok found the company liable by negligence and awarded two thousand ticals in damages to Teo Ah Paeng.

The Bangkok Tramway Company appealed the decision before Justices Wood, Goldney, and Collyer of the British Supreme Court in Singapore claiming "the damages awarded (2,000 ticals) were excessive."[80] Mr. Napier, attorney for the Bangkok Tramway Company, questioned both the accuracy of Teo Ah Paeng's reported lost income during his convalescence after the accident and the medical evidence that Teo Ah Paeng had submitted concerning the seriousness of his injuries. Napier argued that "the injuries [received by the plaintiff] were very slight and the damages claimed, considering the [financial] position of the respondent, were excessive." The crux of the appeal, however, rested on the expert testimony of Dr. T. Heyward Hays, whom Napier introduced as "the leading doctor of Bangkok." Hays submitted what Napier called "conclusive" evidence at the original trial to the effect that the injuries sustained by Teo Ah Paeng were "very slight." Upon hearing Napier's appeal, however, Justice Goldney bluntly interjected: "Doctor Hayes [sic] is the Company's doctor." Napier, perhaps stunned at hearing the Justice's candid appraisal of Hays's bias, retorted:

> There is no evidence of that. The Company simply paid Dr. Hayes [sic] for attending to the plaintiff. Dr. Hayes thought plaintiff was shamming and, on testing plaintiff, was convinced that such was actually the fact. In this case the jury would only grant such injuries as plaintiff actually sustained [i.e. no punitive damages]. The question is "what is his loss?" and for that you have to depend on his own statement, which is uncorroborated. The evidence goes to show that he has a small shop and goes himself or sends his son into the country occasionally. As a matter of fact the plaintiff's son has carried on the business while plaintiff was sick [convalescing]. I submit that the damages are excessive, and such as no reasonable jury would have granted. I submit that your Lordships should order a new trial.[81]

The Justices, however, were not to be swayed by the testimony of a medical doctor who appeared to be on the payroll of the appellant. They conceded that the damages awarded might have been dear, but they refused to overturn the judgment of a jury in an inferior court. While the entanglement of medical expertise and financial interests may not have been an issue in Bangkok, the British Supreme Court in Singapore was unwilling to overlook the issue.

Hays was not alone in this problematic nexus of medical expertise and personal financial interests. The Scottish physician Dr. Peter Gowan, a close friend and sometime business partner of Hays who had formerly served as King Chulalongkorn's personal physician and who also served as an attending physician at Bangrak Hospital, was likewise a shareholder in the Bangkok Tramway Company.[82] Gowan, in fact, was serving as a member of the board of directors for the company in April 1899 when he was called on to amputate the foot of a Siamese man named Nai Wan, whose foot was irreparably damaged by a tramcar.[83] Like Hays, Gowan clearly maintained commercial interests that could at times come into conflict with his role as a medical professional.

Medical expertise presented a challenge in public life as well when claims to authoritative knowledge could be used to avoid legal entanglements. In June 1895, Dr. Hays's horse-drawn carriage struck a Siamese child who was walking in the road accompanied by his mother. Hays immediately alighted from his carriage and gave the child a cursory medical examination on the spot. Perhaps unsurprisingly, Hays deemed the child to be perfectly unscathed in the accident, "and of this he assured the mother."[84] But before Hays could be on his way, a member of the Siamese police force intervened and demanded that Hays accompany him (presumably to the American Legation, where the incident would have to be reported because Hays was a foreign resident under American legal protection). Hays objected, and instead mounted his carriage intending to be on his way, at which time "the constable seized the pony's head and made more demands [of Hays]. This made the Doctor use naughty words—and his whip."[85] In the end, nothing appears to have come of the incident, and the *Bangkok Times* sarcastically notes that the police officer was left "wondering why he cannot perform works of supererogation during the day and remain in his verandah, deaf to all calls, during the weary hours of the night."[86] The incident demonstrates that Hays's medical expertise was operative not only in the context of legal proceedings, but in everyday life as well. In both cases, medical expertise functioned as a shield of sorts, protecting him from liability in cases of accidental injuries. In an era when law was still in formation, the authority of medical expertise could have important consequences both inside and outside the courtroom.

Wheels, Rails, and Flesh

Careful attention to the jurisdictional politics of accidental injury and death in late nineteenth-century Bangkok uncovers the far-reaching work of law mediating the effects of social and technological change in a multicultural environment. It also reveals that the most fundamental notions of civil law remained abstract, ill defined, and actively disputed in the transnational legal context created by extraterritorial law. In the wake of personal misfortune or tragedy, legal actions in Bangkok's plural legal environment were negotiations aimed at finding a consensus on the extent and location of fault and liability. Before liability could be assigned, however, the very legal definitions of social actors were tried and tested. Jurisdictional politics created an arena where even codified corporation law was not the bottom line for isolating the liable party: like foreign subjects residing in Siam, foreign registered corporations had extraterritorial legal rights and the ability to engage in "legal jockeying" to seek out the most favorable jurisdiction.[87] Once the liable party and appropriate jurisdiction were located, however, the subject of negligence and the notion of fault were found to be inconsistent and lacking unanimity. In short, there was no place for the discourse of "justice" when the very metaphysical rudiments of civil law were still very much in doubt.

The disputes discussed in this chapter also demonstrate that legal change is more complex and multifaceted than the historiography of legal change in the (semi-)colonial world has allowed to date. First, the impetus, institutions, and agents involved in these debates all acted independently of the Siamese state. The decentered nature of sociolegal change in Siam thus speaks directly to the question of Siamese sovereignty: crucial decisions over matters pertaining to life and death were adjudicated entirely independently of the will of the Siamese monarch. Second, historians of law in Euro-American jurisdictions and practitioners alike take for granted that legal change occurs in conjunction with and in response to social and technological change.[88] To date, however, scholars have ignored the sociotechnical context of legal change in Siam—as in much of the colonial world—viewing it as a barren field for the "transplanting" of Western legal traditions.[89] When viewed from outside of the overarching narrative of codification, the history of legal change in Siam reveals the same messy evolutionary processes as those that characterize Euro-American jurisdictions. It is therefore relevant to consider parallel legal changes in Britain as law mediated social change in the wake of new technologies and to demonstrate that the same processes held in Siam—but in a complex arena of competing jurisdictions and novel forms of expertise.

Lawyers in late nineteenth-century Bangkok were opportunistic and worked to challenge tacit ideas of loss and liability that informed both legal practices and the tentative consensus shared by the cosmopolitan foreign community. But the legal profession itself was fractious and surprisingly diverse. Medical science, which acted in both a curative and authoritative medicolegal capacity in cases of injury and death, further complicated this already fraught legal environment. In the period under consideration, the plural jurisdictions in Siam were called on to mediate not only the role of medical expertise per se, but peculiar incarnations of medical expertise in the form of social actors with their own interests in the affairs being adjudicated. That is to say, medical experts—in the same manner as legal experts—helped shape the legal context of medicine while also shaping the broader social world.[90]

In addition to making the case for Bangkok as a site of legal evolution in its own right, this chapter has also demonstrated the imbrication of the global and the local in these processes. Local disputes over civil law and liability intersected with ongoing global arguments over the merits of particular nationalist modes of liberal governance. At first glance, these were pragmatic debates over which nation's laws and institutions were best placed to offer protection to expatriate commercial ventures. They corroborate a peculiar sense of "elitist, grieving, [and] nostalgic" nationalism that Will Hanley has dismissed as being typical of a certain narrative strain surrounding cosmopolitanism in turn-of-the-century port cities.[91] Evidence of nationalistic pride underscores the ways in which these debates were likewise a matter of moral concern for foreign residents in cosmopolitan Bangkok. When Danes made anecdotal arguments about the limits of compensatory payments for accidents in their courts, they were making implicit assertions about the virtues of their own national law, which they touted as a system that protected private property and shunned legal entitlements. The arguments and actions of self-interested individuals were grounded in moralistic assertions about the superiority of particular forms of national-cum-imperial legal culture. This is not surprising: technologies participate in particular moral regimes that accompany them like vapor trails as they travel the globe, blurring the distinction between technology as means and morality as ends.[92] In this way, these seemingly idiosyncratic, particular, even punctilious contests over legal liability and the value of human lives and limbs in Bangkok might be said to speak to the global historical context of high imperialism.

Scholars have recently come to recognize the fracturing of a European consensus on Empire in the late nineteenth century, and they have begun to demonstrate the heterogeneity of liberal imperial projects.[93] In addition to land grabs, competitive imperialism in this era was articulated through debates over liberal governance, which was the universalizing political ideology of the day. The transimperial contests discussed in this chapter help to bridge the gap between political theorists of liberal imperialism in the metropole and the agents of empire who inhabited and acted on these ideologies.[94] Such arguments were not limited to the official ideologies of empire that were articulated in the metropole; they were likewise expressed by the nonofficial but still partisan proponents of particular empires linked to European nation-states—members of what Elizabeth Kolsky has called the "third face" of empire—as well as the more blatantly self-interested agents of what Shannon Lee Dawdy has called "rogue colonialism."[95]

In the final analysis, however, despite the global nature of these debates and the fact that they played out primarily in the foreign-language local press and foreign consular courts—venues that were emphatically outside the control of the Siamese state—they are nevertheless indicative of important changes in social life in Bangkok and deserve to be considered as part of the wellspring feeding nascent conversations about legal and political reform in Siam. Quotidian tragedies on the tracks of the Bangkok Tramway Company, along with the jurisdictional politics and competitive debates over legal liberalism that they incited, are a crucial part of the sociohistorical context out of which efforts to construct a national legal system emerged.[96] The public debates over law and liability that occurred in their wake—and especially the contentious and discordant discourses surrounding competing forms of liberalism—are an overlooked part of the discursive context for the project of constructing a national legal system.

By virtue of their very physicality, however, these accidents transcend the confines of discursive analysis. The audible screech of the tramcar's brakes announced the arrival of new forms of technology, social agency, institutions, and forms of expertise in the Siamese capital. And the inevitable collisions of wheels, rails, and flesh wrought new sociohistorical realities that demanded mediation. Mediation often took the form of legal action, but coming to terms with new social and technological realities reached outside the law to touch on everyday conceptions of the causes of human misfortune. These questions are often relegated to legal experts or philosophers, but the following chapter finds that grappling with them was a matter of practical governance and common sense.

CHAPTER 4

Accidental Metaphysics

> Tort law performs an important cultural function
> by "creating" meanings for dutiful relationships,
> risky situations, and attributions of blame for
> "accidents. . . ." Successful tort claims transform
> accidents from "acts of god," beyond anyone's control,
> to socially or personally responsible events. No longer
> a matter of fate, injuries are the consequence of
> accountable, social action.
>
> —Joyce Sterling and Nancy Reichman, "The Cultural
> Agenda of Tort Litigation"

> In every well-drawn code of laws allowance is made
> for what are termed "Acts of God" and for purely
> accidental occurrences.
>
> —"Liability for Criminal Negligence," *Bangkok Times*,
> May 30, 1895

The individual legal subject imbued with rights
is the atomic element in Western legal liberalism. But the system of law that
protects and constrains the individual legal actor consists not only of mandates
and proscriptions; it is also predicated on a distinctive sense of the nature of
causal relations among social actors in the natural world.[1] Which is to say, legal
liberalism possesses its own metaphysics. In spite of its resistance to codification, this backdrop is nonetheless a crucial element of the ideas and institutions that constitute the liberal legal order.[2] The foundations of this
metaphysical system of thought are closely correlated to scientific naturalism
and constitute something like a tacit substrate for making legal sense out of the
actions and engagements of social life. Because of this correlation, the history
of the spread of legal liberalism is also the story of the diffusion of normative

ideas concerning the distinction between the natural and social worlds and the kinds of actions and agency peculiar to each sphere. Bruno Latour has described the inscription of these boundaries as one of many constitutional decisions that help to define the modern world—a notion that highlights the historically and culturally contingent nature of such boundaries.[3]

The notion of the "accident" is just such a boundary marker between the natural and social worlds. While historians have long recognized the accident as an agent of historical change, they have more recently come to consider it as a historical entity in its own right. Roger Cooter, for instance, attempts to locate the genealogical origins of a contemporary culture of the accidental, what he calls the "moment of the accident." Cooter reveals the diverse social and cultural forces that provoked a "deep cultural anxiety" in late Victorian England, which in turn helped produce an explosion in discourse surrounding the accidental.[4] He argues that the generalized sense of social and cultural disorder in late nineteenth-century urban England found expression in a "'civilianization' process" that mobilized military habits of mind and action to confront threatening facets of urban social life. Judith Green offers a competing genealogy of the accident. Instead of teasing out the various threads of "cultural anxiety," Green looks to the shifting strategies and technologies of municipal governance. According to Green, "a watershed moment in the history of 'accidents' came in 1840, when [the epidemiologist William] Farr [1807–1883] recommended an inquiry into the cause of violent death."[5] Farr's search for order in the seemingly random tragedies of daily life in London eventually evolved into "an international system of classification . . . beginning with the 1863 division of accidents that occurred in mines and around railways."[6]

For a moment at the close of the twentieth century, historical scholars in the Anglophone world thought that the historicization of the accident would become its own field, with links to the social history of medicine, labor, and medical jurisprudence. Indeed, valuable studies of related ideas such as "accident proneness" have grown out of a reengagement with the cultural history of the accident and accidental reasoning on the part of scholars in science and technology studies.[7] Continental historical scholars, however, were dismissive of the project from the outset. François Ewald, among the French scholars who claim the closest intellectual affinity to Foucault, objected that the historical "moment of the accident" and its associated metaphysics within liberal legalism were but a transitional moment in the long course of sociopolitical changes associated with the concept of risk as an aspect of governmentality.[8] For Ewald, the moment of the accident was little more than a passing phase on the way to the articulation of the modern welfare state, whereby national solidarity took precedence over personal responsibility as technological and political change spread risk out over a population. But it is premature to dismiss the genealogical study of the accident, particularly since scholars have not yet attempted to consider its history in comparative and cross-cultural contexts.

This chapter provides just such an examination of the moment of the accident in turn-of-the-twentieth-century Siam. This investigation, however, amounts to more than simply a non-European iteration of the Victorian moment of the accident; it is much more than just a "nativist ethnohistory."[9] The appearance of the accident in fin-de-siècle Siam is an indication of the spread of the homogeneous sense of metaphysics associated with Western legal liberalism. The diffusion of the term is corollary to and indicative of the broader reach of a particular historical and cultural iteration of the distinctions between the natural and social worlds, one that remains integral to Western legal thought and practice. The accident therefore deserves to be considered alongside of other "powerful imperial words that moved from West to East" in the late nineteenth century as part of an imperial lexicon.[10]

This genealogy of the accident in Siam will proceed in four parts. First, in the way of context for considering how ideas such as the accident were introduced as part of the metaphysical background of civil legal reasoning, it is necessary to consider earlier and more general efforts to identify and define legal actors and forms of action with legal implications. How were Siamese social actors and actions rendered into a legalistic idiom, and by whom? Second, having established the origins of the civil legal subject and associated actions through etymological and historical linguistic evidence, this chapter offers a cultural and discursive examination of the moment of the accident. The third section examines the genealogy of the accident in practice, which will demonstrate the origins of accidental reasoning as a facet of municipal governance. The final section introduces some of the other salient categories of the metaphysics of civil law and considers evidence of their translation and localization in the Siamese context as part of the introduction of an imperial lexicon of governance.

Translating Tort: The Search for a Subject

Foreign lawyers practicing law in Bangkok attempted to impose order on the chaos of individual misfortune through civil law. The challenge was not only a matter of locating the proper jurisdictional context for civil actions, but more fundamentally of using the categories of Western civil law to interpret the interactions of social life in Siam. In the era before codification, this amounted to an unsystematic search for Siamese analogues to the fundamental principles of Western civil legal traditions. There was no single authority responsible for forging such equivalencies, and the efforts to translate civil law were diverse and inconsistent. Collectively, however, these efforts suggest the novelty of the categories of civil legal reasoning and the outlines of ethnographic knowledge about Siamese social life and metaphysical ideas.

The intellectual labor of Edward Blair Michell, the British barrister who challenged the boundaries of liability in cases of injury and death on the tramway tracks (discussed in chapter 3), provides a window onto the problem of regularizing civil law in late nineteenth-century Siam. In 1892, Michell, a champion rower, boxer, and a renowned expert on falconry who had been called to the Bar by the Middle Temple in 1869, published a bilingual dictionary of the Siamese language. Michell's *A Siamese-English Dictionary for the Use of Students in Both Languages* helps elucidate the process of translation—both literal and cultural—that helped to shape Siamese civil law in the era before codification. Although Michell prefaced his dictionary by remarking that it was intended to be a practical guide for students, and that he had therefore "designedly omitted" "many technical words, especially theological and mythological," his dictionary nevertheless makes a significant intervention in one area of philosophical importance: jurisprudence.[11]

As a practicing barrister in Bangkok, Michell undoubtedly undertook the challenge of finding Siamese analogues for the terms of British civil law as a matter of practical necessity.[12] To translate these ideas, he looked to traditional Siamese terms describing metaphysics and remediation for civil wrongs. When confronted with the task of translating different forms of tort, Michell settled on the Siamese notion of the *khwan*. He identified the *khwan* as the subject of the tort of slander, which he defined as *nintha khwan* (to gossip [against] the *khwan*) and *klao khwan* (to speak [against] the *khwan*). Michell's dictionary likewise associated compensatory actions with the same vernacular metaphysical principles. He equated the Siamese compensatory practices for accidental injury or loss (*tham khwan*), for example, with "reparation, satisfaction" (in the sense of having one's grievances appropriately addressed).[13] His dictionary defines the verb "[*kan-*]*tham khwan*" as "to indemnify," which further substantiates the association between the *khwan* as both the object of civil wrongs and the subject of indemnification or compensation for such wrongs.[14] The appeal to the *khwan* in the act of making compensation for civil wrongs is favored over other vernacular and idiomatic descriptions of compensatory action, such as *"plop jai,"* for instance, which describes the action as an effort to subdue, pacify, or calm the *heart* of a (wronged) individual. Other common contemporary Thai language terms for acts of remediation in the wake of civil loss or wrongs, such as *"chot choei," "chot chai,"* and *"top thaen,"* for example, are entirely missing from Michell's dictionary. *Thot thaen*, another related term, is defined as "reward, recompense," which seems to be a more vernacular term lacking the legal implications of an idea like indemnification. Finally, it is notable that the compensatory actions associated with the *khwan* are also distinct from forms of penal action, such as monetary sanctions (*prap, kha prap*), which Michell translates as "to fine."[15]

In the preface to his dictionary, Michell points to his compatriot Henry Alabaster (1836–1884) as "the only authority" quoted in his work.[16] According to Michell, Alabaster's "'Wheel of the Law' contains a mine of copious and accurate information respecting the meaning of Siamese words, especially bearing upon religious or philosophical learning."[17] Michell's notion of the *khwan* as the subject of civil law, however, is not evidenced in Alabaster's work on Thai Buddhist metaphysics.[18] The discussion of Buddhist metaphysics in Alabaster's work hails from the rationalist reinterpretation of Buddhist doctrine relayed to him by Jao Phraya Thiphakorawong, a member of the Siamese elite. Part 1 of *The Wheel of Law* is in fact a reprint of Alabaster's earlier work, *The Modern Buddhist*, which in turn was a translated and annotated version of Thiphakorawong's own *Nangsue sadaeng kitchanukit* [A book explaining various things].[19]

Thiphakorawong's work, which takes the form of a catechism, is an important testament to changing conceptions of the world from a Buddhist perspective and has been a crucial source for writing the modern intellectual history of Thailand.[20] Following Thiphakorawong, Alabaster's work emphasizes canonical Pali metaphysical terms (in Thai transliteration), notably the *winyan* and *jit*, two of the constituent elements of human consciousness according to Buddhist doctrine.[21] His work eschews vernacular conceptions of the metaphysical components of human life such as the *khwan*, in keeping with the recognizable "Protestant presuppositions" that informed orientalist understandings of Buddhism during the nineteenth century.[22] In spite of his acknowledged debt to Alabaster, Michell's dictionary actually takes a radically different stance on crucial metaphysical questions by favoring vernacular metaphysical ideas. As a practicing barrister, the matter of translating the subject and actions of civil law into the Siamese language was a matter of practical importance for Michell, but other dictionaries from the turn of the twentieth century evince a similar tendency to identify the *khwan* as the subject of civil actions, suggesting that it was more than just an idiosyncratic association forged by one attorney.

The missionary-physician Dr. Samuel J. Smith, a lifelong resident of Siam whose language skills would likely have been far more advanced than Michell's, published his own more comprehensive English-Siamese dictionary in five volumes spanning almost a decade. Like Michell, Smith associates the action of *"tham khwan hai"* and *"kan-tham khwan hai"* with the verb "to indemnify" and "reparation," respectively.[23] Moreover, Smith's work contains other definitions that rely on the same link between aspects of Siamese vernacular metaphysics and emerging patterns of civil legal action. "Compensator [noun]," for instance, is defined as "the person or thing that makes reparations (*tham khwan*) [by offering] means of making amends for an error."[24]

Another dictionary, compiled by George B. McFarland, an American physician and professor of medicine who was employed by the Siamese state, evinces the same association between forms of remediation under civil law and Siamese vernacular metaphysics. McFarland's father was a missionary and educator in Siam, so George spent much of his upbringing there—apart from a sabbatical to complete his higher education in medicine and dentistry in the United States—and appears to have been fluent in the language. Long after his retirement from government service in Siam, McFarland compiled a Siamese language dictionary, based in part on a dictionary that his father had first published in 1865.[25] Although the younger McFarland's dictionary shows a more developed sense of the vocabulary of civil law, it is nevertheless rooted in the kinds of associations first pioneered by Michell, namely, the connection between civil infractions and remediation and the *khwan*. Like Michell, McFarland associates the *khwan* with the torts of slander and libel.[26] (It is perhaps no accident that McFarland follows Michell on this and other counts related to law, since McFarland evidently purchased the rights to Michell's dictionary and incorporated much of it while compiling his own.)[27] In describing compensatory actions, McFarland defines *"bia tham khwan"* as "money or a fine paid by one party to another; in lieu of damages done; amount paid as a compensation."[28] Given its publication date (1941), George B. McFarland's dictionary suggests that this semantic mapping of civil law over vernacular metaphysics was somewhat durable, although it was not the language adopted by the modern civil codes that were promulgated beginning in 1935.[29]

The Moment of the Accident

Among the first instances of the English word "accident" to appear in the archives of Thai history are in the formal contracts that governed transnational commercial life. It was here that Western assumptions about the nature of risk and liability first took root. In these documents, the notion of the accident was primarily related to the fate of investment capital; its use attests to an effort to construct a defined sense of the unforeseen factors that might affect a given commercial venture. Notable examples include the contracts of the royal concessions that established the right to operate a tramcar service in Bangkok (granted in 1887) and the right to produce and sell electrical power (granted in 1898). In the case of the tramway concession, the scope of the "accident" was limited to traffic accidents that might occur along the course of the proposed routes.[30] The Bangkok Electric Company's concession, however, employs the more expansive idea of an "act of God" that might intervene in the company's ability to produce and distribute electricity to its customers.[31] This particular sense of the accident—the idea of an unfortunate event that is beyond the bounds of human intention, foresight, and responsibility—was slow to spread beyond the confines of commercial transactions involving transnational actors.

In terms of its translation, over the course of the second half of the nineteenth century the "accident" gradually began to be associated with a recent Thai neologism, *ubatihet* (along with more elegant forms at a higher register of the language, *upatiwahet* and *upathawahet*). *Ubatihet*, like many of the terms coined to translate foreign concepts and technologies in the nineteenth century, was borrowed from Pali, the language of the Theravada Buddhist canon. According to the Thai Buddhist scholar-monk Ven. Prayut Payutto (*Phra* Bhramagunabhorn), the Thai term comes from the Pali word *"ubattihetu"* (*uppatti* + *hetu*), meaning simply an event that occurs.[32] Margaret Cone defines the Pali *uppatti* as "arising, coming into being, birth."[33] Similarly, according to T. W. Rhys Davids and William Stede, the term signifies "coming forth, product, genesis, origin, rebirth, occasion"; they define *hetu* as "cause, reason, condition."[34] As a dependent determinative compound (Pali: *tappurisa*, Sanskrit: *tatparuṣa*), the Pali term means simply "the cause of an occurrence."[35] Payutto offers an example of how the term might have been used historically in the context of Buddhist monastic life: "one should offer sermons appropriate to events, which is to say that [one should] demonstrate the *dharma* [Buddhist teachings] in such a way that it coheres with *things that happen* [in everyday life]."[36] The Theravada Buddhist commentarial tradition, however, can offer greater insight into the precise meanings and implications of the compound form, *uppattihetu*.

To begin, Rhys Davids and Stede note that in older Pali canonical texts, the use of the term *hetu* is synonymous with *paccaya*, which in philosophical terms meant "reason, cause, ground, motive, means, condition."[37] Over time, however, the meanings of the two terms diverged from each other as evidenced by the *Netti-Pakaraṇa*, which distinguishes between *hetu* as "cause" and *paccaya* as "condition."[38] This distinction seems to conform to efforts to differentiate between moral forms of causation (*hetu*) and natural conditions of causation (*paccaya*).[39] Such philological interventions in the commentarial tradition help to provide a sense of the historical development of notions of causation in the Theravada Buddhist world and hint at the ways in which the lexicon of Buddhist metaphysical thinking was adapted to encompass new and evolving notions of causation.[40]

Returning to the contemporary Thai usages of the term *ubatihet*, Prayut Payutto notes that not only has the orthography of the term changed over time—from the original Pali *uppattihetu* to the Thai *ubatihetu*—but the actual meaning of the word has changed considerably as well.[41] Outside the hermeneutical contexts of the Buddhist commentarial tradition, *ubatihet* came to take on a radically different meaning, which is closer to the English-language sense of an "accident."[42] This should not be surprising, as Wolfgang Schivelbusch has suggested a similar sort of etymological evolution in Europe. The idea of an accident as explicated in sources like Diderot's *Encyclopedie* was primarily "a grammatical and philosophical concept, more or less synonymous with coincidence." According to Schivelbusch, it was only after the industrial revolution altered the size, scale, and frequency of accidents that "accident" came to take on its contemporary connotations.[43]

The novelty—and perhaps rarity—of this particular Thai language neologism in the second half of the nineteenth century is evidenced in part by its absence from bilingual dictionaries that attempted to gloss the English term "accident" in Siamese. *English and Siamese Vocabulary*, a bilingual dictionary published by the American Presbyterian Mission in Bangkok in 1865, offers a periphrastic definition of the term, defining it as an unexpected event—"that which occurs without prior knowledge"—rather than offering a lexical one (i.e., an equivalent term from the Siamese language).[44] When George Bradley McFarland's father, Samuel Gamble McFarland, a missionary who was a longtime resident and educator in Siam, first compiled a vocabulary list of some fourteen thousand terms at around the same time, he omitted the Siamese word for accident altogether.[45] E. B. Michell, who vociferously objected to "the fanciful innovations which some busy-bodies are attempting to introduce into the Siamese language," included an entry for *"upatti"*—which he rightly noted was derived from Pali and translated as "misfortune, ruin"—but did not include an entry for *"ubatihet."*[46]

The newly coined Siamese terms for accident do, however, appear in Monseigneur Jean Baptiste Pallegoix's dictionary, which offers Latin, French, and English translations for Siamese terms. The original edition of Pallegoix's dictionary, which was published in 1854, contains an entry for *"ubati het"* (*sic*: it appears as two distinct words in the subentry under *"ubati,"* "to be born, to issue from"), which it defines as "accident, event."[47] The same entry appears in a later edition of the dictionary, which was edited and published by Pallegoix's successor at the head of the Catholic Archdiocese of Bangkok, Monseigneur Jean-Louis Vey, in 1896.[48] The inclusion of the term, and its definitive association with "accident" at this early date is somewhat anomalous, however, when viewed in light of other historical linguistic evidence from the second half of the nineteenth century and into the early twentieth century. In a Thai-Thai dictionary compiled by the American minister Jesse Caswell and expanded by J. H. Chandler in 1846, for example, there is a single entry for the closely related terms *"upathawa"* and *"ubat,"* which are glossed as "dangerous, as per the Pali [language usage]."[49]

Moreover, other evidence suggests that the "accident" was a novel term or idea for native speakers of the Siamese language as well, not just for longtime foreign residents who acquired it as a second language. When an elite Siamese official, Luang Ratanayatti (secretary of the Siamese legation in London), sat down to compile his own English-Thai dictionary, he evidently did not deem the Siamese neologism *ubatihet* an adequate equivalent to the English idea. Ratanayatti defined "accident" as a matter of happenstance or chance (*"khwam phan oen"*).[50] When King Chulalongkorn surveyed the "causes of premature death" in an essay he contributed to the Thai-language journal *Wachirayan wiset* in 1888, he focused on threats such as inborn disease, intemperance, and illness.[51] The "accident" is conspicuous in its absence. The oversight is perhaps a reflection of the comparatively sheltered life of elite segments of the Siamese population, for whom run-ins with new forms of maiming technology or the mishaps of industrial labor were not a real concern.[52] Yet it also suggests that the idea of a purely "accidental" loss of life was not yet a commonplace idea and that its precise meaning and lexical equivalent were still being negotiated.

The Accident in Practice: Becoming a Social Fact

Although etymological evidence of the "moment of the accident" in Siamese cultural life is somewhat ambivalent, the notion has a clearer provenance within the more confined context of the state bureaucracy. The accident first appears in the archives of the Ministry of the Capital as a new mode of classifying death, arriving in Bangkok from the British colonial world. The moment of the accident in Bangkok implied the naturalization of certain sociotechnical realities in the capital city associated with the arrival of industrial business ventures, steam power, and transportation infrastructure. At the same time, however, it was part and parcel of diffuse efforts to locate and define the limits of negligence and liability for personal misfortune or loss in the nascent civil legal system. This section focuses on the moment of the accident from the perspective of the "investigative modalities" of the modern state.[53] The confluence of British colonial policing strategies and technologies with Siamese municipal governance in the final years of the nineteenth century helped to reify the accident in social life.

The genealogy of the "accident" as a term used in modern Siamese metropolitan governance can be traced back to the arrival of a single bureaucrat. In April 1897, A. J. A. Jardine, a British subject working in the police force of British Burma, was commissioned on loan to serve as inspector general of police for Bangkok. (The loan of British officers to Siam was a relatively common practice; Jardine's successor would arrive through a similar arrangement.) Jardine was hired to bring about the reformation of the municipal police force along the model of British colonial policing in India and Burma. His service in British India began in 1879 when he worked on famine relief in the Bombay Presidency while serving as a lieutenant in the transport department of the military.[54] An opportunity arose in 1882 to enter into the British Indian police force as a probationary officer, and Jardine was appointed. After serving in several different locations, Jardine rose to the position of assistant district superintendent of police for Belgaum in Mysore in April 1884, where he began to make a name for himself through his pursuit of criminal organizations. He quickly rose to prominence in Belgaum for his role in tracking down a gang of thugs ("thuggee"), arresting all but the leader of the group, who absconded across the imperial border into the jurisdiction of the independent Nizam of Hyderabad. In April 1887, Jardine was transferred to British Burma, where he became the first district superintendent of police in Meiktila in central Burma. By 1891, Jardine was said to have effectively rid the city of the dacoits that had long been endemic to the region. After several more successful appointments in Burma, Jardine was transferred to Pegu in January 1897, where he was promoted to deputy commissioner of the Salween district in Lower Burma, his final post before accepting reassignment to the government of King Chulalongkorn in Siam.

When Jardine began his duties as inspector general of police for Bangkok in June 1897, he found himself at the helm of a metropolitan police force that, in his assessment, had apparently "never been trained, or educated in any way."[55] The first order of business for the reformation of the police was to come to a firm statistical grasp of the constitution of the force and the qualifications of its officers. To that end, Jardine conducted a survey of the education of the officers and enlisted men, noting that in Bangkok there were 12 officers (out of a total of 130) and 278 enlisted men (out of 1,247) who were illiterate.[56] His survey divided the personnel at various levels of the police force according to race / ethnicity and religion (rendered in the Thai-language translation of his reports as *chat* and *sasana*, respectively). He recorded, for example, the number of officers and clerks who were followers of Buddha (*sasana phra samana khothama*) versus the prophet Mohammed (*sasana mahamanden*).[57] As a model of action, Jardine clearly looked to the British colonial police force; he effectively imported the same assumptions about race and ethnicity—the ideology of martial races—that were foundational principles in staffing the British colonial military and police forces.[58] Among his first proposals, submitted just days after his tenure began, was to hire "a few experienced European Police Officers in the higher grades of the service . . . [and to establish] a force of 200 natives of India, to be armed and trained so as to cope with riots and demonstrations made by [Chinese] Secret Societies, and to assist in drilling and training the Siamese Police."[59] During the last decade of the nineteenth century, the Bangkok metropolitan police force was increasingly staffed by Sikh and other ethnic South Asians who had served under the British in India.[60] On top of these proposals for reconstituting the force through the recruitment of personnel from abroad, Jardine noted that the metropolitan police did not possess any rules or guidelines for "police officers as to their duty or their powers to arrest and search."[61] He therefore set out to compile a police manual, aimed at establishing procedural rules for the metropolitan police force.[62]

In addition to the British colonial fixation with "martial races" for staffing police and military forces, Jardine also arrived in Bangkok with preconceived ideas about the causes of social disorder, which he had likewise acquired during his time in India and Burma. Looking at the inscrutable muddle of cosmopolitan social life in Siam, Jardine saw analogues for all of the problems that British colonial police had encountered in India and Burma, namely, a focus on banditry and organized crime, which he mapped onto Chinese immigrants and laborers in Siam. Jardine attributed a great deal of the criminal activity in Bangkok—as well as a great deal of the unnatural deaths—to Chinese secret societies (*ang yi*). "Nearly every Chinaman belongs to some Secret Society," according to Jardine, "and there are daily feuds and rows between these societies."[63] More broadly, he noted,

> The Chinese are under very little control, have practically no master, there is no regulation, no census, and no restrictions; they are lighter taxed than the [native] people of the country, and in most cases when employed in large numbers are a terror to their employers. . . . The numerous gambling dens, opium dens, and drinking shops and public

brothels, especially in the Chinese quarter of Sampeng [Sampheng], are the cause of a good many violent crimes.[64]

His description of the Chinese in Siam is redolent of British views of "thug-gee," dacoits, and other threats to the British colonial state in India and Burma and therefore suggests how imperial taxonomies of problematic forms of social life were transferred to Siam through policing.[65]

Perhaps even more troubling than the dismal state of the police force, in Jardine's assessment, was the state of legal affairs in the Siamese capital. Bangkok was in effect a colonial port city where foreign residents enjoyed extraterritorial legal privileges. In addition to the difficulties created by a transnational and plural legal system, however, there was also a glaring lack of authority in matters of law or procedure for Siamese subjects. After almost two years on the job, in 1899, Jardine lamented that there was still "no regular Criminal Procedure Code, or a Penal Code," and that although "the old Police Act is supposed to be in force . . . I have failed to get an official reply as to whether I can enforce it."[66] To address this quandary, Jardine made a series of recommendations for the reformation of the legal grounds of the metropolitan police force, including specific regulations governing police work, inquests, relations between police and local authorities within the capital, traffic, weapons, and rules of criminal procedure.[67] Jardine submitted his recommendations concerning the legal foundations of policing the capital city directly to the head of the Ministry of the Capital, Prince Naret Worarit (1855–1925, figure 8). (He likewise voiced his disappointment directly to Naret when he observed that his proposals had failed to make any sort of impact on the prince's administration.)[68] Jardine apparently understood—quite rightly—that judicial and executive powers were conflated in the role of Minister of the Capital and had not yet become the concern of a national judiciary body or the nascent Ministry of Justice, which had been created only a few years before his arrival.[69]

Beyond the issues of personnel and legal institutions, Jardine's model of efficient police administration was also crucially concerned with the introduction of documentary practices. As the head of the Bangkok Metropolitan Police, Jardine counted the keeping of records and the compilation of statistics as among his primary duties. In this regard, his *Report on the Police Administration of Bangkok, Suburbs, and Railway Divisions for 1898–1899* was an integral part of his efforts to overhaul the organization of the metropolitan police force. He intended the ninety-two-page document, which he touted as "the first report of its kind ever submitted" in Siam, to be the foundation of a new archive that would be capable of producing "statistics which can be relied on,

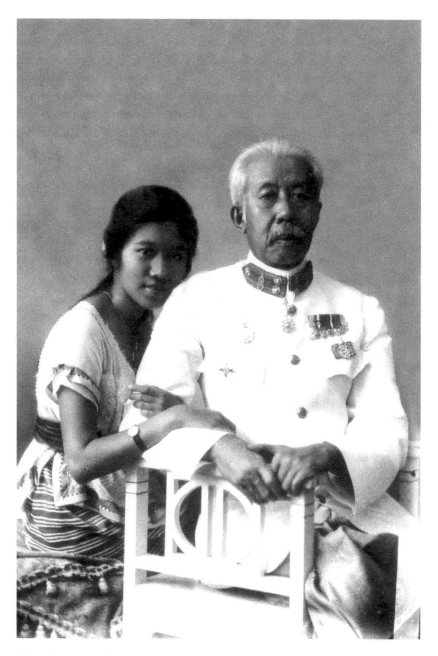

Figure 8. Portrait of Prince Naret Worarit (1855–1925), head of the Ministry of the Capital (*krasuang nakhornban*), with his daughter. National Archives of Thailand, image # 13M.00016.

and will then be able to show a true record of crime and the working of the Police Force under my control, and from which the [effects of] government or otherwise in the administration will be easily seen."[70] This documentary impulse reflects more than simply a desire for the greater bureaucratization of the police force; it indicates the spread of what has been called a European "culture of fact"—epistemological trends toward statistical and probabilistic thinking that were reflected in the application of risk calculation at the level of population.[71]

Jardine's documentary impulse amounted to a desire to compile a taxonomy of aspects of social life in the capital. As a police administrator, his chief concern was with criminal actions under his jurisdiction, so he began by compiling records of such activity in quarterly and annual increments. But not all events were easily identifiable as the result of criminal actions. British common law, for instance, had long recognized the need to investigate forms of death that were deemed "unnatural."[72] When calculating the number of victims of violent crime in the city each year, Jardine also had to take into account cases of "unnatural death," since he suspected that "a good many of these are victims of Secret Societies"—who were adept at making violent deaths appear natural or accidental—"and therefore [evidence of foul play was] hard to detect."[73] Jardine's death registry for the year 1898–99 included figures for murder (thirty-three), drowning (twenty-two), and "other causes" (twenty-nine), which included those who "die in the streets from opium eater's-dysentry [sic]."[74]

In the following year's report, however, Jardine noticed some glaring discrepancies in his new system of classifying and counting deaths. The most pronounced among the year-on-year deviations were increases of eighteen in the number of recorded suicides and twenty-three in the number of "accidental deaths."[75] According to Jardine, the fluctuations could be explained as a clerical error, whereby the district inspectors responsible for Bangkok, the Railway, and the Suburbs, had all included suicides in their total number of accidental deaths.[76] There were other inaccuracies in Jardine's figures; he noted, for instance, "It is surprising to find that there was not a single fatal carriage accident, or case of being run over by the tram in Bangkok during the past year."[77] In actuality, there had been at least one deadly accident on the tramway tracks: a Chinese man was run over and killed near Sam Yaek in May of that year (the new year began in April according to the Siamese calendar).[78] Clerical errors aside, the report suggests something of the novel nature of this governmental project of discerning among different forms of death and calculating statistics applicable to the entire population of the capital and surrounding environs.

When Jardine's report was translated into the Thai language, the registry of accidental deaths appeared as a table with the title "Registry of people who died by 'accident' in the year 118"—with the English word "accident" transliterated into the Thai alphabet and set apart with quotation marks.[79] For a time, the accident referred to a certain kind of fatality that existed in the Siamese language only in transliterated form in the Siamese language translation of the annual reports submitted by Inspector General Jardine to Prince Naret. It was utilized by those in positions of executive power to describe a particular category of the loss of human life. Significantly, the term was employed by two officials of the Siamese state with extensive experience abroad: Jardine, an officer on loan from the British Indian Constabulary, and Prince Naret, who had worked in the Siamese legation in London. The use of the English term transliterated into the Thai alphabet reveals the process whereby foreign ideas were mapped onto indigenous social reality.

The moment of the accident in Siamese metropolitan governance is related to efforts to gain statistical control over life and death in the European metropole that have been described as part of a new form of biopolitics.[80] Over the course of the nineteenth century in Britain, figures like William Farr and John Snow helped to usher in a revolution in statistical knowledge of the body politic.[81] Advances in statistical and geographical reasoning helped advance epidemiological knowledge, which in turn transformed individual deaths into a matter of concern for the agents and institutions of municipal governance. Subsequent revisions of the mortality figures in Victorian Britain would eventually result in a standard classification of types of deaths, including a detailed classification of accidental deaths that tried to account for differential risks according to occupation.[82] Jardine's attempts to grapple with the criminal and accidental loss of human life in Bangkok were part of a broader shift in the nature of sovereign governmental power in Siam, one that witnessed the emergence of a modern state focused simultaneously on the geographical extent of its will and the biological strength of its populace. Counting violent and accidental deaths is one small facet of what Michel Foucault called "the entry of life into history," one instance of a broader trend whereby sovereign power transformed into the "manager of 'the biological existence of a population.'"[83]

Jardine did not perceive his efforts as part of a watershed in the nature of governance in the Siamese capital. In fact, at the time when he submitted his first report circa April 1899, he was becoming increasingly frustrated with the lack of traction and attention that his proposals concerning police personnel, laws, and procedures had garnered to date. In spite of his optimism for the future of Bangkok once a European-modeled police force—and European officers—had arrived, he concluded the report on a dejected note: "owing to none of my proposed [legal] Acts being passed, the work is not encouraging, and I am inclined to stop going outside my ordinary duty when I find it does no good, and is not appreciated, or taken any notice of."[84] What Jardine could not know was that some of his strategies and efforts were taking root in more subtle ways. Jardine helped to usher in the use of these bureaucratic technologies for accounting for life and death at the level of the population. Under his tenure, a new decree regarding the registration of deaths in Bangkok was announced on April 18, 1900.[85] Moreover, his efforts to impose a taxonomy on the loss of life in the capital was part of the broader transformation of Siamese social life, under the converging trends of new forms of governance and legal reasoning.

Distilling Agency: Accidents and Negligence

At the same time as the notion of accidental occurrences was rising to prominence as part of early trends in governmentality in the Siamese capital, more diffuse ideas about the nature and limits of human agency were beginning to surface. As in British common law during the early nineteenth century, the earlier fatalistic or transcendental views of the causes of individual misfortune were beginning to coalesce into a mundane continuum of human fault (as described in chapter 3). This continuum, which was marked by human intention on the one end and accidental occurrences belonging to the natural world at the other, was likewise being translated into a corresponding spectrum of liability in the context of the nascent Siamese justice system. This period might be likened to the process of distillation, whereby the metaphysics of liberal legal culture was reducing and concentrating—distilling—received notions of the limits of human agency. Cases of injury and death involving the Bangkok Tramway Company are again instructive here; they help to reveal how patterns of discourse surrounding such events were gradually shifting alongside of changing governmental strategies.

As suggested at the start of this chapter, the metaphysics of civil law constituted an implied backdrop for making sense of the interactions of human social life. The notion of the accident was a crucial part of the taxonomy for making sense of personal misfortunes and liability, but not all accidents were created equal. Some accidental occurrences were more readily identifiable than others. Commentary in the English-language press suggests that this gradation was a matter of broad consensus and became a part of public discourse in the wake of tragic misfortunes along the tramway tracks. By the turn of the twentieth century, however, even sheer or "pure" accidents required some adjudication as quotidian tragedies on the tramway tracks persisted, inciting a widespread desire for new forms of accountability.

On the morning of August 21, 1901, "a child had its leg cut off by being run over by an electric [tram]car" at Sam Yaek intersection on the New Road line.[86] The driver of the tramcar, a Siamese man named Nai Choi, had recently been involved in another incident when the tramcar he was driving had run "over and killed a Chinese beggar" in Banthawai district. The *Bangkok Times* did not explicitly make the connection, but it seems that this recent history contributed to the desire to see Nai Choi arraigned on (unspecified) criminal charges before the municipal police court. At the arraignment, however, "The Court, after characterising the affair as a pure accident, dismissed the accused."[87] For the accident-prone driver at least, identifying "pure" accidents was beginning to become a matter for the magistrates.[88] In other cases, the drivers themselves helped to differentiate between "pure" and other kinds of accidents through their own actions.

Even an ostensibly "pure" accident became a legal matter when the driver fled the scene. In the early evening hours of September 17, 1901, as a Chinese man was crossing the New Road near the intersection with Oriental Avenue in Bangrak, he was caught by the wheel guard on the front of a passing tramcar and knocked to the ground.[89] The tramcar passed over his head and one of his hands, "death of course being instantaneous."[90] Unfortunately, since the spate of tramcar accidents had recently provoked the ire of the police and nascent criminal justice system in the Siamese capital, drivers had taken to fleeing the scene in the chaotic aftermath of tragedy. "As in the previous fatal accident of a similar nature," the *Bangkok Times* reported, "the driver of the car on seeing what had occurred took off his [company-issued] hat and coat and bolted."[91] Although "the affair" was apparently deemed to have been "a pure accident," the act of fleeing constituted a challenge to the public verdict of a "pure" accident, and a warrant was issued for the driver's arrest.

If "pure" accidents defined one pole of the emerging spectrum of the causes of human misfortune, with intentional actions at the other extreme, the idea of negligence occupied the intermediate ground. Negligence was a crucial intermediary in the creation of a legal distinction between misfortune wrought by natural causes and those caused by human agency. Jardine introduced the accident as part of a governmental reckoning with social life in the Siamese capital, but it was his successor, Eric St. J. Lawson, who intervened in cases of death and dismemberment to articulate a new form of liability: criminal negligence. Here, too, the Bangkok Tramway Company and its accidents provides a useful lens. At the turn of the twentieth century, the emerging governmental techniques in Bangkok converged into a new taxonomy for interpreting the loss of life and limb on the tramway tracks as negligence was criminalized. But extraterritoriality and limited liability continued to definitively shape new efforts to locate and define responsibility for individual misfortune. Efforts to criminalize negligent behavior were prompted by the public discourse over the need for accountability, on the one hand, and the challenges posed by the corporate and extraterritorial legal rights of the Bangkok Tramway Company, on the other.

One of the more prominent incidents that prompted this negotiation happened not on the tramway tracks but outside of the company's power generation station for the New Road Line tramway at Ames Bridge. In early February 1899, two Siamese laborers unloaded a delivery of wood at the power plant from their boat, which was anchored in the New Canal (*khlong khut mai*). In what became known in the press as the latest "Tramway Horror," an employee of the Bangkok Tramway Company opened the exhaust vents on the boilers that supplied electrical power to the tramcars, spewing steam and boiling water into the canal.[92] The two deliverymen, who were resting unawares in their boat after the morning's hard labor, were grievously scalded in the incident and later died at Bangrak Hospital.[93] The *Bangkok Times* noted with outrage, "There have already been too many accidents of this sort, and nobody has inquired too curiously if anybody is directly responsible."[94] With no small hint of facetiousness, the paper then stated what had become a truism in cases involving the Bangkok Tramway Company: "Of course no blame attaches actually to Europeans, but the Tramway authorities would seem now to consider that by a payment to the relatives of poor people killed or injured their responsibility [in cases of accidental injury and death] ceases."[95] The *Bangkok Times* pushed for "extradition" [*sic*] of the Danish subject who was apparently at fault in the case. It asserted—without attribution—"The Acting Consul-General for Denmark will hand the accused over, if proof of his guilt is furnished."[96]

Such public discourses about liability were beginning to coalesce around a novel sense of human culpability for seemingly accidental loss and misfortune. Etymologically, there is some evidence to suggest that the introduction of a new sense of liability through negligence can be dated to the turn of the twentieth century. Pallegoix's dictionary (1854) contains several Siamese language entries that he associates with "negligence," but in each case they refer to a vernacular sense of the term, as in careless or shoddy work. Examples include *"e aen"* ("Negligent.—To act with negligence.—To stagger in walking, not straight"), *"loe"* ("Negligent; negligence"; related terms, including *loen loe*, are defined "Without precaution, negligent, imprudent"), *"tabit taboi"* ("To act with negligence"), and *"talip taloi"* ("To work with negligence").[97]

Moreover, in other instances where Pallegoix translates colloquial (non-Pali/Sanskrit) Siamese words using "negligence" or the French term "negligence," none seem to imply legal implications for careless actions.[98] Similarly, in Msgr. Vey's redaction of Pallegoix's dictionary (1896), *pramat*, the term that has come to mean "negligence" in contemporary Thai, is defined as a matter of social indiscretion: "To presume, to dare, to have confidence in one's self, to despise."[99] Vey also glosses the term according to a more colloquial register, associated with clumsiness or carelessness, as, for example, *"pramat luem ton*: to forget one's self."[100] Even in attorney E. B. Michell's dictionary (1892), which includes an entry for *pramat*, the term is defined in vernacular—as opposed to legalistic—terms, as "careless, besotted, stupid."[101]

It is not until Luang Ratanayatti's English-Thai dictionary (1901) that we begin to see the possibility of a more legalistic sense of negligence beginning to emerge. Ratanayatti's dictionary offers two Thai-language equivalents for the English term: *khwam mai ao jai sai, khwam loen loe*. The former is a colloquial rendering suggesting lack of attention, while the latter might suggest a more legalistic understanding, since *"loen loe"* is often appended to *"pramat"* in order to convey the full legal sense of criminal negligence.[102] The dictionary of Rev. Dr. Samuel Smith offers the first instance of *"pramat"* together with *"loen loe,"* and might therefore be the earliest instance of the contemporary legalistic sense of *pramat loen loe* as "criminal negligence," which dates to 1905.[103] The development of a legal language for describing criminal negligence roughly paralleled police efforts to legally enforce the new taxonomy of culpability.

On the morning of March 5, 1900, the newly installed police inspector, Eric St. J. Lawson, charged two drivers in the employ of the Bangkok Tramway Company with "rash and furious driving" that had resulted in the injury of a man named Ishmael.[104] The charges were filed in the metropolitan Police Court (*san polisapha*), which was an anomalous venue for hearing a case of criminal negligence, since the court was in effect a small claims court dealing with petty criminal and civil offenses.[105] Moreover, the case against the drivers was further hampered by the fact that there were no legal standards concerning the driving of the tramcars, so a finding of criminal negligence against the drivers would have had to rely on the subjective opinion of the magistrate(s). Given these conditions, the case against the drivers must be viewed as a preliminary stage in efforts to criminalize negligent conduct. Indeed, Lawson's true intention in filing the charges seems to have been geared toward obtaining some kind of legislative provision governing the speed of the tramcars. After evidence had been presented in the case, "Mr. Lawson asked the Court to make an order, or give an opinion, that the cars should not travel faster than

6 or 7 miles an hour. This was about the pace of [horse-drawn] carriages driving, and should be enough for the tramcars."[106]

While the city awaited a verdict in the case, rumors circulated that the magistrates of the Police Court would refuse to pass judgment on the drivers on
account of (a) the limited mandate of their court and (b) the lack of any formal laws governing the speed of tramcars.[107] The magistrates, however, surprised observers when they ruled that although legally "the [tram]cars may
be driven at any speed, however fast, . . . they may not be driven as to inflict
bodily injury on any one."[108] The ruling appears to be based on the original
concession granted to the Bangkok Tramway Company, which included language concerning negligent operation resulting in injuries to "other vehicles
or persons using the same roads or places."[109] The judgment of criminal negligence against the two drivers meant, according to the *Bangkok Times*, that
employees of the Bangkok Tramway Company would have some degree of
"personal responsibility" for cases of injury and death.[110] Although the finding resulted in only a "small" fine against the drivers, the case was celebrated
as a landmark decision in the press insofar as it was seen as a check—however
small—against a company that appeared increasingly untouchable. The *Bangkok Times* opined,

> If the Borispah [*sic*: "*Polisapha*," Police] Court had decided that it was
> powerless in the matter, the only remedy in such cases [of injury and
> death on the tramway tracks] would have lain in suing the Tramways
> Company. And unfortunately that Company is able practically to put it
> out of the power of nine-tenths of possible claimants to get judgment
> one way or the other. [As a registered corporation under Danish law,]
> the Company has a right to insist on any action against it being tried in
> Copenhagen. We do not say that they would do so, but a limited liabil-
> ity company has very little soul; its first duty is, or ought to be, to its
> shareholders; and it is not well that it should have such a power, practi-
> cally putting it, if desired, beyond the reach of the law in the majority
> of cases. It is satisfactory therefore that the law in Bangkok has been able
> to reach the employees of the Company.[111]

In short, findings of criminal negligence against Siamese drivers in the employ
of the Bangkok Tramway Company had become a (somewhat toothless) proxy
for efforts to hold accountable a transnational limited liability corporation.

Similarly, when a Chinese man was killed on the tramway tracks on September 17, 1901, the (aptly named) chief police inspector, Sheriff, delivered
the driver to the Police Court and filed charges of "negligent and furious driving" against him. Some two months later, on November 13, the driver was

found guilty and sentenced to one year in prison. The *Bangkok Times* again celebrated, suggesting, "This decision should be useful 'pour encourager les autres.'"[112] (In spite of the persistent anti-French tone of the newspaper, the editors of the *Bangkok Times* evidently found the French language to be most appropriate when it came to discussing issues of public safety. The paper often switched to French when providing sardonic commentary on aspects of the *"mission civilisatrice."* The same idiom appears in commentary on similar legal cases involving subaltern Siamese subjects, including in reference to the above "Tramway Horror.")[113] The case confirms the discernible trend whereby the civil liabilities of a transnational corporation had become the criminal liabilities of its Siamese employees.

Lawson's efforts to criminalize negligent driving are redolent of the same sort of constitutional decision making that had helped to define the accident during Jardine's tenure. The idea of the "pure" accident had the effect of normalizing—and naturalizing, in the sense of making them a part of the natural world outside of human control—tragedies and misfortunes along the tramway tracks. The criminalization of the driver's negligent behavior, on the other hand, was an attempt to identify some form of human agency and culpability in certain kinds of tragic events. It represented a pragmatic negotiation with the realities of limited liability corporation law in an extraterritorial legal arena.

Accidents of Empire

The accident is a defining feature of a certain kind of secular reasoning with important repercussions in the realm of law. This is one sense of the titular notion of "accidental metaphysics"—the metaphysics *of* the accident—namely, the idea that the accident is an operational term in defining the world in which human lives take place. It names and frames a sphere of action that can impinge on human life—in consequential and often tragic ways—without any implication of human responsibility. There is, however, a second and more critical sense of the term, which refers to the historically and culturally contingent nature of the metaphysical decisions surrounding the notion of the accident.

The accident as we understand it is not the only conceivable boundary marker between the natural and social worlds. Ethnographies attest to any number of alternative configurations, the notion of witchcraft being a preeminent example of the ways in which human intentionality can cross over into the realms of natural causation.[114] Buddhist ideas surrounding karma similarly trouble any easy distinction between the social and natural worlds by high-lighting metaphysical remnants of past lives as a principle of causality behind present misfortune.[115] As a response to these alternative conceptions of the world, the accident might be understood as a technology of secularization: it purifies (in the Latourian sense) the conjoined arena of the natural and social worlds by erecting a boundary between the two and by denying the efficacy of supernatural forces—or at least negating any efforts to make sense of such forces, as in the case of "acts of God."[116]

In spite of their resistance to codification, accidental metaphysics are not abstract matters best relegated to religious or philosophical treatises. Instead, this chapter has demonstrated that they are practical matters decided by attorneys and bureaucrats whose labors required them to make sense of social life in a cosmopolitan treaty port. Long before modern civil legal codes and institutions could be promulgated to govern social life, lawyers had to identify Siamese analogues for the agents and actions of civil law. This was a matter of practical necessity for foreign lawyers attempting to carve out a sphere of civil legal reasoning from the chaos of social life. The practical work of coming to terms with the muddle of social life in the Siamese capital also characterized the work of police officials, who arrived in Siam from the British colonial world and attempted to transpose the ideologies and habits of imperial policing on social life in the Siamese capital. These disparate efforts were united by a common metaphysics: a shared sense of the boundaries between social life and agency on the one hand, and the natural world and its independent forces on the other, as well as a concerted denial of any forces that might be said to transgress these boundaries. For this reason, this chapter might aptly be titled "Everyday Metaphysics" insofar as it locates Latour's constitutional decisions regarding the boundaries between nature and culture in the quotidian labors of attorneys and bureaucrats.

Bernard Cohn has identified the ways in which the colonial world was "not only a territory but an epistemological space as well."[117] In South Asia, British colonial administrators looked to discover "self-evident" "facts" about Indian society that would allow for efficient governance. In Cohn's analysis, "The British believed they could explore and conquer this space through translation: establishing correspondence could make the unknown and the strange knowable."[118] In Siam, foreign residents, administrators, and consular officials were likewise seeking ways to render social life more recognizable and manageable. The accident was just such a device: it constituted part of a normative metaphysical grid for understanding social interactions. Of course, like so many other fundamental categories of European political modernity, its application was problematic. In practice, the new metaphysics of liberal legalism had to be translated and reconfigured in the face of seemingly incommensurate "concepts, categories, institutions, and practices."[119] Moreover, like the forms of knowledge produced by Orientalist scholar-administrators in colonial India, the accident was part of an inherently conservative grammar of rule. Although the notion of the accident had the effect of helping to codify the definition of a Siamese legal subject, it did so without introducing a new regime of legal rights: the subject of civil law in Siam was therefore defined negatively, through a constrained sense of agency, rather than positively as part of a broader effort to articulate legal rights.

For all their contingency and practicality, the imposition of accidental metaphysics should be understood as part of a broader epistemological project aimed at bringing order to social life in Siam. Just as was the case with the loss of life and limb on the tramway tracks, here again injury and death constituted the crucial context for ushering in modernity through civil legal institutions and governmental tactics. The notion of the accident bisected indigenous notions about bad death (*tai hong*); it created on the one hand a realm of human misfortune that was deemed natural and without human intention or responsibility, and on the other a sphere of death that was to be treated as the outcome of intentional (or criminally negligent) human action. Thus, in symmetry with the burgeoning field of legal action and discourse surrounding accidents came a concomitant rise in medico-legal and forensic interest in death. And it is precisely those forms of interest and expertise that are the subject of the following chapter.

CHAPTER 5

Morbid Subjects

> The crisis consists precisely in the fact that the old is
> dying and the new cannot be born; in this interregnum
> a great variety of morbid symptoms appear.
>
> —Antonio Gramsci, *Prison Notebooks*

> The emergence of the human as a political subject was
> intimately tied to its emergence as an *injured* subject.
>
> —Steven Pierce and Anupama Rao, *Discipline and the
> Other Body*

On March 25, 1884, two representatives of the Siamese government paid a visit to Ernest Satow, the British consul to Siam. According to Satow's account of the meeting, the Siamese officials, including Phraya Thep Phlu of the Bangkok metropolitan police, came to inquire about legal proceedings against a British subject who was suspected of having caused physical harm to a Siamese subject, which resulted in death. One of the Siamese officials complained to Satow that "sufficient notice had not been given to him to send down an officer to the inquiry at the Agency [the British Consul] this morning."[1] Satow informed them that the legal proceedings that day were "merely a preliminary inquiry, & that if it appeared necessary to indite [*sic*] the accused for manslaughter, a trial w[ou]ld take place with assessors [(a jury)], presided over by myself when due notice sh[ou]ld be given to" the Siamese state. On the matter of procedure, Satow then

> told him [Thep Phlu] it is necessary to get Drs. Gowan & Deuntzer [foreign physicians in the employ of the Siamese state] to make a postmortem in order to ascertain the real cause of death, w[h]ich ought to have been done at once (the deceased died on the 21st), & that if the assault was of such a serious nature as alleged, a complaint sh[ou]ld have been made [to British consular officials] at once.

The Siamese officials, according to Satow's account, "agreed to get the doctors to hold a postmortem exam[inatio]n & then to decide whether he [they] w[ou]ld ask for a prosecution for manslaughter" in the British consular court.

By invoking the standards of medicolegal evidence upheld by the British consular court in order to protect a British subject suspected of involvement in the death of a Siamese subject, Satow helped to politicize unnatural death in Bangkok. He signaled to Siamese officials that in the absence of clear forensic evidence, British consular officials would not allow the Siamese state to pursue criminal charges against British subjects in British consular court. The encounter therefore revealed medical jurisprudence as a new field of contestation between the Siamese state and foreign powers. Taking up such legal cases and the correspondence of Siamese government ministers, this chapter reveals how medicolegal scrutiny transformed dead Siamese bodies into politicized subjects of transnational concern in the final decades of the nineteenth century.

The link between forensic medicine and politics is not as obscure at it might seem. In British history, for example, the medicolegal investigation of cases of unnatural death, an institution known as the inquest, is deeply imbricated in the history of constitutional politics. Although inquests initially began as a safeguard for the king's financial interests in cases of unnatural death, the institution eventually became a part of civic life and a guard against the excesses of autocratic rule.[2] British inquests were held in public spaces, usually a pub, and allowed for a sort of local sovereignty over the legal and economic repercussions of cases of unnatural death. By the early nineteenth century, the inquest had come to be viewed as a crucial facet of constitutional politics and a central feature in radical democratic political rhetoric, as candidates for the office of coroner like Thomas Wakley used it as a signpost for advancing the cause of popular liberties.[3] The relationship between forensic medicine and politics was even more salient in the colonial world, however, where arguments about European racial and moral superiority were substantiated through medical discourses about indigenous bodies.[4] Medicine was thus a seemingly objective means of giving voice to politicized and racialized "truths" about native bodies.[5] Racialized medical knowledge was not simply a matter of discourse, however: it came to life in colonial legal institutions, where the testimony of forensic experts could mitigate "European criminal culpability in murder trials" by transforming a criminal act of homicidal violence into an "accidental" death.[6]

The history of forensic medicine in late nineteenth-century Siam differs in crucial respects from that of both metropolitan and colonial British history.

Officials in the Siamese state first confronted Western medical jurisprudence as one facet of the state's ongoing and asymmetrical engagement with foreign imperial powers. The Anglo-Siamese Bowring Treaty (1855) and other unequal trade treaties signed in its wake established extraterritorial legal exemptions for foreign subjects residing in Siam.[7] In cases where foreign residents were accused of having caused physical harm to a Siamese subject, foreign consular officials could appeal to forensic evidence to protect their subjects, as evidenced by the incident in Satow's journal. In the final years of the nineteenth century, as the ranks of foreign residents grew and political status became malleable in a context of increasingly fraught imperial competition, the pursuit of justice in cases of unnatural death was effectively transformed into a matter of transnational political concern. In this distinctive social, legal, and political environment, the standards of evidence recognized by foreign consular courts became hegemonic, and officials in the Siamese Ministry of the Capital were ultimately forced to try and assimilate foreign (primarily British) standards and practices for the investigation of cases of unnatural death in the capital city. The early history of forensic medicine in Siam thus elucidates the practical ways in which law and medicine figured in contests over Siamese sovereignty.

More broadly, this history provides important and often unexpected insights into the nature of race, science, and society in the colonial world. In the first instance, it demonstrates the ways in which the presumably objective realm of medicolegal science was inherently politicized: race was a subtle but persistent consideration both in the examination of the dead and in assessing the credibility of forensic evidence. Moreover, the study of legal debates over forensic evidence in a plural legal arena also provides a unique vantage on the unsettled relations between racial and political belonging in the colonial world. As Britain and France sought demographic supremacy in Siam through the enrollment of Asian subjects as protégés, they seem to have elevated the bonds of political subjectivity over the dividing lines of racial difference. Finally, while the history of legal medicine has been linked to crucial developments in civil society in the metropolitan world, this chapter plots a very different trajectory, one that challenges the emancipatory prospects of medical jurisprudence. Reforms in the arena of legal medicine were not intended to secure justice for the masses, but rather to meet the practical challenges faced by the Siamese elite in their ongoing engagement with imperial powers. The result was a form of necropolitics, in the general sense of discursive and practical actions oriented around dead bodies.[8] This sense of necropolitics differs in important respects from the canonical understanding, which focuses on "the power and the capacity to dictate who may live and who must die."[9] I use it here to signify the process whereby medicolegal expertise forged direct bonds between the state and the bodies of its subjects. Those bodies, in turn, became the morbid subjects of a sovereign necropolis.

Before delving into the efforts of the Siamese state to implement forensic medical investigations into cases of unnatural death, it is necessary to consider the broader conditions that helped to make unnatural death and forensic medicine a forum for political contestation in Siam. The following discussion highlights two such factors: (1) extraterritorial legal rights and the associated problem of differential standards of medicolegal evidence in foreign consular courts and (2) the registration of Asian immigrants in Siam as the political subjects of foreign powers. Both cases offer surprising evidence suggesting that under certain conditions political affiliation transcended racial difference in the colonial world.

Evidence on Trial: Extraterritoriality and Consular Courts

Extraterritoriality gave the European imperial powers "the right to protect their citizens according to their own forms and process of law and [to] treat them as if they resided within territory actually subject to their jurisdiction."[10] Extraterritorial legal privileges in Siam (as elsewhere in the colonial world) were conferred based on the political status of the individual. Foreign residents who registered as political subjects with the consulates of any of the imperial powers who had signed unequal trade treaties with Siam were eligible for extraterritorial legal status while residing in Siam. In practice, the extraterritorial rights of a foreign resident were protected by consular officials and legal institutions established by their home nation. In the event that a protected foreigner was named as a defendant in a criminal or civil action, any legal proceedings would have to take place in a foreign consular court. Foreign consular courts are therefore one important factor in explaining how forensic medicine rose to prominence as a matter of political concern in late nineteenth-century Siam. The trial of an ethnic Malay man named Salim, who was living in Siam under British legal protection, is a case in point.

In August 1892, Salim was brought before the British consular court in Bangkok on charges of having murdered a Siamese subject.[11] Salim's defense counsel, none other than British attorney E. B. Michell—who challenged the protections of corporate law in chapter 3 and helped to articulate the metaphysics of civil law in chapter 4—mounted a vigorous attack on the standards of medicolegal evidence and expertise recognized and employed by the Siamese state. Witnesses providing testimony on the nature of the injuries sustained by the deceased included the Siamese district official (*nai amphoe*), who admitted that he "made a *post-mortem* examination because he was told to do so by the authorities [his superiors]," but he personally possessed "no medical knowledge." An unidentified Siamese woman (likely a bystander or relative of the deceased) gave similarly nonexpert evidence concerning the cause of death. Finally, a Chinese man named Duan, who was employed by the Siamese state as the wound "dresser" at Bangrak Hospital, noted a broken wrist, a cut to the head, and an injured bladder when describing the injuries sustained by the deceased. Duan also testified that the abdomen and side of the deceased's body were discolored, and, according to the account published in the *Bangkok Times*, he asserted, "These injuries were the cause of death." Under cross-examination, Michell attacked Duan's credentials, revealing that although he had been working as a wound dresser for seven years, he lacked any formal medical training or certification. By holding up Siamese forensic evidence against the standards for expert testimony demanded in the British consular court, Michell made quick work of the Siamese state's case against Salim. But Michell was not finished yet.

The crux of Michell's defense came when he argued before the five British-born jurors selected to hear the case that when deciding a case as serious as murder, definitive forensic evidence was required to determine the cause of death.[12] In his closing remarks, Michell "dwelt at length on the necessity for clear proof of such a serious charge before convicting. [According to him,] there had been no reasonable proof of the cause of death—no *post mortem* examination—nothing to show that death was not due to the excessive use of opium or any act of the deceased's own."[13] Michell's appeal to opium as a latent cause of death is just one way in which notions of race and morality were smuggled into the apparently objective science of forensic medicine; native bodies were assumed to be diseased bodies. Here Michell perhaps relied upon Norman Chevers's canonical text on medical jurisprudence in British India. "In commencing his search for the cause of death in any case where the operation of violence is suspected," according to Chevers, "the Surgeon must determine to satisfy himself upon three points," namely, whether the injury was itself mortal, whether the deceased suffered from any preexisting "organic disease of any important organ," and finally, the extent to which the death could be said to be the result of the injury, the disease, or a combination of both. Chevers further specifies that "intemperate persons suffering from organic disease" of the organs in the abdominal cavity are more susceptible to hemorrhage from relatively slight injury.[14] There were, however, limits to such racialized disparities.

In the end, the attorney Michell and likewise the panel of five British-born jurors evidently favored Salim's political status as a compatriot over his racial status as a native-born Malay. With Salim's fate in the balance, the jury found him not guilty of murder, and likewise of the lesser charges of manslaughter and aiding and abetting. The verdict in the case became a de facto referendum on the standards of medicolegal evidence in Siam. The jurors appended a brief statement to the verdict, noting "The jury wish to express their opinion that it would have been very much better if there had been some medical testimony as to the cause of death" presented in the case. A postscript to the trial report in the *Bangkok Times* reads: "In consequence of the report on this verdict made by Chief [Police] Inspector Sheriff to the [Siamese] authorities, we understand, the police officials have been authorized to call in regular medical men in future, in cases where Siamese subjects have died from injuries supposed to be inflicted by foreigners."

Transnational legal cases such as the trial of Salim were the backdrop for conversations among Siamese officials concerning the need for higher standards of medicolegal evidence in Siam. The early years of Siamese police inquests into cases of unnatural death were characterized by a high degree of executive authority over the meaning and outcome of cases of unnatural death, as discussed in chapter 1. By the last decade of the nineteenth century, however, extraterritorial law and foreign consular courts began to make an impression on the Siamese officials who governed the capital city. Cases such as the trial of Salim demonstrated the need for a new form of medicolegal expertise in the investigation of unnatural deaths above and beyond the executive authority of Siamese officials. The fact that Salim was Malay points to another important factor in the rise of forensic medicine as an authoritative form of knowledge: the enrollment of Asian subjects as foreign residents with extraterritorial legal privileges.

Western Subjects, Asian Bodies: The Demographics of Extraterritoriality

The unequal trade treaties that instituted extraterritorial legal privileges for foreign residents also increased commercial activity in Siam by granting residential rights to foreign merchants, and standardizing duties on goods for import and export.[15] Siam thus became a desirable destination for a diverse group of immigrants from across South and East Asia. In the ensuing half-century after the first treaty was signed in 1855, a huge influx of laborers and merchants from British colonial territories in Asia and from coastal regions of southern China added to the cosmopolitan composition of Bangkok.[16] More-over, the British annexation of Upper Burma in 1886, and the creation of French Indochina in 1887, brought a dramatic surge in the number of Asian immigrants who could potentially claim extraterritorial legal status as the subjects of foreign powers. These changing demographics are crucial for understanding the rise of forensic medicine as a "political science" in fin-de-siècle Bangkok.

The English-language press kept tabs on the growing ranks of French legal subjects of Asian ethnicity. In August 1896, the *Bangkok Times* wryly noted, "The manufacturing of FRENCH SUBJECTS goes on at a merry rate. This morning the neighborhood of Custom House Lane [outside of the French consulate in the Bangrak area] was crowded with aspirants for that honour."[17] Ironically, although British officials in Siam and in London were fixated on the threat of the increasing numbers of French protégés in Siam, the British had far more foreign subjects in Siam than the French. Between 1887 and 1895, British consular officials added 9,281 new British subjects to their rosters (only 381 of these had been born in Siam, the vast majority being immigrants from territories under the authority of the Government of British India).[18] In addi-tion, there were untold numbers who had failed to register formally but who would nevertheless claim extraterritorial privileges if involved in legal proceed-ings. "Asiatic" British subjects in Siam quickly came to outnumber those of British birth: by 1902, there were 2,198 Asiatic British subjects recognized by the British Consulate in Bangkok, no more than 350 of whom were of Euro-pean provenance.[19] The dramatic increases in the number of registered for-eign residents in Siam became a bone of contention between the British and French, who had opposing views on the question of extraterritoriality and how best to leverage it in their relations with Siam—and with each other. The de-mographic disparity between the British and French and their subjects in Siam was likely outweighed by the French tendency to assert their privileges accord-ing to the most liberal reading of the treaties.

The French maintained a legalistic and expansive interpretation of their rights under extraterritoriality, which they applied to the process of register-ing new legal subjects.[20] This was especially true after the French took con-trol of former Siamese territories on the west bank of the Mekong River in 1893. By 1895, they had established consular offices in the northern and east-ern Siamese regions of Nan and Korat, which the British feared they would use as "centers from which large numbers of Siamese subjects of Cambodian or Annamite stock might be registered as French protégés to hinder Siamese authority."[21] From the British perspective, French registration had turned Siam into the stage for a kind of imperial battle by proxy waged through the logic of demographics, with the enrollment of legal subjects as armaments. Each new French Asiatic subject became a de facto outpost of French jurisdiction, and therefore an extension of its demographic—if not territorial—influence in Siam. Evidence suggests that this was indeed the explicit strategy of the French for confronting what they perceived to be British predominance in Siam.[22]

The British, in contrast, adopted a more conciliatory stance, hoping to ingratiate themselves to the Siamese. As early as 1884–85, Satow, who would soon be appointed the British minister to Siam, expressed in a private memorandum his desire to effect "the limitation of British protection to such persons as are actually entitled to it."[23] Satow's sense of entitlement was likely a matter of both racial belonging and cultural competency. In August 1895, Maurice de Bunsen, the ranking British official in Siam at the time, observed, "it cannot but be extremely galling to the self-respect of Siam to be deprived of jurisdiction over a large proportion of its entire population, made up by Asiatics, who, by birth, are as far removed as the Siamese themselves are from European ideals of justice."[24] De Bunsen also questioned the logic of allowing Asian immigrants living under British protection in Siam to transfer extraterritorial privileges to their descendants indefinitely, given that they would presumably become assimilated in Siam over successive generations.

Of course, the relatively conservative British position on the question of extraterritorial rights was also a matter of sheer economy: asserting extraterritorial rights for the vast numbers of Shan, Burmese, and Indian laborers who had emigrated from Burma to northern Siam to work in the teak logging industry would have overrun the limited resources of the British consular court in Bangkok.[25] For this reason, the British acquiesced to Siamese proposals to institute a "mixed court" in the north, known as the International Court at Chiang Mai, with jurisdiction over civil cases involving Siamese and British subjects residing there. The move was not an unqualified relinquishing of extraterritorial rights, but it was a step toward greater jurisdictional sovereignty for Siam.[26] The French objected to the International Court—which they saw as a challenge to the institution of extraterritoriality—and lamented the fact that the British had given up their claims to extraterritoriality for so many of their subjects in Siam.

Extraterritoriality undoubtedly represented a "stigma of inferiority" for Siam and was "a major preoccupation" for its leaders in the late nineteenth and early twentieth centuries.[27] Although it was not a part of the explicit discourse of state officials surrounding legal medicine and justice in turn-of-the-twentieth-century Siam, these shifting demographics of political belonging also help to explain how forensic medicine rose to prominence as a new form of authoritative knowledge. The registration of Asian residents in Siam as legal subjects of European imperial powers—so-called protégés—effectively blurred the racial and ethnic lines that had previously helped to define political belonging and its correlate, legal subjectivity. When it came to legal matters in British India, for example, complexion mattered. Jordanna Bailkin has argued that although "the judicial methods for establishing the racial identity (and thus the legal privileges) of defendants" in British imperial courts "were never systematic," "the defendant's plea that he was a European British subject was accepted by the High Court if it were satisfied by his physical appearance that his claim was true."[28] Contemporary observers in Siam were similarly attentive to racial difference in death; a typical report in the *Bangkok Times*, for instance, notes, "The dead body of a fair-skinned female child was seen floating in the river, past Messrs Kiam Hoa Heng's, yesterday."[29] Moreover, corpses were commonly identified as "Chinese" in the press, perhaps by the telltale queue hairstyle that men wore as a sign of allegiance to the Qing Dynasty.[30] When foreign consular officials in Siam extended the extraterritorial legal privileges enjoyed by European- and American-born residents to Asian immigrants, it had the unintended effect of projecting the inequities of differential legal rights onto the dead: no longer could a dead Asian body be presumed to be a Siamese subject.

This situation—the possibility of Western legal subjects inhabiting Asian bodies—heightened the need for expertise in dealing with the dead. It called for the intervention of forensic expertise to ensure that the rights of the dead were adequately protected. In Siam at least, the enrollment of foreign protégés by the imperial powers elevated political subjectivity over racial or ethnic identity, confirming Ann Stoler's findings that "the *quality* and *intensity* of racism . . . varied enormously in different contexts and at different moments in any particular colonial encounter."[31] In a variation on the old adage, extraterritoriality, it seems, made strange political bedfellows, provoking sentiments of alliance and affiliation that transgressed apparent racial boundaries in favor of the assertion of imperial interests. These conditions conspired to make forensic expertise an essential form of authoritative knowledge in adjudicating matters of death in the cosmopolitan port city. Implementing the new standards of expertise fell to senior officials in the Siamese state, who had to come to terms with and try to assimilate the new standards of forensic evidence.

Charnel Knowledge and Imperial Power

On December 7, 1892, Minister of the Capital Prince Naret Worarit painted a vivid picture of the landscape of extraterritorial jurisdiction in Siam in a letter addressed to his counterpart in the Siamese Ministry of Religious Affairs.

The letter begins by underlining the issue of legal complaints filed by Siamese subjects against foreign residents enjoying the legal protections of extraterritoriality. Naret observed, "These days, legal cases often arise whereby people under foreign protection kill people under Siamese protection (*khon fai sayam*). In such cases, those under Siamese protection have to file a complaint [against the perpetrator] in consular court according to the dictates of the foreign treaties."[32] Thus far, the letter seems to introduce a general complaint against the system of extraterritorial law in Siam. In the final decade of the nineteenth century, however, Siamese government ministers were well accustomed to the system, and they understood that a daunting series of comprehensive legal reforms would be needed before they might hope to challenge it. (By this time, it was generally understood that the Siamese state would have to adopt a system of law modeled on Western principles, codes, and institutions before the issue of extraterritorial rights would be reexamined by European powers.)[33] Naret's letter, however, goes beyond the general injustice of extraterritorial law to name a much more specific point of contention: the shortcomings of the Siamese state's manner of dealing with certain kinds of death.

The subject of Prince Naret's letter is in fact the emerging disparity between the standards of forensic evidence observed and implemented by the Siamese state versus those employed by foreign consular courts in Bangkok. "The foreign legations, which abide by the standards of international law" in deliberating evidence and deciding whether or not to try a criminal case, "do not accept the testimony of [Siamese] district officials (*phanak ngan amphoe*) regarding postmortem examinations as evidence because those officials cannot clearly state the cause of death."[34] In cases of unnatural death, Naret observed, foreign consular courts would only accept the forensic testimony of a medical doctor in the Western tradition (*phaet*) who had conducted an autopsy in order to determine the precise cause of death. The implication, Naret realized, was that "in cases where the Siamese side does not send a physician to inspect the corpse [and] conduct an autopsy revealing the cause of death, the [foreign] consular courts simply throw the matter out."[35] Foreign legations in Bangkok were well within their rights to simply dismiss cases of suspected foul play against their subjects in the event that the Siamese state was unable to arrange for an autopsy performed by a medical doctor to determine the cause of death. In these instances, relatives of the deceased Siamese subject would have no further legal recourse. "This state of affairs," Prince Naret rightly observed, "has been to the detriment of the Siamese side."[36]

In the coming months, as ministerial discussions over the standards of evidence employed by the Siamese versus the foreign consular courts would escalate, the notion of people on the "Siamese side" "losing advantage" to foreign residents in Siam would become a refrain, and at times a rallying cry, for efforts intended to overcome the inequities of the plural legal system created by extraterritorial law.[37] This imbalance of justice between the vast majority of Bangkok's residents and the few who enjoyed privileged political and legal status as foreign residents helped consolidate a sense of Siamese subjectivity based on the recognition of collective disadvantage. Armed with this insight into the evolving effects of extraterritorial law on Siamese subjects, Prince Naret turned to forensic medicine as a means of addressing the injustice.

Bureaucratizing Death Investigations

The social and political realities of late nineteenth-century Siam—including extraterritoriality, foreign consular courts, and the growing ranks of Asiatic protégés—all conspired to make forensic medicine a significant form of authoritative knowledge. On the one hand, the standards of medicolegal evidence upheld by foreign consular courts became the last line of defense for foreign residents accused of harming Siamese subjects. On the other hand, Siamese state officials realized that forensic investigative procedures might be utilized in order to challenge and overcome the obstacles that prevented Siam from obtaining justice in foreign consular courts. But while forensic medicine was touted as the answer to some of the inequities instituted by extraterritorial law, the question of how to actually implement this new form of expertise remained. To understand how forensic medicine was implemented in this period, we must look to Naret and his role within the rapidly changing state bureaucracy. These conditions helped to determine both the extent to which forensic medicine was implemented by the Siamese state and likewise the nature of elite interest in dead and injured Siamese subjects.

Prince Naret's letter (December 7, 1892) to Jao Phraya Phasakorawong, which lays out the contentious matter of political subjectivity under extraterritorial law and provides evidence of a consolidation of notions of political belonging in Siam, also points to the potential solution to the problem. According to Naret, the solution lay in reforming the standards of forensic evidence in Siamese courts and introducing forensic medicine as part of the Siamese police inquest. He called for "royal permission to have the [Metropolitan] Police Division summon a physician along with the district official in order to inspect [and] conduct a surgical autopsy of corpses that bore evidence of foul play where a foreign subject [is suspected of having] harmed a Siamese subject."[38] Not wanting to burden the state with the added expense of dealing with the remains, Naret suggested that once the autopsy was completed, the relatives of the deceased (literally, the "corpse's owners," *jao khong sop*) could come and take the body away for burial or cremation. The evidence produced by these procedures would be preserved by police in the event of a legal inquiry into the death (presumably requested by the Siamese state in a foreign consular court). The crux of Prince Naret's letter, however, is the question of who could be called on to conduct autopsies for the Siamese police in cases of unnatural death that would meet the evidentiary standards of foreign consular courts.

The fact that Naret's letter was addressed to Phasakorawong, head of the Ministry of Religious Affairs, suggests that he had already come up with a solution. In December 1892—in the wake of the recent reformation of the government ministries in April of the same year—the Hospital Department (*krom phayaban*), which was responsible for overseeing physicians who were hired by the Siamese state, was still an administrative division under the Ministry of Religious Affairs.[39] Foreign physicians employed by the Hospital Department served as doctors and hospital inspectors, but they were also responsible for the education of medical students at the newly founded medical college. The doctors were educators, and the Hospital Department was therefore housed within the Ministry of Religious Affairs, which was responsible for education.[40] If Naret wanted an economical solution to the challenge of meeting the standards of medicolegal evidence established in the foreign consular courts, he needed the help of Phasakorawong in reassigning a physician in the employ of the state to the task of conducting autopsies. Naret had one particular physician in mind: the American Dr. T. Heyward Hays.

Dr. Hays was the obvious candidate for several reasons. First, and perhaps most important, he was already in Bangkok, working under contract on a fixed salary for the Hospital Department as superintendent of government hospitals.[41] Naret understood the terms of Hays's contract with the Hospital Department to be sufficiently vague as to allow them to add autopsies to his workload without incurring any additional expense. According to Naret, performing autopsies in cases of unnatural death was "the responsibility of Dr. Hays on account of his salaried appointment with the [Siamese] Hospital Department, which was charged with caring for the injuries and illnesses of the people."[42] In cases where a foreign subject was suspected of having killed a Siamese subject, Naret proposed that the police would summon Dr. Hays, who would then go and inspect the corpse (at the scene) and later conduct a surgical autopsy (presumably at a government hospital) to determine the exact cause of death. Hays would then compile an inquest report and give a copy of the report to police officials, who would preserve it as evidence in the event of any legal case that might arise in the consular courts. The plan had the virtue of thrift. Unfortunately, the very thrift of the plan would be its downfall, hampering the progress of forensic science and medicine in Bangkok for several years and leading to revealing conversations about who was qualified to present forensic testimony before the consular courts.

Days after Naret submitted his plan to Phasakorawong, it was clear that Dr. Hays was unwilling to accept the new role as coroner to the Siamese state. When informed of the state's plans, Hays submitted a counterproposal to the Hospital Department through an official named Khun Phisitsaphawijan.[43] Hays reported that "there are many students at the [newly founded Siamese] medical college who have sufficient knowledge to be able to" conduct postmortem examinations and autopsies in cases of unnatural death and that "the students should therefore be made to conduct autopsies as requested by the Ministry of the Capital."[44] According to Hays, there were four students in particular who had been trained in surgery and were capable of performing the duties. Hays further proposed that the students might share the duties of inspecting corpses as needed by the Ministry of the Capital on a rotating basis. He did, however, add one concession to Prince Naret's original plan: if a particular case should prove too difficult for the medical students, then Dr. Hays would accompany them and supervise in the examination.

The original proposal that reached the ears of Dr. Hays was geared toward addressing the specific problem of reforming Siamese inquest procedures in such a way that they would produce evidence that met the standards of foreign consular courts. The Siamese police needed to produce appropriate documentary evidence in cases of unnatural death so that foreign courts could no longer simply dismiss criminal complaints against foreign residents suspected of having harmed Siamese subjects. The proposal arrived in a period of significant changes in the Siamese government, however, and Dr. Hays seems to have misunderstood the scope of the proposed changes, which were essentially an attempt to reform the standards of Siamese evidence law in practice without addressing the question in theory.[45] In his response to Prince Naret, Hays stated that he would not be able to perform both his current duties as superintendent of government hospitals and the additional responsibilities of the newly proposed role, which he understood to be that of a "regular medical officer of the court" (*mo prajam samrap san*). Hays reiterated his offer to recommend students from the medical college to fulfill the role of coroner and suggested that, "in important cases," he "or another European physician could be assigned to assist in the investigation."[46] Yet Hays's recommendations went still further, overstepping the ambitions of Prince Naret and helping to demonstrate the precise nature of the Siamese state's interest in forensic medicine at the time.

Hays suggested that the Ministry of the Capital might institute inquest procedures for *all* cases of unnatural death—"not just in cases where foreigners killed Thai people [*khon thai*], but in all cases including even the lowliest serf."[47] If such a system were put in place, Hays thought that the graduates of the newly established Siamese royal medical college would be able to fill this new role, which required a person knowledgeable in (Western) medicine (*phu ru wicha phaet*). Medical students would sign a contract as part of their enrollment in the new college that required them to work as civil servants for the government for a period of three years after their graduation.[48] Since many of the students were unable to find appropriate medical work within the Siamese government upon graduation, he reasoned, they might each be given a district where they could support themselves through fees charged to the state for each autopsy (and presumably other medical services provided to the populace at large). In effect, Hays's proposal called for the application of forensic medicine at the level of population governance in a normative sense; he advocated extending forensic investigation to all cases of unnatural death in Siam. Discussions within the Siamese state over forensic medicine, however, trended in the opposite direction. Juxtaposing Hay's proposal with the ensuing plans made by Naret reveals a point of inflection in the relations between medical science and Siamese political life in the last decade of the nineteenth century.

For Naret and other elite Siamese officials, the emerging question of their political responsibility to a group of people who were, by default, Siamese legal subjects was still determined by the exigencies of imperial politics. Naret was interested in forensic medicine only insofar as it might be useful in addressing the conditions of the Siamese state's diminished sovereignty. For him, forensic medicine provided an important form of leverage in rare but consequential cases of unnatural death that had the potential for transnational legal repercussions. An autopsy allowed the Siamese state to present expert medicolegal evidence against foreign residents suspected of having injured or killed a Siamese subject. This pragmatic, transactional arrangement with a new form of expertise was not indicative of a shift toward a broader, more encompassing sense of political solidarity and responsibility to the Siamese body politic. In many ways, it corresponded to long-standing patterns of elite interest in new and foreign sources of knowledge.[49] By calling attention to the (dead) bodies of Siamese subjects, forensic medicine did not level or undermine the hierarchical nature of social and political life in Siam. Instead, it seems to have reinforced it by allowing Siamese elites to martial Siamese bodies more effectively in the course of political projects intended to bolster the state's claims to sovereignty.

The consolidated sense of Siamese subjectivity that emerged from the engagement with forensic medicine is emphatically not the sort associated with individual agency and the constitution of political life that normative understandings of civil society would have us expect.[50] Forensic medicine did not become a vehicle for popular democratic challenges to autocratic power as it had in nineteenth-century Britain.[51] Nor did it foster a sense of self-identification among subaltern Siamese subjects themselves. Rather, what we see in Naret's burgeoning interest in medical jurisprudence is an elite bureaucrat finding concrete terms for confronting an ongoing political challenge to the state. While Naret sought to implement forensic medical concern for the dead and injured bodies of Siamese subjects, he did so in order to invoke those bodies in the arena of imperial politics. The interests of the subaltern dead were passed over in favor of those of the state and its elite agents. This transaction created a new political constituency of morbid subjects—that is, mute bodies, *objects* that in spite of the intervention of medicolegal expertise were emphatically not able "to *object*" to the claims made on their behalf.[52] Even in light of the relatively constrained scope of Naret's initiative, however, conforming to the new standards of medicolegal expertise would nevertheless prove to be a much more vexing issue than the Siamese government ministers realized.

A Question of Credentials?: Race, Objectivity, and Expertise

Hays's subtle but steadfast refusal to accept new responsibilities as a coroner sparked a new conversation among Siamese officials about the nature of medicolegal expertise. Based on his letters, Prince Naret obviously did not view the question of expertise and medicolegal evidence in foreign consular courts as a matter permitting racial bias or discrimination. When asked by Phasakorawong whether he thought that the Siamese state should employ a foreign or Siamese physician to conduct autopsies, Naret replied that he had "no preference in the matter whatsoever, so long as the doctor who performs the autopsies has sufficient knowledge to be able to speak to the symptomatic causes of death so that the foreign consular courts will believe him."[53] Initially, Naret's sole concern was that the person appointed be sufficiently credible "so that the consular courts will not overrule the cause of death and throw out the case as has happened before."[54] His thoughts on the issue of medical credentials for graduates of the newly founded Siamese medical college clearly support this view of medical expertise.

It was paramount, Naret cautioned, that the Ministry of Religious Affairs, which was responsible for medical education, administer the qualifying examinations at the medical college and the medical licensing process (*ok nangsue samkhan jaeng khwam-ru phaet*) in such a way that foreigners would trust in it. Until such standards were in place, however, Naret insisted that Dr. Hays accept the added responsibilities of performing autopsies in cases of unnatural death involving foreign subjects and compiling reports of his findings to be submitted to the foreign consular courts.[55] Perhaps out of compromise in the face of Hays's repeated refusals, Naret suggested that Hays might bring medical students along with him when called to perform an autopsy, which would lighten his burden somewhat and provide an educational opportunity for advanced medical students. He stressed, however, that Dr. Hays should perform all the documentation duties himself so that the consular courts would accept the evidence provided by the Siamese police and justice would be served for Siamese subjects murdered at the hands of foreigners.[56] Naret's reservations about appointing Siamese medical students to conduct autopsies concerned the relatively manageable issues of credentials and experience, not the more indelible problem of racial prejudice. But for the time being, the unresolved issue of finding a physician to conduct autopsies in cases of unnatural death would continue to fester.

Sometime in late May 1893, a fight broke out at a rice mill between two employees, a Siamese man named Nai Khram and a South Asian (*khaek*) named Ali, who was living in Siam under British legal protection.[57] Three days later, Nai Khram died after a bout of uncontrollable vomiting. The Siamese doctors treating the man concluded that he had died as a result of some underlying illness, and not from injuries sustained in the fight. (The victim in this case exhibited what a layman today might recognize as classic symptoms of brain trauma [concussion] as the result of a blow to the head. The physicians, however, attributed the death to illness and not the wounds sustained during the altercation.) Lacking other options, the Siamese police summoned Dr. Hays to perform an autopsy and determine the cause of death. Hays acquiesced, and he too attributed the death to an unspecified illness. He then resumed his demands for extra compensation for performing the autopsy.[58]

Naret accepted the doctor's judgment that this particular case involved an underlying chronic illness and not a fatal injury inflicted by a foreign subject, but the case nevertheless prompted a renewed discussion of Naret's earlier proposals regarding the appointment of a physician to conduct autopsies. First, although Naret accepted Hays's judgment in the case, he nevertheless criticized his forensic investigation and the knowledge it produced as not worth the expense.[59] Second, Naret noted that in cases of death that involve bodily injury, "it is absolutely essential to quickly appoint a physician to inspect the body, so that there would be no doubt. Otherwise, conditions will result in the loss"—presumably of evidence and medicolegal certainty, but also of the opportunity to file charges in consular courts.[60] But Naret was tired of dealing with Hays's repeated refusals and what he regarded as his extravagant demands for compensation for conducting autopsies. Naret therefore began to look around for other options, a move that would highlight a new facet of the transnational debates over medicolegal expertise.

In his frustration with Hays, Naret asked Phasakorawong to appoint a Siamese physician, Luang Damrong Phaetyakhun, to take over the duties of medical examiner.[61] Phasakorawong responded that the idea of appointing "Luang Damrong to take over the duties of inspecting corpses and conducting autopsies instead of Dr. Hays seems like a good one," but he had one reservation.[62] Phasakorawong was afraid that "even though it is true that Damrong Phaetyakhun was indeed trained and certified in medicine he was also a Thai and a servant of the King" of Siam.[63] Phasakorawong feared that because of this, foreign consular courts might not accept forensic medical evidence that was produced and attested to by Luang Damrong. He suggested that they might instead try to hire another European physician who had recently entered the service of the Ministry of the Palace, whom the foreign legations might view as more trustworthy than a Siamese subject.

This exchange reveals that although much of the debate remained unchanged from the time of Prince Naret's first proposal to address the growing gap in medicolegal standards of evidence in December 1892, the intervening months had seen some significant developments in the efforts of the Siamese state to reform forensic investigations in Bangkok. Naret continued to insist on finding the most economical solution to the state's problem of insufficient medicolegal expertise; his persistence in trying to enlist Dr. Hays to examine cases of unnatural death attests to this. At the same time, however, Naret was beginning to grasp the key issue of speed in inspecting bodies and determining the cause of death. He realized that carrying out the autopsy in a timely manner was just as important as having a qualified physician determine the cause of death. Promptness, along with appropriate medical credentials and documentation, was added to the growing list of requisites for medicolegal evidence that would meet the standards of the foreign consular courts. But just as the Siamese officials came to terms with the essentials of forensic medical investigations, the parameters of authority and credibility seemed to be shifting, as Phasakorawong astutely suspected.

The plural legal regime created by extraterritorial law in Siam meant that the Siamese state had to conform to the standards of evidence upheld by the foreign consular courts if they hoped to pursue criminal charges against foreign subjects residing in Siam. The discourses of modern legal medicine and the tacit standards of evidence in the foreign consular courts had thus become hegemonic. Yet Phasakorawong realized—well before Naret—that there were other, extrajudicial factors involved when foreign consular courts assessed evidence in a case of unnatural death and deliberated whether to bring charges against a foreign resident. Not all medical credentials were created equal, and the professional credentials of Siamese physicians did not guarantee that consular courts would recognize their authority. In recognizing that the race of the physician mattered when it came to inspecting bodies and submitting medicolegal evidence to the foreign consular courts, Siamese officials were coming to terms with one of the most pervasive features of knowledge production in the colonial world. As Pauline Kusiak has argued, "debates about what counted as knowledge, and about who counted as legitimate knowledge producers, were written into the very fabric of colonial socio-technical systems."[64]

Moreover, despite the discourse of scientific objectivity, and the belief that a physician could ascertain the exact cause of death through forensic investigation, when assessing forensic evidence consular courts also seemed to take into account the political affiliations of its producers. This amounted to another strike against Siamese physicians who would submit forensic evidence against a foreign subject before a consular court. To participate in the new system of authoritative expert knowledge—and to protect their subjects from the injustices of extraterritorial law—the Siamese state would have to hire foreign medical professionals and ensure proper documentation in cases of unnatural death. A Siamese physician such as Luang Damrong simply would not do. The Siamese state eventually turned instead to a British physician, Dr. P. A. Nightingale, to try and institute medicolegal evidentiary procedures that would meet the standards of foreign consular officials and their courts.

Semi-colonial Necropolitics

Forensic medicine was a science peculiarly suited to the social and political milieu of turn-of-the-twentieth-century Siam. As in other imperial contexts, it served as a technology of indemnification for foreign residents who might be implicated in the wrongful death of a Siamese subject. At the same time, forensic medicine was also deployed by members of the Siamese elite in service of their ongoing efforts to challenge the perceived injustices of extraterritorial law. Arguing that debates over medical jurisprudence provided a vehicle for elite Siamese officials to contest extraterritorial law, however, does not negate the objectifying power of forensic medical science. Unlike in Britain, the medicolegal investigation of cases of unnatural death in Siam did not correspond to political movements aimed at constitutional reform or popular liberties. Forensic medicine in Siam was infused from the start with elite political agendas. Its epistemology was not one of civic "truth," but rather one of leverage: using the dead to support the political agenda of the Siamese elite. Forensic medicine did not empower political subjects. The early history of forensic medicine in Siam therefore does not mesh with genealogies of democratic politics, nor does it conform to histories of colonial law and medicine as technologies of domination and control, let alone with celebratory narratives about the rise of professional medicine. It does, however, offer insights into the nature of race, science, and society in the colonial world and contributes to our understanding of the practical ways in which law and medicine figured in debates over Siamese sovereignty, thereby helping to reconfigure political life.

First, respecting race, science, and society, the history of forensic medicine in Siam demonstrates the ways in which the presumably objective realm of medicolegal science was inherently politicized. Race was an operative category both in the examination of the dead and in assessing the credibility of forensic evidence and expertise. As foreign powers enrolled Asian immigrants to Siam as protégés who enjoyed the same extraterritorial privileges as Europeans, they effectively blurred tacit assumptions about the affinity between racial and political identity.[65] These confusions were in turn projected onto the dead: if some Asian bodies were invested with forms of political identity and legal privilege usually associated with European bodies, then every unidentified corpse necessitated expert intervention. Forensic medicine thus became a peculiarly political science, one that—like other "travelling sciences"—helped to "(re)constitute" race as a category of social and political analysis.[66] These developments intersected in important ways with broader efforts on the part of the Siamese elite to reconfigure Siam from a multiethnic kingdom to a homogeneous nation-state populated by Thais.[67]

Second, the state's newfound forensic interest in the bodies of its subjects had profound implications for the development of Thai political culture. The forensic turn in Thai history occurred at a transitional moment when the personal ties of patron-client relations, which had long served as intermediary links between the state and its subjects, began to fray.[68] Scholars attentive to these developments have argued that the dissolution of hierarchical feudal ties resulted in a new form of political subjectivity, which David Wyatt has described as "a compromise or amalgam between the old concept of the 'subject,' stripped of the intermediaries that stood between the king and the peasant, and the modern concept of the 'citizen.'"[69] Wyatt's amalgam suggests the ambiguity and heterogeneity of the new sense of political subjectivity that was emerging in this transitional era—and likewise hints ominously at the potential for the continual postponement of this transformation from subject to citizen—but it fails to capture the peculiar morbidity of the state's new concern for its subjects.

Although forensic interest constituted a mode of direct relations between the state and its subjects, the resulting form of political recognition did not result in the empowerment of subjects as citizens imbued with rights. Instead, it created morbid subjects, a political constituency that seemed to demand expert forms of attention and intervention, and which acquiesced to the legal and political claims made on its behalf. Medicolegal concern bestowed on Siam's morbid subjects a problematic form of both political and ontic status, one that bears a striking resemblance to Achille Mbembe's notion of the necropolitical subject of the postcolony, which occupies a liminal space between life and death, one that in ontic terms constitutes a "third zone between subjecthood and objecthood."[70] Necropolitics in late nineteenth-century Siam, however, was not a matter of enacting violence—whether according to the racial ethos of war articulated by Foucault and Mbembe, or in the classical sense of sovereignty as the monopoly of violence within a defined territory.[71] Rather, Siamese necropolitics was part and parcel of a practical engagement with conditions of constrained sovereignty, most notably extraterritorial law. The following chapter follows the corpse into the morgue in order to ground this somewhat diffuse vision of necropolitics in the physical modalities of forensic practice—both surgical and documentary.

CHAPTER 6

Incisions and Inscriptions

> All of the different modes of intervention and the
> heterogeneous forms of work that are carried out
> around the dead constitute ways of being "with and
> apart"—of reconfiguring evidential relations as much
> as personal relationships, of entering into some modes
> of discourse and abjuring others.
>
> —Zoë Crossland, Epilogue to *Necropolitics: Mass Graves*
> *and Exhumations in the Age of Human Rights*

On May 24, 1896, members of a Siamese family
heard a ruckus coming from the quarters of their servant, a twenty-five-year-
old debt slave named Amdaeng Si.[1] Rushing to the room, they found her list-
less and incoherent. They summoned a doctor, who tried to care for her, but
she could not speak, and their efforts were in vain: eventually her heart stopped,
and she died. At first glance, the case of Amdaeng Si is entirely unremarkable
within the context of the "Death by various causes" files of the Ministry of
the Capital. It was simply another case of the death of a Siamese subject under
unnatural but not unduly suspicious conditions. With further investigation,
the police might have collected witness statements and other clues to suggest
that—as in so many other cases—the deceased had been suffering from chronic
disease or had chosen drugs as an escape from the oppressive conditions of a
life in debt bondage. This case, however, would be different. What distinguishes
the inquest into the death of Amdaeng Si from the dozens of others that came
before since the state began to investigate unnatural death was the intervention of forensic medicine: hers was the first documented case of unnatural
death to receive an autopsy and a full medical forensic investigation conducted
by physicians working for the Siamese state in conjunction with the metropolitan police force.

Beginning in May 1896, corpses were moved out of temples and public
space and into the morgue at the Bangkok Police Hospital, where doctors—

as opposed to witnesses, district officials, and police—were charged with identifying the cause of death. These changes amounted to a significant shift in the meaning and practice of handling unnatural death in the Siamese capital, as the executive authority of elite officials gave way to the medical expertise of physicians and the medicolegal judgment of the courts. Who were the practitioners of forensic medicine that wielded this new form of authority over death? How did they fit into the larger context of professional medicine in turn-of-the-twentieth-century Siam? And, more important, how was medicolegal authority over death enacted in practice within the bureaucratic logic of the Siamese state? This chapter addresses these questions through an examination of the social constitution and mediation of forensic medicine within the confines of state bureaucracy.

Entering the Morgue

According to Mo Meng Yim, one of the physicians in attendance at the autopsy of Amdaeng Si, the procedure began just after 8:00 a.m. on Friday, May 25, the morning after she died.[2] The autopsy took place in the morgue of the police hospital located near Sam Yaek—where New Road forks near Lamphunchai Road in central Bangkok. After the initial surgical incisions had been made, Dr. P. A. Nightingale, the other physician in attendance, performed a thorough investigation, "inspecting the body in every manner."[3] Dr. Nightingale then took the extra step of removing the stomach from the body and placing it inside a wide-mouthed glass jar, which he intended to take home for further consideration. (It is not clear exactly what procedures Nightingale planned to use, but he likely intended to try and identify harmful substances in the contents of the stomach.) In this early era of forensic medicine, the chain of custody and an antiseptic laboratory space were luxuries, and the chemical analysis of stomach contents readily became homework.

There are notable discrepancies in the documentation surrounding the forensic medical procedures conducted during the investigation into the death of Amdaeng Si. The first hint that something was amiss in the investigation is that the documents appear in two separate places in the "Death by various causes" files, suggesting that there was some delay in the production and submission of the documents.[4] This oversight might be accounted for by considering the time that had elapsed between the autopsy procedure and compilation of the original English autopsy report by Dr. Nightingale and the subsequent preparation of a Thai-language translation of the documents by Mo Meng Yim. A closer reading of the documents, however, reveals that there were other reasons for the delay in ascertaining the cause of death. The Thai-language death certificate (dated May 28, 1896) concludes, "when the autopsy was conducted, I [Nightingale] discovered the symptoms of disease in the deceased, who died as a result of disease in the lungs and heart."[5] In the police report, however, two senior police officials, Phraya Intharathibodi and Phra Thep Phlu, note that at the time of the autopsy Dr. Nightingale was unable to determine the cause of death. According to their report, having finished the autopsy, but without a cause of death to enter in the death certificate, Nightingale decided to remove the deceased's stomach for further testing.[6] If Nightingale discovered anything in the course of testing the stomach contents, they concluded, he would submit an additional report to the Ministry of the Capital, which oversaw the Siamese police and compiled archival records of police investigations into cases of unnatural death.

The death certificate of Amdaeng Si states with conviction that evidence of (presumably fatal) symptoms of disease was discovered during the initial autopsy, but the police report suggests that no cause of death was discovered at that time. Was this contradiction perhaps evidence of a conflict between police officials and the vanguard of forensic medicine in Bangkok? Or is it simply evidence of a failure in the practice of forensic medicine? A careful study of the realities of forensic medicine in the service of the Siamese state in this period reveals that such inconsistencies were not unique. In fact, irregularities in practice and incongruities in documentation were typical of the early implementation of forensic medicine in Siam. They are indicative of the peculiar challenges of mediating a new form of expertise—challenges that went well beyond internecine disputes within the investigative and medical arms of the Siamese police force, as this chapter demonstrates. Dr. Nightingale, failing to find a cause of death during the initial autopsy, hypothesized that the cause of death might yet be discovered residing among the contents of Amdaeng Si's stomach. When his theory failed to pan out, however, Nightingale was forced to amend the autopsy report and proclaim symptoms of disease— possibly fabricated—as the cause of death. In this case at least, the juridical need for certainty in discerning a cause of death apparently trumped the empirical maxim of "seeing with one's own eyes" during the autopsy.[7] Clearly, at its outset, this new form of authoritative medical knowledge left much to be desired.

In spite of these shortcomings, the case of Amdaeng Si nevertheless marks a significant break with earlier police investigations into cases of unnatural death, which relied on witness testimony and the observations of police and district officials who possessed no medical expertise whatsoever. But the moment when corpses entered the morgue at the police hospital likewise marked the end of the system of executive authority over the meaning of unnatural death in Bangkok. By appealing to medical expertise, Siamese officials were acknowledging that it was no longer sufficient for them to forge meaning out of the cacophony of colloquial discourses on death found in witness testimony and vernacular investigational techniques into unnatural death in the capital. (The din of voices, idioms, and registers in the colloquial witness statements and the efforts of Siamese officials to create authoritative meaning out of them were discussed in chapter 1.) In May 1896, officials in the Siamese state effectively elected to adopt the standards of evidence of the foreign consular courts and to accept the authority of medical expertise in its investigations. This chapter examines the implications of this decision in practice. It introduces the practitioners as well as the other forms of social agency that both constructed the assemblage of forensic medicine in turn-of-the-twentieth-century Bangkok and ultimately undermined it.

Mediator Deathworkers: The Practitioners of Early Forensic Medicine

If May 1896 marks the start of a new epistemic era in Siam, when elite officials abdicated their authority in cases of unnatural death to the certainty of forensic medicine, then it is essential to consider the practitioners of this new science.[8] In theory and in discourse, medicolegal expertise was a matter of scientific objectivity and professional credentials. In practice, however, Siamese officials understood that there were significant barriers to entry for those who would submit scientific evidence to consular courts (as discussed in chapter 5). For foreign legations in Siam it was clear that the credibility of evidence submitted by Siamese subjects was compromised by their political allegiances and diminished by their Siamese medical credentials. The only viable option for the Siamese state, it seemed, was to capitulate and hire a foreign physician to conduct medical examinations as part of police investigations into cases of unnatural death. But forensic medicine was a new form of authoritative knowledge in Bangkok, one that required a significant degree of mediation for the Siamese royal elites, who were about to relinquish their authority over the semantics of death. Meeting the standards of evidence of foreign consular courts therefore meant hiring a foreign physician capable of producing authoritative readings of dead bodies and finding a translator with sufficient medical knowledge to be able to mediate the new form of expertise to Siamese officials.

Mo Meng Yim, who helped to conduct the autopsy in the case of Amdaeng Si, makes his first appearance as a civil servant in the employ of the Siamese state in 1892. On Saturday, August 27 of that year, Meng Yim was introduced by Minister of the Capital Prince Naret as the attending physician at the opening of the new police hospital at Sam Yaek on New Road.[9] *The Bangkok Times* credited Luang Visudhborihan (also known as Captain Plian), the superintendent of police, with organizing the hospital, which was located on property seized from a Chinese secret society (*ang yi*).[10] Meng Yim's role at the police hospital was initially a therapeutic one; he oversaw the medical care of injured and ill police officers.[11] Forensic medicine had not yet become a priority for the police or the Ministry of the Capital. (Indeed, even six years later, when a new police hospital opened, press coverage focused on the number of policemen being treated there.)[12] At the time of his appointment, postmortem examinations were still conducted at the site of death or on the grounds of the nearest temple—often in the open air—by police and district officials, and corpses were then sent to the temple cemetery for burial or cremation, not the morgue.

There is no record of Meng Yim's qualifications for the role of attending physician at the hospital, nor of his medical credentials—though he is fairly consistently referred to as *mo* (doctor) in documents compiled by the Ministry of the Capital. Moreover, in his autopsy reports Meng Yim identifies himself as the "head physician" (*phaet thi nueng*) at the police hospital. His name betrays his Chinese ancestry, but Meng Yim's language skills—he was fluent in English and in the Thai language (as discussed below in relation to his duties as translator)—suggest that he was raised in a multilingual environment in cosmopolitan Bangkok. Judging by his language skills and medical education alone, it seems likely that Meng Yim was from a family of some financial means. (It is also possible that like other wealthy Chinese in Bangkok, he may have enjoyed extraterritorial legal rights as a registered foreign resident under French or, more likely in his case given his English-language skills, British protection.) Whatever Meng Yim's credentials were, he served as physician at the police hospital for several years before corpses began to arrive at the morgue as part of standard police procedure in cases of unnatural death and forensic medicine began to occupy more of his time. At that point, however proficient he might have been in meeting the medical needs of the Siamese police force, Meng Yim's Asian ancestry and Siamese-language skills marked him as unsuited for the task of compiling medicolegal evidence in cases of unnatural death. The Ministry of the Capital therefore needed a foreign presence to document the procedures in the morgue at the police hospital.

Dr. P. A. (Percy Athelstan) Nightingale, an English physician, was eventually hired by the Ministry of the Capital to join Meng Yim in the morgue of the police hospital. Born in 1867, Nightingale hailed from a long line of British nobility. His family had held the baronet of Newport Pond in Essex County since its creation in 1628. (One of his predecessors, Sir Robert Nightingale [d. 1722], the fourth baronet, had served as director of the East India Company some two hundred years before, perhaps setting the precedent for traveling abroad in search of one's fortune.)[13] Percy Nightingale studied medicine at what was perhaps the premier institution at the time, the University of Edinburgh Medical School. After receiving his doctorate, he set off for Bangkok, arriving in late May 1894 at the age of twenty-seven, intending to start a private practice.[14] Soon after his arrival, however, Nightingale learned that the position of physician in attendance to the British legation in Bangkok was vacant, and he applied for the post.[15] His application was successful, and he was appointed to that position at the end of July 1894 at a salary of £300 per year.[16] At around the same time, Nightingale also entered into a partnership with a British entrepreneur named G. Kennedy Reid, serving as "consulting physician" at the English pharmacy in Bangkok.[17]

Not long after his appointment as physician to the British legation, Nightingale's credentials would be tested in his new role as de facto medical examiner. In September 1894, he became embroiled in a public debate over the proper circumstances for ordering an autopsy in cases of unnatural death. In late August of that year, a British subject living in Siam named J. J. Grant had gone missing from his riverside home during the middle of the night.[18] Grant worked for the opium tax farm in the city, and given the nature of that business, it was natural to suspect that foul play might have been involved in his disappearance.[19] The corpse was finally recovered several days later—after some tribulations due to the actions of local villagers who objected to police efforts to retrieve it—floating naked in the river downstream at Samut Prakan (*pak nam*).

The *Siam Free Press*, a local newspaper that was widely regarded as being anti-Siamese, anti-British, and pro-French, pounced on the opportunity to criticize the investigational practices of the Siamese police and British officials alike.[20] According to the *Bangkok Times*, the *Siam Free Press* was in the habit of using "every incident, capable of being put to such use, as a weapon against officials, whether English or Siamese."[21] During the final decade of the nineteenth century, political tensions between pro-British and pro-French interests in Siam ran high. Disputes between the two factions would often converge over the actions of the Siamese police, which the French regarded as a de facto arm of the British military, owing to the high numbers of officers recruited from British India—primarily consisting of British administrators and Sikh officers.[22] Although the disputes would reach an all-time high during the Pak Nam Incident of 1893 (when the French sent an envoy of gunboats to exact territorial concessions from Siam), they would reverberate for some years to come, often finding expression in the local press.[23]

In the case of Grant's death, the *Free Press* lambasted officials for not conducting a postmortem examination of the body. They editorialized that "a grave omission has been clearly evident in the treatment of this case, and a lamentable want of consideration and foresight on the part of our Consular Officials, who cannot feel very surprised if their conduct does not meet with general approval among the British community."[24] The *Free Press* accused the British—incorrectly, as it happens—of failing to even dispatch a medical examiner to the scene once the body had been retrieved from the river. In fact, according to the *Bangkok Times*, Dr. Nightingale, in his capacity as physician to the British legation, had been summoned to the scene; it was quickly determined, however, that "no examination of the body in the state of decomposition in which it was found, would have availed anything." The *Bangkok Times* concluded, "the Doctor exercised, in our opinion, a wise discretion in advising immediate burial."[25]

The disputes surrounding the procedures involved in investigating Grant's death highlight the differential nature of investigations into cases of unnatural death in colonial-era Bangkok. In this one case involving the death of a foreign resident, no fewer than three separate investigations were conducted. First, according to the *Bangkok Times*, there was an investigation carried out by the Siamese police at the request of the British consulate. The paper does not report on the investigative techniques that were employed by the Siamese police, but they likely amounted to interviewing Grant's household servants and a cursory search of the surrounding area for the body. Second, Grant's employer, the holder of the opium tax farm, commissioned a private investigation that involved interviews with Grant's household servants, his neighbors, and his landlord, all of whom testified that they had not heard any noise during the night that Grant disappeared. Finally, the British consulate conducted its own independent investigation, which included retrieving the body and calling on Dr. Nightingale to perform a postmortem examination—which he declined on account of the advanced state of decomposition of the body. (It seems possible, however, that Nightingale might never have actually seen the body, which had already been sealed in a coffin by the time he arrived at the scene.)[26]

In the end, despite the furor in the *Siam Free Press*, forensic medicine was something of an afterthought in the case of J. J. Grant. Only one of the three independent investigations—that carried out by the officials of the British consulate—even attempted to use forensic medicine to gather evidence in the case. Given the contemporary standards of medicolegal evidentiary laws in England, it comes as no surprise that public debates did not include discussion of Nightingale's qualifications to act as a forensic pathologist. In this era, standard medical training and proximity alone were sufficient to qualify a physician as expert medical witness.[27]

In the aftermath of the debates prompted by the death of Grant, the authorities of the British legation in Bangkok would call on Nightingale in his role as medical attendant to perform postmortem examinations in several other cases. Nightingale assisted Dr. Hans Adamsen, a physician in the employ of the Siamese Hospital Department, with a postmortem examination in the case of a shooting in Chinatown (*sampheng*) in February 1895.[28] He was also called on by the Siamese government to care for Siamese subjects in police custody on at least one occasion before he had entered the employment of the Ministry of the Capital.[29] Some time before January 1896, Nightingale was appointed by the Siamese government as "inspector to control the slaughtering of cattle for food," and he began to appear in newspaper reports concerning the surprisingly contentious issue of the inspection of livestock at privately owned slaughterhouses in the city.[30] (Although Nightingale's credentials to work as a forensic pathologist would go unquestioned during his time in Bangkok, his qualifications to serve as a cattle inspector and veterinary surgeon for the Siamese government would not. In a few years' time, Nightingale would leave Bangkok in the aftermath of a legal battle related to this issue, as discussed later.)

Nightingale was formally appointed by the Siamese state to the position of Chief Doctor of the Police Department—or, as the role was more often called (after the British office), Medical Officer of Health—in March 1896, and it was in that capacity that he oversaw the autopsy of Amdaeng Si, the first documented case of a surgical autopsy conducted by the Siamese state, alongside Mo Meng Yim in the morgue at the police hospital.[31] In spite of these new responsibilities working on behalf of the Siamese government, Nightingale retained his appointment as medical attendant to the British legation.[32] In fact, it is quite possible that it was precisely his standing with the British legation that recommended Nightingale to officials in the Siamese state as they confronted the challenges posed by extraterritoriality and the differential standards of evidence employed by foreign consular courts.

Doctors Meng Yim and Nightingale likely shared a similar sense of both the potential and limitations of forensic medicine in the waning years of the nineteenth century. They understood that medical training and credentials gave them a distinct advantage over Siamese police and the officials of the Ministry of the Capital in ascertaining the cause of death in cases of unnatural death. They also understood the importance of properly documenting the procedures in order that their conclusions might serve as evidence in the foreign consular courts of the Siamese capital. But their tacit sense of the nature of forensic medicine at the turn of the twentieth century had to be communicated to officials in the Siamese government who had their own ideas and expectations. In that respect, translation was essential to the localization of medicolegal science in treaty port Bangkok.

Documenting Death

From the earliest proposals to reform forensic investigation in Siam, the issue of documentation was crucial. Even Minister of the Capital Prince Naret, who did not initially grasp the necessity of hiring foreign physicians to conduct autopsies, came to understand the gravity of properly documenting postmortem examination procedures and their findings. As discussed previously, Naret tried to implement a procedure whereby a foreign doctor, T. Heyward Hays, would be present at the autopsy and responsible for documenting the procedures and findings in cases where a foreign subject killed a Siamese subject. He came to understand that proper documentation was the only chance of obtaining a fair hearing for criminal allegations against foreign residents in their respective consular courts. Thus, when police investigations into cases of unnatural death were finally routed through the morgue at the police hospital beginning in May 1896, documentation was a preeminent concern.

For the Siamese state to provide the kind of forensic evidence that would meet the standards of foreign consular courts in Bangkok, it needed to hire a foreign physician to conduct postmortem examinations that would produce a definitive statement of the cause of death. The cause of death had to be articulated in the terminology of Western medical science—in the English language—in the form of a death certificate. Dr. Nightingale's presence in the morgue at the police hospital lent the requisite sense of expertise to the proceedings, and his signature on the death certificate authorized the findings as to the cause of death in a manner that conformed with the standards of the foreign legations and their consular courts.

While English-language certificates of death matched the expectations of foreign consular courts, the forensic medical investigations conducted by the metropolitan police had another crucial audience: Siamese officials. For this reason, when an autopsy was performed at the morgue of the police hospital, the resulting death certificate had to be translated into the Thai language as well. In official documents, "death certificate"—rendered into Thai through a mixture of translation and transliteration as *"nangsue soe te fi ket"* (certificate letter)—quickly replaced the diverse and unwieldy terms that had previously been used to describe reports of postmortem examinations submitted by police, district officials, and witnesses. The very novelty and foreign nature of this new bureaucratic medium is revealed by the long-standing use of the transliterated term in official reports originating at the morgue of the police hospital. (The garbled pronunciation and misspellings of the word, including references to a *"sio li ket"* a year after the introduction of autopsies and death certificates, likewise attests to this.)[33] The vernacular practice of the postmortem examination (*kan-chanasut phlik sop*) and its associated documentation, which was conducted by police, officials, and witnesses alike, was no longer adequate. Causes of death in cases of unnatural death had to be determined with a greater degree of certainty in the sequestered space of the morgue and under the auspices of medical expertise. The death certificate recorded the findings of the surgical autopsy (*kan-pha sop*) and was authored by a foreign physician. In this transitional period, Meng Yim also referred to the forensic medical investigation into cases of unnatural death as "surgical investigation" (*kan-chanasut pha sop*), which combines the terms for the vernacular investigation conducted by police (*kan-chanasut*) with the surgical methods of postmortem examination (*kan-pha sop*).[34] The death certificate was thus an object imported from a different culture, a signifier in a different semantics of death. For these reasons, it required mediation and translation.

Each certificate of death was introduced by an autopsy report (*nangsue rai ngan*) in the Thai language authored by Mo Meng Yim. In addition to documenting the autopsy procedures themselves, Meng Yim's reports served as a brief for the officials at the Ministry of the Capital who would review and file the documents. At the same time, the autopsy reports chronicle the chain of custody in the case, from the discovery of the body to its arrival at the morgue, through the autopsy procedure, and finally, the arrangements made for the disposal of the corpse. In this respect, Meng Yim's reports also served to link the proceedings in the morgue at the police hospital with the realm of legal medicine and the evidentiary standards in the foreign consular courts.

Despite their formulaic nature, Meng Yim's autopsy reports constitute important evidence for deconstructing the ethos of forensic medical investigation in late nineteenth-century Bangkok. Their stock sequencing and phrasing suggest that Meng Yim and the officials at the Ministry of the Capital understood the importance of chronology in documenting forensic evidence. They also demonstrate the superior position of the foreign physician, Dr. Nightingale, both in the proceedings at the morgue and in the documentary record that officials hoped to compile for cases of unnatural death. Each report begins with the arrival of the corpse at the morgue, with Meng Yim recording the date and time as well as the names of the police officers who delivered the corpse. Next, the reports offer a brief account of the nature of the death in question and the circumstances that merited a postmortem examination as related to Meng Yim by the police. The reports then stress that Meng Yim "right away" (*than dai*) summoned Dr. P. A. Nightingale to conduct the autopsy. In some cases, Dr. Nightingale was able to attend to the autopsy promptly, but in other cases he wrote back to Meng Yim appointing a later time for the procedure to take place. In every case, Meng Yim is careful to report that the two physicians arrived "simultaneously" (*phrom duai*) at the morgue to conduct the autopsy.[35] This aspect of the autopsy reports suggests that Meng Yim had some awareness of the importance of the chain of custody of evidence in conducting forensic investigations. Officials in the Ministry of the Capital likewise must have understood that consular courts would throw out forensic medical evidence if it were revealed that Nightingale was not present at the time of the autopsy. Such strict adherence to the principle of the chain of custody of evidence is in stark contrast to the case of Amdaeng Si and the forensic analysis of her stomach. These procedural developments might therefore be taken as evidence of the performative nature of forensic medicine in this period, as the Siamese state and its agents aspired to meet the standards set by the foreign consular courts. In Siam, as in other colonial contexts, medicine "was not a tool of the colonial state, but a set of practices through which the state was performed," often by indigenous subordinates.[36]

After the autopsy procedure was completed (the reports do not describe the surgical aspects of the examinations in great detail), Meng Yim records that he requested a death certificate (*nangsue soe te fi ket*) from Nightingale, which would be "preserved as evidence" (*wai pen lak than*). Although Meng Yim refers to himself as the "head physician [of the police hospital]" (*phaet thi nueng*), this portion of his autopsy reports shows his deference to Dr. Nightingale, who is clearly in charge of the proceedings in the morgue. Next, the autopsy reports note that Meng Yim translated the original English-language death certificate and submitted the original and his translation along with his autopsy report.[37] Meng Yim's reports inevitably end with a preemptive apology for any inaccuracies in his translation. He seems keenly aware of the possibility of error—not at the level of vocabulary, but rather in terms of semantic elements (*nuea khwam*) that might have been lost in translation (*ja khlat khluean prakan dai*).

Finally, Meng Yim documents what became of the corpse after the autopsy. The financial burden of disposing of the corpse most often fell to Mo Meng Yim (who was presumably reimbursed by the Siamese government). This includes both cases of unidentified corpses and cases in which family members came to the morgue to plead poverty and ask for his help in paying for funerary costs. Standard burial costs amounted to four Baht, which included hiring the undertaker of a local temple (usually Wat Phlap phla Chai) to cart the body away and bury it at the temple cemetery, where the bones would be disinterred and cremated en masse at a later date.

Meng Yim's autopsy reports were an important part of the process of documenting cases of unnatural death in late nineteenth-century Bangkok. They provided context for the Siamese officials in the Ministry of the Capital, including Prince Naret and his subordinates, who would review the files and preserve them as evidence. The reports also helped to couple the forensic medical practices of the Siamese metropolitan police with the requirements of legal medicine as practiced in the consular courts. They established a chronology of the inquest and detailed the chain of custody for the corpse, the focus of the forensic medical investigation, while specifying the chain of command in the conduct of the forensic medical investigation. But for all the insight that these documents provide into the institutional practice of forensic medicine, they are clearly secondary to the English-language death certificate, the authoritative statement of medical science in cases of unnatural death.

Translating Authority

When Siamese officials first awakened to the problem of different standards of evidence between Siamese and foreign consular courts in Bangkok in the final decade of the nineteenth century, they saw forensic medicine as one potential solution. Once the morgue at the police hospital opened, however, the Siamese elite may have been disappointed to learn that the supposed authority of forensic medicine was not as advertised. Early cases reveal evidence of indeterminacy and ambiguity in the original English-language death certificates composed by Dr. Nightingale. Instead of a straightforward record of the surgical procedure and a definitive statement of the medical examiner's findings about the cause of death, many of the certificates hedged. In other cases, Nightingale's certificates included extraneous observations that had no clear basis in forensic pathology. Translation played a crucial role in reconciling the expectations of the Siamese elite with the realities of forensic medicine as a discipline that was still in its infancy. It also functioned as mediator between Western and Siamese medical systems, as Mo Meng Yim worked to render Nightingale's death certificates in an idiom that would be intelligible to his superiors in the Ministry of the Capital.

Documents concerning the death of a prostitute named Amdaeng Wan (also referred to as "Ing" by Nightingale) from a suspected drug overdose in January 1897 merit close consideration for what they reveal about the cross-cultural translation of medical authority.[38] After conducting an autopsy, Dr. Nightingale acknowledged the ambivalence of his findings in the death certificate. The original English-language death certificate summarizes the physical condition of the deceased based on the state of her internal organs, noting "both lungs were slightly diseased and the heart was fatty, while the various abdominal organs were much congested and irritated."[39] Nightingale cites these general physical symptoms of pathology in the clinical language of Western anatomy, but he plainly acknowledges his inability to determine the exact cause of death. Dismissing witness accounts that suggested an opium overdose, Nightingale revealed that "the contents of the stomach were examined, but no trace of opium could be found. I am of opinion that death was due to some irritant poison, though I could not determine its exact nature."[40] Nightingale's death certificate contested the findings of the original police investigation, but it failed to offer a definitive conclusion based on medical science. For the officials of the Ministry of the Capital, the death certificate would clearly have failed to instill confidence in the methods employed by the medical examiner.

Mo Meng Yim, in his role as translator, had to work to conceal the authoritative breaches in the original English versions of some death certificates while rendering the findings of the autopsy into a medical cosmology more familiar to his superiors. Where Nightingale unapologetically announced his lack of conviction regarding the outcome of an autopsy, Meng Yim intervened in translation to reassure the Siamese authorities of the certitude of forensic medicine. In the case of Amdaeng Wan, Meng Yim editorializes in his translation, making Nightingale's uncertainty sound like an aberration. In his Thai translation of the death certificate, Meng Yim also admits the absence of evidence of opium use, but he is not so cavalier in admitting the failings of the medical investigation. Meng Yim interpolates, "I [Nightingale] am of the opinion that the symptoms causing death were related to a disorder of the fire element, which was poisoned by some substance. Unfortunately, as of yet, I am unable to state [the cause of death] with absolute certainty in the usual manner."[41] The reference to the "fire element" is a clear deviation from the Western medical terminology that characterizes the original document. It refers to Siamese traditional medicine, which identified four elements that make up the human constitution, illness being a result of imbalance of these elements.[42] Meng Yim's translation departs from the strictly physiological basis of Nightingale's forensic examination and reverts to a more recognizably Siamese idiom for conveying the cause of death. But beyond rendering Nightingale's findings in the terms of traditional Siamese medical cosmology, Meng Yim's translation also claims exceptionality for this particular case, as a deviation from the "usual manner" in which forensic inquiry is able to render an exact cause of death. It is also possible that evoking the elemental theory of health was likewise a strategy for Meng Yim to avoid the admission of inconclusive physiological evidence from a Western medical perspective.

In addition to such authoritative breaches, Nightingale's English-language death certificates challenged the skill of his translator in other ways. Some documents, for example, contain elaborate grammatical constructions that would have required a high degree of fluency to translate. In the case of a young Chinese beggar who dropped dead outside of a Chinese theater, for example, Nightingale's death certificate records plainly that "I made a postmortem examination on the body of a Chinaman at the Police Mortuary, and found that death was due to disease of the lungs and liver."[43] Nightingale ventures beyond the confines of the morgue and the empirical findings of the postmortem examination, however, adding that "the man had probably been a confirmed opium smoker."[44] (Such interpolations regarding the issue of drug use are likewise indicative of the troubling ways in which race and ethnicity infiltrated the supposedly objective scientific practices of assessing the cause of death. As scholars have noted in other colonial jurisdictions, European racial and moral superiority was substantiated through medical discourses about indigenous bodies.)[45] Mo Meng Yim skillfully translates the supposition in his Thai-language version of the death certificate: "The individual shows symptoms suggesting that it is possible that [. . .] he was an opium smoker."[46] Meng Yim's fluency is beyond doubt, and yet he inevitably included the preemptive apology in his autopsy reports for any potential deficiencies in his translations— perhaps suggesting to his superiors the opaqueness of the English-language death certificate, the crucial medium of forensic medicine. Whatever Meng Yim's medical credentials, perhaps his most crucial role was as a mediator helping to present an image of forensic medicine to his superiors as accessible and authoritative at a time when it was anything but.

The translations produced in the morgue reveal that the death certificate could at times function as a "boundary object," allowing those who inhabited different sociocultural worlds to engage differentially with the knowledge created by a single form of scientific practice.[47] Foreign physicians in the employ of the Siamese state inhabited the world of forensic science comfortably; they understood the expectations of foreign consular courts and yet were aware of and seemingly untroubled by the limitations of forensic medicine in practice. Agents of the Siamese state, by contrast, experienced the individual failings of forensic medical expertise as a threat to the authority of medicolegal science and certainty. They therefore worked to conceal authoritative breaches in the knowledge produced in the morgue.

The English-language death certificate—along with its Thai translation—did not replace the colloquial witness accounts and the reports of the vernacular police investigations into cases of unnatural death. All three types of documents continue to appear in the "Death by various causes" files of the Ministry of the Capital after the introduction of forensic medicine in May 1896. Nor did autopsies replace police work at the scene of death. In fact, autopsies were conducted in a relatively small number of reported cases of unnatural death.[48] Death certificates did, however, bring a new kind of closure to the investigations. They constituted an authoritative conclusion that was often lacking in cases documented in the early years of Siamese police inquests as documented in the "Death by various causes" files. Moreover, there can be no doubt that the finality of the death certificate served to displace other voices within the case files. Witnesses with their peculiar concerns for the locality of the death, police fixated on external signs of violence, and district officials made aware of the limitations of their own knowledge would all be muted by the authoritative findings recorded by the hand of a foreign physician in the morgue of the police hospital.

Marginalia in the "Death by various causes" files attest to this process whereby Siamese officials came to accept the authority of forensic medical findings in cases of unnatural death. The case of Amdaeng Wan is again instructive in this context. When the documents concerning her death reached the authorities in the Ministry of the Capital, it entered the "Death by various causes" files as something of an enigma. Prince Naret reviewed the documents, but there was no definitive cause of death to be found in either the witness statements gathered by police or the death certificates produced by Drs. Nightingale and Meng Yim. Both the vernacular investigative techniques of the police and the scientific tactics of the physicians had failed to identify the cause of death. Faced with conflicting evidence, Naret sided with the findings of the forensic medical investigation over those of police and witnesses. He dismissed the consensus opinion of numerous witness accounts that Amdaeng Wan had taken opium on the grounds that the medical investigation yielded no evidence of opium in her stomach. Naret reasoned that if she had died as a result of ingesting drugs, "then whatever she had consumed would either appear in the contents of her stomach or [would appear] in the harmful effects that it had wrought on her stomach and intestines," and there was no such evidence in Dr. Nightingale's investigation.[49] "Deaths that occur under suspicious circumstances such as this," Prince Naret's marginal note continues, "require that we investigate the facts thoroughly, because death [sic: murder?] is a capital offense."[50] Prince Naret then ordered Phraya Intharathibodi and the police to investigate the matter further and to obtain more detailed testimony from the witnesses involved, including Amdaeng Wan's lover and the wife of her lover.

Although the forensic medical investigation into the death of Amdaeng Wan had not produced any definitive conclusions and there was no latitude for furthering that investigation after the disposal of the corpse, Prince Naret nevertheless sided with the authority of modern medicine in the case. His verdict in the matter reflects an implicit trust in the ability of forensic medicine to root out the cause of death, despite the fact that the findings of physicians in the morgue of the police hospital had been anything but definitive to date. Naret's verdict further corroborates the shift whereby Siamese officials abdicated the privilege of executive authority in favor of the expertise of medicolegal science, effectively ushering in a new regime of authoritative knowledge in cases of unnatural death.

"Table for Two?": The Social Nature of Forensic Medicine

During the two years that Drs. Nightingale and Meng Yim worked together conducting autopsies in the morgue at the police hospital, they helped to establish forensic medicine as a central part of the investigation and documentation of cases of unnatural death in the Siamese capital. Through a confluence of credentials, expertise, and skillful translations, they displaced forensic investigations from the public arena of the temple cemetery and the jurisdiction of executive authority into the sequestered space of the morgue under the auspices of professional Western medicine. It was no longer necessary— or viable—for Siamese authorities to collate and edit colloquial witness testimony and vernacular police investigations into a coherent narrative of death. Thereafter, the practitioners of medical science would provide their own definitive narrative as cases of unnatural death entered a new era of medicolegal jurisdiction. But the era would prove to be short-lived, and the progress made in medicolegal science was revealed to be dependent on the fragile working relationship of Drs. Nightingale and Meng Yim over the autopsy table. When their partnership ended, the new habits of investigation and documentation of cases of unnatural death quickly unwound.

After two years of working with Meng Yim in the morgue at the police hospital, Nightingale took an extended leave of absence from his office and returned to England. He left Bangkok on April 25, 1898, four months after having lost a libel case that he had brought against the proprietor of the *Bangkok Times*. The case hinged on Nightingale's competence to act as a cattle inspector and veterinary surgeon for the Siamese government. Charles Thorne, the editor of the *Bangkok Times*, had questioned Nightingale's credentials in print—pointing out that he was not, in fact, a veterinarian—and Nightingale had filed suit in the British consular court.[51] Thorne won the suit, but he would later apologize—in print—to Nightingale for his comments.[52] After losing the highly public case, Nightingale apparently decided to spend some time away from Bangkok, and he booked his passage home. With Nightingale gone, another British physician, Dr. H. Campbell Highet, took over the duties of medical officer of health for the Siamese government. Highet also filled in for Nightingale alongside Mo Meng Yim as medical examiner in the morgue of the police hospital, but it was not to be a lasting partnership.

According to Meng Yim's account, when Highet first arrived at the police hospital (likely in late April or May 1898), the two physicians worked together in the same manner as Meng Yim and Nightingale had before.[53] But then, sometime in early September 1898, in the presence of the inspector general of police (A. J. A. Jardine), Highet introduced administrative changes at the police hospital and informed Meng Yim that he would be transferred to a new branch. Just a few months after Nightingale's departure, on September 9, a new police hospital had opened at Sala Daeng (at the eastern end of Silom Road), a few kilometers from the first location at Sam Yaek on New Road.[54] Meng Yim, who had been working as the head physician at the original location for six years, was not happy with the transfer order.[55] (In those days, long before the skytrain and the elevated expressway, this would have been a formidable commute, and it would have made Meng Yim's habit of lunching at home impossible.) Meng Yim informed Highet that it would be a hardship for him to move his family to the vicinity of the Sala Daeng police hospital and that since he could see no benefit from the move, he refused the transfer order. It is not clear whether Highet proposed the transfer as a result of friction between himself and Meng Yim (to which the latter was apparently blind), but from that moment on their working relationship quickly deteriorated.

In a letter of complaint addressed to Prince Naret, Meng Yim claimed that from that day forward, Highet continually accused him of insubordinate behavior.[56] For his part, Meng Yim maintained that he continued to perform his duties at the police hospital as before. After Meng Yim's initial refusal to accept his new post, Highet told him that he would speak with Jardine, the inspector general of police, to see if they could allocate money to cover the cost of Meng Yim's commuting expenses so that he would not have to move his family. Placated by the gesture and the promised commuting allowance, Meng Yim accepted the transfer and began reporting to work at the new police hospital at Sala Daeng. For a time, he worked mornings at the police hospital and afternoons at the office of the Department of Local Sanitation. Meng Yim claimed that although he never disobeyed Highet's orders, Highet remained dissatisfied with him and continually threatened to fire him and find a replacement.[57] At his wit's end, and with no other recourse, Meng Yim wrote to Prince Naret to request a transfer within the Department of Local Sanitation and outside the authority of Highet.[58]

Nothing seems to have come of the tussle during Nightingale's absence, but he returned the following year to find a letter from Meng Yim outlining his troubles with Highet. Meng Yim's entreaty, dated July 27, 1899, recounts the entire episode that had played out in Nightingale's sabbatical and is worth quoting at length. He writes, with perhaps undue humility,

> Sir, As Dr. Highet expressed himself this morning of being very sick of me, and used very indecent language such as the word damn was given to me many times, Such word I should think with my little education, is fit to be used only with coolies, and not expressed by a Dr. who holds a position such as Dr. Highet. Previous to your return from Europe he has many times befraned [sic: defamed?] to me in the same manner, and expressed himself so far as to get a new man for my place. May I now be allowed to approached [sic] you with a request for your Kind permission to allow me not to attend the police hospital [at *Sala Daeng*] any further for which service I do not feel inclined to spend any more money [for commuting costs] out of my own pocket for which I receive no returns [sic: added compensation?] and for which I am not paid [reimbursed] for, and in return of which I receive nothing was [sic: but] damn. Hoping you will not refuse to favor me with the requested permission otherwise I will be obliged to apply to the higher authority.[59]

In a dramatic departure from his customary signature, Meng Yim signs his letter, "Yours most obediently, Chin [*Jin*] Meng Yim," using the ethnic marker for a Chinese man rather than referring to his credentials as a medical doctor or his rank as head physician of the police hospital.

A week later, on August 3, 1899, Nightingale wrote directly to Prince Naret, dismissing Meng Yim's allegations and presumably denying his request for a transfer.[60] Meng Yim had apparently stopped going to work at the police hospital after submitting his most recent transfer request to Nightingale. Nightingale informed Prince Naret of Meng Yim's absence for the past week and repudiated his allegations against Highet, calling them "a piece of impertinence."[61] Moreover, Nightingale seems to have accepted Highet's evaluation of Meng Yim's work, adding "Dr. Highet has reported to me that [Meng] Yim is quite useless to him, as he not only constantly neglects his duties, but on more than one occasion has come in a state quite unfit to even try and perform them."[62] Although Meng Yim staunchly defended his professionalism in the face of Highet's complaints, there is evidence to suggest that he had perhaps lost interest in his work in the morgue at the police hospital.

One day in early September 1898, several months after Nightingale had left Bangkok, the metropolitan police found the body of a Chinese beggar lying dead on the side of the road.[63] The police examined the physical condition of the corpse and on finding it emaciated in the manner of opium addicts (*rang kai phom haeng*), they surmised that he had likely died of opium withdrawal, a condition known as opium eater's dysentery (*pen rok long daeng tai*).[64] Unable to locate any relatives—who would presumably take custody of the body and make burial arrangements—the senior police official, Luang Wisutborihan, ordered police officers to take the body to the police hospital so that Mo Meng Yim could perform an autopsy. (In cases such as this, where police had good reason to suspect drug use as the cause of death—and in the absence of clear evidence of violence—it is possible that the police looked to the police hospital as little more than an expedient means of disposing of the body.) When the body arrived at the morgue, however, Meng Yim refused delivery. Instead, he gave the police officers a letter to take back to their superiors.

Meng Yim's letter (dated September 7, 1898) is a marvel of bureaucratic obstruction and a testament to the Kafkaesque muddle into which forensic medicine had stumbled during Nightingale's absence.[65] It was likely written in the days following Highet's announcement that Meng Yim would be transferred to the new branch of the police hospital at Sala Daeng, and it clearly suggests Meng Yim's state of mind. He begins by explaining, "At this time, I have yet to receive word of any sort of formal authorization respecting the inspection of corpses or the conduct of autopsies."[66] "If, therefore," the note continues, "events [cases of unnatural death] should happen to occur in your district, Luang [Wisutborihan], I would advise you to make your own arrangements according to government protocol."[67] Meng Yim signed the note and then added a postscript: "Moreover, the autopsy table and the instruments used for conducting autopsies and various other items have all been sent together to the [newly built] Sala Daeng Hospital."[68] The body of the Chinese beggar had arrived in the midst of the opening of the new branch of the police hospital, and it gave Meng Yim an opportunity to voice his displeasure over the newly proposed changes through an act of bureaucratic civil disobedience. Without calling attention to his own plight, Meng Yim focused on issues of protocol and the tools of the trade, specifically the autopsy table.

When word of the incident reached the higher offices of the Ministry of the Capital, the officials in charge were perplexed. Phraya Thoraninarubet, a senior police official who oversaw inquests for a time instead of Prince Naret, wrote to both Luang Wisutborihan and Inspector General of Police Jardine and asked what had become of the standing order to deliver corpses to the morgue for an autopsy in cases of unnatural death.[69] Thoraninarubet suspected that the problem was simply a matter of outdated protocol: "the autopsy table had already been taken to [the] Sala Daeng [branch of the police hospital], but the old standing order [to deliver corpses to the main branch at Sam Yaek] had not yet been rescinded."[70] Reinstating forensic medical practice in the Bangkok metropolitan police, however, would not be as simple as rerouting bodies to the new morgue. The sociotechnical network that had facilitated the development of forensic medical expertise in late nineteenth-century Bangkok had undoubtedly suffered due to Nightingale's departure. In his absence, Highet had failed to cultivate harmonious working relations with Meng Yim, and Nightingale showed no signs of willingness to repair those relations. But what might be said of the other partners in the scientific endeavor? What of the autopsy table?

Bruno Latour has pointed out the tendency of sociologists to "invoke the power of social explanations" without acknowledging the inherently fragile and transitory nature of social relations.[71] He argues that theories of social power are always already predicated on a broader definition of the social, which includes the material (nonhuman) elements that allow congeries of social relations to endure and project power. Latour's response is actor-network-theory (ANT), which insistently asks, "Since every sociologist loads *things* into social ties to give them enough weight to account for their durability and extension, why not do this explicitly instead of doing it on the sly?"[72] From the perspective of ANT, the autopsy table-in-transit provides an opportunity to reflect on the delicate nature of scientific expertise. Forensic medical expertise in late nineteenth-century Bangkok was contingent on the (already quite fragile) working relationship of Drs. Nightingale and Meng Yim and their documentary habits, which allowed them to project the authority of postmortem examinations outside of the morgue—both to the foreign consular courts but also up the chain of command within the Siamese Ministry of the Capital. But in addition to these conditions of possibility, the project of constructing and projecting forensic medical expertise was likewise made possible by the autopsy table and associated instruments with which incisions were made, organs inspected, and medicolegal evidence created. All of these must be regarded as essential nodes in the new semantics of death that emerged from the morgue of the police hospital.

Although the autopsy table and equipment would eventually arrive, and a morgue was established at the new branch of the police hospital at Sala Daeng, the procedures and documentation habits previously practiced by Drs. Night-ingale and Meng Yim did not. After the transfer to the new hospital, autopsy reports and death certificates no longer appear in the "Death by various causes" files of the Ministry of the Capital. Forensic investigation into cases of unnat-ural death once again became the domain of untrained police officers—sometimes aided by the undertaker of the local temple—performing vernacular forms of investigation at the scene.[73] Some of the files contain references to autopsies being performed, but there is no documentation of the procedures—whether in Thai or English. Absent too are the death certificates that had be-come the authoritative document in the inquest files, linking Siamese police investigations to the standards of legal medicine practiced in the foreign con-sular courts.[74] In their place, the executive authority of the Siamese officials over cases of unnatural death seems to have reasserted itself, along with the ad hoc practices of making meaning out of the scant evidence assembled by Siamese police in their investigations. The tentative inroads made by modern forensic medicine into the realm of unnatural death in the Siamese capital had given way once more to the authority of elite officials. And this reversal in the fortunes of medicolegal expertise was, perhaps, not coincidental. The concern for justice in the plural legal environment created by extraterritorial law had driven the forensic investigation of cases of unnatural death, but a new form of concern was in ascendance, and it would provoke a new regime of state interest in the dead.

Assembling Science

As corpses moved from the chaotic and crowded spaces of vernacular foren-sic interventions—the grounds of the nearest Buddhist temple—to the seques-tered and presumably more sterile environs of the morgue, medical expertise took precedence. This transition was in effect mandated by the plural legal arena in treaty port Bangkok, as the Siamese state worked to address the dis-advantaged status of Siamese legal subjects vis-à-vis foreign residents and their consular institutions by implementing forensic investigations into cases of un-natural death. It would be shortsighted, however, to regard this development as a simple victory of modern medical science. Like other forms of knowl-edge transfer in the colonial world, the implementation of medicolegal sci-ence in Siam was an asymmetrical affair.[75] Asymmetries in the construction of forensic expertise began with the very conditions of extraterritoriality. By virtue of the unequal trade treaties that established extraterritorial legal priv-ileges for foreign residents in Siam, the Siamese state was forced to try to conform to the standards of evidence recognized in the foreign consular courts. Forensic medicine might thus be said to have inhabited a peculiar institutional ecology in the plural legal arena of turn-of-the-twentieth-century Siam. Moreover, like other forms of scientific expertise, it was also inherently rooted in the collaborative work of social actors.[76]

Archival evidence attests to the ways in which the rise of forensic expertise was ultimately the product of documentary habits and delicate social relations; it is a tale not of scientific achievement, but of social mediation in "the brokered world."[77] In practice, forensic medicine in Siam depended on the working relationship of a foreign physician and a Siamese subordinate. Meng Yim worked alongside Nightingale in the confines of the morgue, assisting in the forensic examination of corpses and in the production of documentary forms of evidence that would be admissible in foreign consular courts. Meng Yim's remit, however, extended far beyond the immediacy of morbid labors in the morgue; he was also tasked with mediating their work for the benefit of their superiors within the Siamese Ministry of the Capital.

Death certificates, the documentary fruits of their labors, attest to the quintessential role of translation and mediation in the production of forensic science. They reveal how Meng Yim worked both to translate Western etiologies into a distinctively Siamese idiom and to conceal lacunae in the forensic findings. Meng Yim was a translator who was capable of both participating in the production of forensic knowledge and rendering it legible to the Siamese officials who oversaw affairs in the capital. The documentary existence of unnatural death in Siam, particularly in the legible form of the death certificate, thus helped to mediate between its various social and institutional lives. For a time, forensic medicine successfully "embrace[d] a wide variety of incompatible components" and constituted an epistemic field that was capable of being mobilized in support of divergent social and political interests.[78] But undermined by the inherent fragility of social relations and the shifting sands of political concern, it would not prove to be a durable assemblage.

Conclusion

> Sovereignty has been a place that only the dead
> can inhabit.
>
> —Claudio Lomnitz, *Death and the Idea of Mexico*

        Whatever the cause of Mo Meng Yim's falling
out with Dr. Highet and his superiors in the Ministry of the Capital, his fall
from grace marked the end of an era—albeit a brief one—in forensic medicine in Siam. It is not clear what became of Meng Yim in the aftermath, but it
seems likely that his tenure in the Hospital Department ended soon after.
Nightingale resigned from his positions at the British legation and as medical
officer of health to the Ministry of the Capital in December 1901.[1] Dr. Highet
replaced him as the Chief Medical Officer of Health—as well as the chief medical attendant to the British Legation.[2] Highet, however, was a new breed of
physician whose training and interests lay more in public health and the British field of "medical policing" than medical jurisprudence. As he noted in his
letter of application for the position of Chief Medical Officer of Health, "be-
sides my usual Medical qualifications I hold the London Degree of Doctor of
Public Health, a degree which entitles me to hold a similar position in any city
in England."[3] Under his tenure, the Ministry of the Capital would adopt a more
interventionist agenda into matters of public well-being. Thus, the brief rise
and fall of forensic medical authority in Siam might be said to have corresponded with the arrival of a new paradigm of state consideration for the
dead.

    In the ensuing years, concerns over obtaining justice for Siamese subjects
in the plural legal arena created by extraterritorial law gave way dramatically

to a new fixation on the threat of contagious disease in an increasingly inter-connected world. Reported outbreaks of bubonic plague in India and in the ports of Hong Kong and Canton in southern China had alarmed Siamese of-ficials and Bangkok residents since at least 1894.[4] The Siamese state instituted quarantine procedures for arriving ships and built a hospital on Ko Phai, an island in the Gulf of Siam, to handle suspected cases of plague on those ves-sels.[5] In May 1898, rumors circulated the city, eventually ending up in the press, that plague had arrived in Bangkok.[6] Plague, however, was not the only po-tential scourge: beriberi (*rok nep cha* or *rok buam*), which at the time was mis-takenly considered a contagious disease, was likewise a focus of public health officials.[7] State officials were equally concerned with outbreaks of contagious disease among livestock too, including rinderpest, foot and mouth, and an-thrax.[8] While the plague case would eventually prove to be a false diagnosis, the fear of an outbreak of contagious disease was very real, and it had pro-found effects on the nature of state medicine in Siam.[9]

From that point forward, experience with contagious disease became one of the primary prerequisites for hiring new medical personnel from abroad. When Highet appointed a new medical officer in 1904, for example, he noted that the appointee, Dr. Modern Carthew, "has seen a great deal of plague in India."[10] Moreover, the new primacy of public health expertise is evidenced by unsolicited applications from physicians seeking an appointment in public health administration. A Dr. Richard Harding Brewridge, for example, touted, "I can therefore claim both by experience and my qualifications to be very fully equipped to carry out all medical examinations both before and after death; also to discover the origin and cause of Epidemic disease."[11] In the end, it was not a concern for (in)justice that would prompt greater state oversight of death in the capital, but concern for the spread of disease.[12]

Within two years, the Siamese state would adopt new procedures for re-cording every death within the capital city along with its cause. The announce-ment in the *Bangkok Times* reads, "We heard that by direction of His Majesty instructions have been given to the police to report to Headquarters all deaths that occur within the districts of the different stations in Bangkok, with the cause of death in each case. This should be the beginning of a proper regis-tration of death."[13] State concern for the dead had shifted from the necrop-olitics of forensic concern in a plural legal arena to the biopolitics of concern for health at the level of population.[14] From that moment on the dead would be counted.

The dead, of course, as we have seen, already *did* count in turn-of-the-century Bangkok. A central argument of this study has been that the peculiar conditions of constrained sovereignty imposed on the Siamese state had the effect of politicizing dead and injured bodies. In her study of another colonial-era port city, Ruth Rogaski developed the idea of the hypercolony as a theoretical model capable of encapsulating "the potential implications that arise when one urban space is divided among multiple imperialisms."[15] Like the Chinese port city of Tianjin, turn-of-the-twentieth-century Bangkok was subject to a plurality of imperialisms. In Siam, however, the dividing lines between these multiple imperial projects were demographic rather than territorial. Unequal trade treaties signed with foreign imperial powers granted extraterritorial legal privileges to foreigners residing in Siam. Their ranks included a growing number of Asians who claimed protected subject status as "protégés" of the foreign powers; they too were exempted from Siamese law and enjoyed the protection of foreign consular officials and legal institutions.

From the perspective of the imperial powers, each of these legal subjects constituted a de facto outpost of imperial jurisdiction, and therefore an extension of its demographic—if not territorial—influence. For the Siamese, they were a testament to the kingdom's constrained sovereignty: each foreign subject was a living, breathing check on the rule of Siamese law and the jurisdiction of the sovereign. In every social and commercial interaction, they troubled and teased at the limits of Siamese jurisdiction. Such privileged legal actors were a common feature of the plural legal arenas that took shape across the colonial world as part of the "culture of legalities" that constituted the colonial order.[16] In life, these resident aliens were subject to different regimes of rights than those of indigenous peoples. It has been little noted, however, that legal status extended beyond life as well. It was precisely this projection of legal difference onto the dead body that demanded the adoption of legal and medicolegal forms of expertise as a means of distinguishing between bodies that inhabited the same urban space but that belonged to very different legal and political worlds.

The real implications of these social, political, and legal arrangements can best be perceived through the accidental juxtapositions of daily urban life. Thus, I have endeavored to create a sense of historicity in my depiction of life—and especially death—in turn-of-the-century Bangkok. This more encompassing historical vision has revealed the Siamese capital to be a city crowded with actors and forms of agency that do not figure in normative accounts of Thai history. In addition to the subaltern dead, the sovereign necropolis was a city full of doctors, lawyers, newspapermen, judges, and jurors, but also limited liability corporations, managers, shareholders, and the forms of technology that foreign capital bestowed on the city's few crowded and pitted streets. Together, through their uneasy and often antagonistic interactions, these figures helped to shape social life in Siam.

The stories of death and dismemberment in these pages attest to the ways in which "scientific and technological developments slice into settled social relationships and compel a redefinition, through law, of established rights and duties."[17] By focusing on the Bangkok Tramway Company as a legal actor, this book has attempted to contribute to ongoing efforts in the history of capitalism to interrogate what Dan Bouk has called "evidence of financial power transmuting into cultural power."[18] Corporate ethnographic interest in Siamese deathways forged an uneasy and unprecedented combination of extrajudicial compensatory action with legal indemnification that served to codify disparities between lives that were legally privileged and lives that were redeemable in the sense of being readily exchanged for compensatory payments.[19]

Of course, it was not just the representatives and institutions of foreign states, experts, and transnational flows of capital, commerce, and expertise that helped give rise to the sovereign necropolis. The new iterations of Siamese legal and political subjectivity that emerged around the turn of the twentieth century were likewise shaped by the indigenous sociocultural world. These factors perhaps included the sovereign's sense of his jurisdiction over the living and the dead—as suggested by King Chulalongkorn's letter to his subordinates discussed in the opening pages of this book. They most certainly included, however, remnants of the hierarchical feudal social order, on the one hand, and everyday forms of logic and practice through which the cosmopolitan populace of Siam made sense of death, on the other.

I have argued in this study that the confluence of these traditional forms of social, cultural, and political life with new legal and medicolegal institutions and forms of concern adopted by the Siamese state had the effect of reinscribing feudal forms of social difference onto the lives of its subjects. The morbid subjects of the sovereign necropolis were lives that were indelibly marked not by *sakdina*, the traditional Thai scale of feudal social ranking, nor by the transcendent sense of value that liberal legal regimes claim to impart to human life.[20] Instead, they were lives whose identity was indexed in crucial ways to one facet of their metaphysical constitution, the *khwan*. They were, in short, lives that *mattered* differently, and their historical constitution is yet another indicator of the ways in which Thai modernity might be regarded as alternative—a challenge to the normative developmental trajectories that have plotted Eurocentric visions of modernity.[21] The prominent place of the dead and injured in the Siamese polity as documented in this study constitutes a seminal feature of this alterity, with direct bearing on the relations between state and subject and the historical transition from royal subject to citizen.

In an early attempt to sketch out this transition, David K. Wyatt pointed to changes in religious culture and education that gave birth to a "new civic sense," which was reinforced through enrollment in new state institutions and contact with government officials.[22] The result, he argued, was a communal awakening to "the idea that all inhabitants of Siam were subjects of a single king, members of a single body politic."[23] Of course, the end result, as Wyatt acknowledged, was not exactly the modern sense of liberal democratic "citizenship," but rather "a compromise or amalgam between the old concept of the 'subject,' stripped of the intermediaries that stood between the king and the peasant, and the modern concept of the 'citizen.'"[24] This amalgam, however, was an uneasy one, and Wyatt recognized that its inherent contradictions would persist and trouble Thai history.

In this book, I have sought to contribute to our understanding of this historical transition from subject to citizen in a way that overcomes the limits of Eurocentric visions of modernizing legal and political change. Attending to the dense archival accretions concerning the dead and injured has paved the way for a radically inductive reenvisioning of the Siamese polity. In the process, this study has revealed a crucial but overlooked facet of Thai modernity at a formative historical moment: namely, the prominent place of the dead. These findings suggest that the presumption of a rights-bearing citizen waiting to emerge from under the weight of a feudal social order and an absolute monarchy is fundamentally misplaced. Eschewing such teleological temptations, I have endeavored to take the Siamese sovereign and his ministers at their word as they began to recognize the dead and injured as their constituents. As the state assented to shifting civil legal practices surrounding death and injury and invested in medicolegal expertise, it helped to create novel forms of legal and political subjectivity. Through such pragmatic actions, the Siamese state both asserted its sovereignty and helped to reconstitute the Thai polity as one peopled by morbid subjects, silent witnesses to elite agendas and interests.

Theoretical studies of law in colonial contexts have tended to privilege positive law as articulated in codes and institutions. The best of these studies, such as Samera Esmeir's *Juridical Humanity*, explore these developments in order to reveal the troubled history of "humanitarian" legal interventions. They provide challenging reappraisals of how the social world is defined in opposition to the natural and the ways in which humanity itself is yoked to legal instruments. *Sovereign Necropolis* provides a similar narrative, one that consciously makes room for a broader vision of social agency while prioritizing the social and cultural implications of practical legal arrangements ahead of positive law. In the course of doing so, it identifies a central paradox in the evolution of liberal legalism in Thailand. On the one hand, law works as a secularizing technology: it eradicates the spirits and transcendent forms of agency that might be said to cause human misfortune in favor of a purified, secular vision of the social world. On the other hand, and in a troubling sleight of hand, some social actors within that newly profane world are identified not by the imminent markings of social identity—nor by the liberal shibboleth of human life above all else—but rather according to a metaphysical principle most closely associated with states of injury and death. Their lives are thus rendered ephemeral and ethereal. Legally—and arguably politically—they are *khwan*: lives that bear silent witness; lives that are eminently redeemable. While the modern state legal system has exorcised any vestiges of the traditional metaphysical notions of personhood in favor of a secular legal subject, the epilogue suggests ways in which these metaphysical remnants continue to haunt the Thai justice system. What was true in the era of tramcars, extraterritoriality, and absolute monarchy is substantially true in the age of Mercedes-Benz, global finance capital, and abrogation of democratic rule.

The very act of recognizing the dead as a political constituency marks a radical departure from and challenge to normative post-Enlightenment accounts of political development, which privilege the rights and obligations imbued in the living as the foundation of democratic politics. This classical conception has been challenged from a number of directions, including archeological analysis highlighting the material foundations of political association, as well as studies that work to "deemphasize questions of elite intellectual culture and formal politics" in order to attend to the illegible, the inarticulate, and the ordinary.[25] The revisionist challenge made in this study is equally in tune with the efforts of postcolonial thinkers to articulate histories that resist and trouble Eurocentric models of historical development and with recent historical and anthropological work in death studies. And while this is hardly an uplifting theory of political life, I nevertheless maintain that the sovereign necropolis constitutes a more accurate starting point for making sense of modern Thai politics. By considering the ways in which subaltern subjects were constituted as lives lived-in-death, mute witnesses to claims made on their behalf, we gain insight into the fundamental historical conditions that allow factions of society to continue to delay, diminish, and depreciate the democratic process.

Epilogue

Spirits in a Material World

> The historical limits of capitalist relations appear in those traumatic events that fall outside the economic realm of commercial exchange and contractual agreement, but whose material impact on human lives, in cases of accidental injury, . . . nevertheless valorizes new debt relations that the modern social order must somehow realize in the form of monetary value.
>
> —William Pietz, "Death of the Deodand: Accursed Objects and the Money Value of Human Life"

> And just as they seem to be occupied with revolution-izing themselves and things, creating something that did not exist before, precisely in such epochs of revolutionary crisis they anxiously conjure up the spirits of the past to their service.
>
> —Karl Marx, "The Eighteenth Brumaire of Louis Bonaparte"

Red and blue lights flash and a spotlight illu-minates the wreckage of a police car at 3:00 a.m. at the side of a Bangkok thoroughfare. A British-Thai B-movie actress named Anna Reese (Anna Hamblaouris) paces the scene in a soiled summer jumper, distraught. She kneels on the passenger seat of the police car, pleading with the corpse of the slain police officer, asking *"tham mai?"* (Why?). Staggering around the car, she mumbles *"pen pai mai dai"* (It can't be). Her relatives, among the first to arrive at the scene, divert her as police try to question her. Standing in front of the body, her hand holding the open car door, Reese refuses to give her account to the police, telling them that her own family will not understand what has happened, that they will jump to the wrong conclusions. A soft-spoken police officer, notebook in hand to record her statement, can be heard consoling the actress: *"ubatihet mi koet khuen samoe"* (Accidents happen. [They] happen all the time).[1]

Reese did not go the police station that night. Citing the emotional trauma of the accident—she suffered only minor physical injuries—she refused to co-operate and left the scene in the company of relatives. She surrendered to police some twelve hours later and submitted to blood tests for drugs and alcohol—both of which would have been of dubious value after so much time had elapsed.[2] Even without a positive test for intoxicants, Reese faced potential charges including reckless driving causing death and escaping arrest. She was released by police on her own recognizance, however, after assuring them that she was prepared to make restitution to the family of the deceased officer. In the Thai justice system, where allegations of wrongful death have to be filed by the injured party rather than state prosecutors, it is common practice for the two parties to reach a settlement that precludes further legal action. The Thai justice system encourages parties to enter mediation in order to agree on such settlements, especially in cases where the accused possesses substantial means.[3]

Days later, Reese attended the officer's funeral service. During the ceremony, a woman in the audience signaled that she was being possessed by the spirit of the deceased officer, and she called out for Reese. By the time Reese reached her side, however, the spirit had already departed and Reese had to learn of the spirit's wishes through those seated in the vicinity of the woman. When pressed by reporters after the encounter, Reese disclosed that the spirit of the slain officer asked his family to forgive her. She offered a paraphrase of what she understood to be the spirit's message: "'Don't hold her [Anna] guilty, she is already very sad for what happened, forgive her'—something like that."[4] Soon after the ceremony, Reese invited the press to observe her temporary ordination as a Buddhist nun so that she could accrue merit for the spirit of the deceased officer.

It would be months still, however, before the two parties would agree on a compensatory arrangement amid sometimes heated negotiations. The Thai police oversaw the proceedings, which took place at the Prawet district police station near where the accident occurred. After some initial deliberation, the officer's widow requested compensation totaling 6.2 million baht (approximately $180,000) based on a calculation of her husband's projected future earnings and the fact that he left behind two young daughters. Although her insurance company had already agreed to pay 1.2 million baht of the settlement, Reese objected and walked out. She reiterated her stance that she would pay no more than 2 million baht ($58,000)—a number that was very likely less than the value of the car she was driving.[5] They would later settle on an undisclosed sum, after which Reese reported that she once again intended to ordain temporarily as a Buddhist nun in order to make merit for the officer.[6]

Reese effectively received two forms of acquittal for her role in the death: the absolution of an apparition on the one hand, and the amnesty of the accident on the other. Forensic anthropologists and pathologists alike attest to the fact that the dead can speak and that "they always speak truthfully, challenging lies and misinformation about their lives and deaths."[7] Zoë Crossland has identified this belief as part of a widely held "folk theory of agency at the heart of the assertively scientific fields of forensics."[8] But while the dead speak volumes about past traumas, and they do so without fault, there are limitations: "theirs is a constrained and descriptive field of speech that does not deal with feelings, wishes, or desires."[9] For that, we must look to other channels through which the dead might communicate. In contemporary Thailand, however—where the dead are commonly thought to voice their wishes through mediums—their speech can sometimes seem to stretch the limits of credulity. The dead, it seems, are eager to forgive and anxious to quell the grudges of the living.

The second form of acquittal came from the police officer at the scene, who helped to mitigate Reese's culpability in the death through an appeal to "accidental reasoning." While we might concede that accidents do indeed happen all the time *today*, this study has suggested that this was not always the case. To accept the accident as a natural fact is to participate in a particular vision of the world, one with a distinct historical provenance that is not without moral implications.

In many ways, the two acquittals are utterly at odds with each other. Accidental reasoning implies a secular vision of the natural world, as well as a historically and culturally specific mode of defining the limitations of human agency and responsibility. It is a world where social conflicts are handled through the rule of law, rather than through interpersonal and communal modes of expiation. The absolution of the apparition, in contrast, implies a social world that is rife with spiritual presence and transcendent forms of agency—where supernatural beings help to dictate the actions and fates of the living.[10] It is only in the latter world that it makes sense for Reese—or other parties—to undertake *kan-tham khwan*, the action of making amends for a lost life through a compensatory payment made to the spirit of the deceased.

But, as has been shown in this study, *kan-tham khwan* might be seen as a gesture capable of bridging these two seemingly irreconcilable worlds. Insofar as it masquerades as a payment made to placate the spirit of the deceased, *kan-tham khwan* conforms to the logic and spirit of traditional forms of reme-diation for lost life. It is a testament to the survival of customary modes of action in an age of ostensibly normalized and homogeneous forms of law and order. At the same time, however, it is a form of action that imparts indemni-fication or legal protection for the injurer or culpable party. In this respect, *kan-tham khwan* participates in the long-standing logic of noblesse oblige, whereby social superiors are entitled to make amends for potentially wrong-ful actions that cost the lives of their subordinates.

In the context of the Thai justice system, the Reese affair is not especially remarkable. One could easily cite other examples of wealthy individuals com-mitting vehicular homicide and walking away physically uninjured and le-gally unscathed, their only penalty being an ex gratia payment—a death benefit that in many cases amounted to far less than the value of the imported car they were driving. In recent years alone, one might cite the cases of Kanpithak "Moo Ham" Patchimsawat, who drove his Mercedes into a bus queue, killing one and gravely injuring several others in 2007; Orachorn "Praewa" The-phasadin Na Ayudhya, who was driving underage and without a license when she killed nine in an expressway accident in 2010; Peerapol Thaksinthaweesap, the son of a prominent Bangkok businessman, who dismembered a seventeen-year-old Lao girl named Kambai Inthilat in 2011 while driving his father's Porsche Cayman; Vorayuth "Boss" Yoovidya, grandson of the founder of the Red Bull energy drink empire, whose Ferrari struck and killed a police officer in 2012; Patchuda Jayruan, a university student who killed three cyclists while driving drunk in Chiang Mai in 2015; and Janepob Verraporn, who walked away unharmed when his speeding Mercedes crashed into a Ford Fiesta, leav-ing two graduate students dead in 2016.[11] Indeed, Reese herself recently re-prised her role as "speeding lady"—though fortunately with less tragic consequences.[12]

In addition to compensatory payments, such cases often produce public displays of remorse and mercy. Picture Peerapol Thaksinthaweesap, the humbled scion, lowering his head in deep prostration before the mother of Kambai Inthilat, for example; or Anna Reese, wearing the white garments of a lay renunciant, taking to her knees in order to offer a respectful *wai* (a ges-ture of respect involving a slight bow with hands pressed together as in prayer) before the widow of the deceased officer. Such images depict the lev-eling of social privilege in the face of human tragedy. They are a testament to the idea that no matter one's social status, the supreme dignity of human life is unassailable. (Contrition, however, is not the only possibility; other cases have produced very different images. Social media images documenting the international travels of Vorayuth Yoovidya—seen snowboarding in Japan or trackside at Formula One racing events while evading arrest warrants at home—made the rounds on message boards and stoked local anger over the apparent impunity of the rich.)[13]

And yet, these scenes of remorse and reconciliation are troubled by the reality of the legal machinations that accompany them. Absent in many cases are criminal charges, legal proceedings, or correctional outcomes—at least not to the degree that average Thais insist would befit such serious offenses. Though the injurers often remain subject to lesser charges of reckless driving and leaving the scene of an accident, these settlements spare the wealthy offenders from having to serve time in jail for the more serious offense of vehicular homicide. Instead, the scenes are figuratively captioned by announcements of compensatory agreements with the injured parties or relatives of the deceased, often with the express support of the police and representatives of state legal institutions.[14]

Such cases provide an obvious window onto issues of social and economic inequality in contemporary Thailand. Stories of imported luxury automobiles and wealthy untouchables speak to gross disparities in income and wealth distribution that have had profound implications for political life in the new millennium.[15] Unconnected, they are too easily dismissed as "senseless tragedies," "accidents," or—more fittingly though still insufficiently—evidence of the carelessness and callousness of "rich kids." Collectively, however, these events are more than just fodder for tabloids and gossip mills. More troublingly and more fundamentally, they suggest real discrepancies within the justice system as well as discernible differences in the valuation of human lives. A closer reading, one aimed at an inductive understanding of these disparate "deaths by various causes" (*tai duai het tang tang*), reveals important analogues with historical developments in turn-of-the-twentieth-century Siam.

The case of Anna Reese, and others like it, is suggestive of the ways in which the historical configurations that took shape during the era of the sovereign necropolis endure. While the *khwan* often goes unmentioned—at least in the public discourse about such compensatory practices—the victims nevertheless bear a strong resemblance to the morbid subjects of the sovereign necropolis: they are lives that seem in some ways eminently redeemable in exchange for compensatory payments and actions. The spirits of the deceased are treated as silent witnesses to the injustices surrounding their death—or worse, they are invoked in order to authorize death payments and acquit the culpable parties.

Sociolegal research in contemporary northern Thailand suggests that the *khwan* remains essential to the ways in which Thai legal subjects make sense of both personal misfortune and processes of remediation. As one of several causal registers for making sense of personal loss, the *khwan* continues to be invoked alongside other traditional cosmological principles when Thais meet with misfortune.[16] This is true even as the broader social and cultural fabric that helped to reinforce the associated extrajudicial modes of remediation has begun to disintegrate under the impacts of urbanization and secularization.[17] David and Jaruwan Engel have argued that this insistence on the assertion of such metaphysical principles as integral parts of the injured party's identity has helped produce a distinctive sense of legal subjectivity in contemporary northern Thailand, one that eschews legal entanglements and tends to view injury as the responsibility of the injured person.[18] This study has uncovered the colonial-era genealogy for such troubling forms of legal subjectivity in the morbid subjects of the sovereign necropolis. And each day brings new tragedies—demonstrations of socioeconomic inequality and the persistent rendering of the lives of the many as lives "lived in death." Thus, it can be said that although the *khwan* did not find its way into modern Thai legal codes, these particular ghosts continue to haunt the Thai justice system and the subaltern legal subject alike.

ACKNOWLEDGMENTS

I received financial support from several sources for the research, writing, and publication of this book. These include the Andrew W. Mellon Foundation and the Institute for International Education; at Cornell University, the Southeast Asia Program, Department of History, and the Graduate School; the Thai Studies Institute of Chulalongkorn University; and the Office of the Provost and Dean of Faculties, Boston College. Foreign Language and Area Studies (FLAS) funding from the U.S. Department of Education supported Thai-language study at the Southeast Asian Summer Studies Institute (SEASSI) at the University of Wisconsin-Madison, at the Advanced Study of Thai (AST) Program in Chiang Mai, Thailand, and at Cornell University. Along the way, I had the good fortune to work with creative and passionate Thai-language instructors, including Sidhorn Sangdhanoo (SEASSI), members of the Faculty of Humanities at Chiang Mai University (AST), and especially Ngampit Jagacinski (Cornell).

The research for this book would not have been possible without the permission of the National Research Council of Thailand and the support of the History Department at Chulalongkorn University. Special thanks to Chalong Soontravanich, Suwimon Roongcharoen, and Thanaphol Limapichart, who provided logistical and moral support, plus good humor when it was most needed. Research seminars at Walailak and Chulalongkorn Universities in February 2012 provided the first occasions to present my research findings. I am grateful to the generous audiences at both venues—especially Davisakd Puaksom, who endured both presentations and later read the completed manuscript. During the course of my research and writing, I benefited from the hard work and professionalism of the staff at several libraries and research institutes, including the Prince Damrong Rajanuphap Library, the Archives of Siriraj Hospital, and the National Health Archive and Museum at the Ministry of Public Health (thanks to Nopphanat Anuphongphat), but the staff of the National Archives of Thailand deserve special recognition (especially Khun Tai). Finally, thanks to Arwut (Meng) Teeraeak, who helped me begin to reframe this project over an impromptu lunch across the street from the National Archives in June 2015, and then pointed me toward the perfect source to help me do so.

At Cornell, I was fortunate to find two homes: McGraw Hall, home of the History Department, and the Kahin Center, home of the Southeast Asia Program (SEAP). Friends and colleagues in both places helped to shape my thinking through reading groups, writing groups, colloquia, brown bag lunches, and hallway banter. Many have continued to do so long after I left Ithaca. While those debts are too many to name, special thanks go to Daniel Ahlquist, Andrew Amstutz, Claudine Ang, Ernesto Bassi, Dave Blome, Bernardo Brown, Becky Butler, Jack Chia, Vivian Choi, Rishad Choudhury, Lawrence Chua, Pamela Corey, Mari Crabtree, Ray Craib, Brian Cuddy, Abi Fisher, Amanda Flaim, Sinja Graf, Greg Green, Carter Higgins, Kate Horning, Itsie Hull, Hayden Kantor, Amy Kohout, Samson Lim, Michael Lynch, Kaya McGowan, Rose Metro, Daegan Miller, Matt Minarchek, Anto Mohsin, Lorraine Paterson, Tom Patton, John Phan, Josh Savala, Suman Seth, Ivan Small, Popy Suthiwan, Eileen Vo, Alexis Walker, Yuanchong Wang, Chika Watanabe, Rachel Weil, and Jon Young. Special thanks also to Daena Funahashi and Andrew Johnson for a timely conversation about bad death over good Isan food in Bangkok in 2011 and to Matthew Reeder for insightful comments during a meeting in Bangkok in June 2015.

During the course of research, writing, and revision, this work benefited from critical discussion in a number of venues. I thank the attendees and especially the organizers and respondents at the following meetings: the 2013 and 2018 meetings of the Association for Asian Studies (Tamara Loos and Tyrell Haberkorn, respectively); the 2013 New York and 2018 New England Regional meetings of the Association for Asian Studies (Mitch Aso and Karen Teoh); the Means of Transport workshop at the Joint Center for History and Economics, Harvard University (Victor Seow and Clapperton Mavhunga); the Law & Society Association's Early Career Workshop 2015 (where I was fortunate to find Nate Holdren among my cohort); the 2016 Annual Asian Studies Summer Institute on the theme of "Decolonizing Science in Asia" at Penn State University (organizers: Prakash Kumar, Projit Mukharji, and Amit Prasad; participants: Dwai Banerjee, Nicole Barnes, Burton Cleetus, Lijing Jiang, Gabriela Soto Laveaga, Lan Li, Juno Parreñas, Charu Singh, and Bharat Venkat); the Mellon Seminar Conference on Violence / Non-Violence at the Mahindra Humanities Center (Jacqueline Bhabha); and the 2018 meeting of the History of Science Society (Anthony Medrano and Warwick Anderson). Christopher Hamlin provided helpful feedback on my presentation at the 2015 annual meeting of the American Association for the History of Medicine and then invited me to attend the workshop "Locating Forensic Science and Medicine" in London later that summer. My thanks to Chris and the attendees of that conference for advice and encouragement since, especially Daniel Asen, Binyamin Blum, Ian Burney, Projit Mukharji, and Mitra Sharafi. Portions of chapter 5 first appeared in print as "Morbid Subjects: Forensic Medicine and Sovereignty in Siam," *Modern Asian Studies* 52, no. 2 (March 2018): 394–420 and are reprinted herein with the permission of Cambridge University Press.

A research fellowship at the Mahindra Humanities Center, Harvard University in 2015–16 allowed me to make significant progress on revisions to the manuscript. I am grateful to Homi Bhabha and Steven Biel for the opportunity to join in the center's Andrew W. Mellon Foundation Seminar on Violence and Non-Violence, and to the fantastic staff (Neal Akatsuka, Mary Halpenny-Killip, Sarah Razor, and Andrea Volpe) for making it feel like home. My Mahindra compatriots, Konstanze Baron, Matthew Baxter, Nils Bock, Zain Lakhani, Mira Rai Waits, and Mónica Salas-Landa were a constant source of advice, encouragement, and collegiality. I would also like to thank the organizers and participants of the Thai Studies Seminar at Harvard, including Michael Herzfeld, Jay Rosengard, Joe Harris, Scott Stonington, Sittithep Eaksittipong, and Jutathorn Pravattiyagul.

At Boston College, I have found a temporary home in a vibrant department surrounded by an exciting cohort of VAPs, including Ramaesh Bhagirat, Matthew Delvaux, Craig Gallagher, Evan Hepler-Smith, Ingu Hwang, Felix Jiménez, Steve Pieragastini, Jenna Tonn, Carolyn Twomey, Catherine Warner, and Andrea Wenz. Our intrepid leader, Sarah Ross, helped keep me on task during the revision process with her warm (and persistent!) invitations to "QFAW!" (Quit 'Fooling' Around and Write!).

At Cornell University Press, Emily Andrew graciously welcomed even my strangest queries with good humor. Thanks as well to Bethany Wasik, and to Robert Griffin and Kate Gibson of Westchester Publishing Services for their expert assistance with copyediting. I am indebted to the two anonymous reviewers who provided detailed reports that allowed me to correct a few glaring issues and hopefully make the book more accessible. Any remaining flaws, of course, are my own.

A few colleagues warrant special thanks for the time and energy they expended helping me to wrangle this project into shape. First among them are the members of my dissertation committee at Cornell. Tamara Loos, Durba Ghosh, and Anne Blackburn were expecting a very different project when I left for the archives, yet the training they provided prepared me to be attentive to the stories of death and dismemberment that I encountered there. They each offered seminal insights to help me make better sense of them after I returned. At every stage in my graduate training, research, and writing, Samson

Lim has gone above and beyond to offer advice and encouragement; he also generously read and commented on several chapter drafts. Mónica Salas-Landa had no idea what she was getting herself into when I proposed a "book boot camp" in summer 2016, but she tirelessly read (and often reread) every chapter and helped me make peace with my own vision for the project. Daniel Asen, Michael Herzfeld, James McHugh, and Thongchai Winichakul also read and commented on portions of the manuscript at various stages.

My very first and most enduring debts are to my parents and siblings. My most profound are to Su-Ping. Though she may very well never make it through the book, Su-Ping is happier than anyone to see me send off this manuscript. And it is her patience, love, and labor, more than anyone else, that have made it possible for me to finish it. Finally, my heartfelt thanks to Quinn (aka Tong Tong, aka the Puzzle Master) and Josephine (Jojo) for their blissful disinterest.

T. P.
Jamaica Plain, MA

Bad Death: Metaphysics and Making Amends

The Siamese concept of *tai hong* ("inauspicious" or bad death) constitutes a wide-ranging system of beliefs and practices for dealing with the aftermath of sudden or unforeseen losses of human life. For an introduction to these ideas and practices in particular regional contexts, see Stanley J. Tambiah, *Buddhism and the Spirit Cults in North-East Thailand*, 189–94, and 312–26; and Phra Khru Anusaranasasanakiarti and Charles F. Keyes, "Funerary Rites and the Buddhist Meaning of Death: An Interpretive Text from Northern Thailand," *Journal of the Siam Society* 68, no. 1 (1980).

The beliefs and practices surrounding inauspicious death in late nineteenth-century Siam do not correspond to any single religious tradition or canon and must therefore be reconstructed based on contemporary survivals and ethnographic evidence that is highly politicized. With respect to the latter, there are two genres of early literature on spirits left behind by the departed. The first are rationalist accounts penned by members of the sociocultural elite intent on debunking the widespread beliefs in such spirits. Important examples of the rationalist literature include Chao Phraya Thiphakorawong's *Nangsue sadaeng kittchanukit* [A book explaining various things] (Bangkok: Khuru Sapha, 1971 [1867]) and Prince Si Saowaphang's *Wa duai amnat phi lae phi lok* [On the power of spirits] (Krungthep: Rong phim luang nai phra borom maha ratchawang, 2464 [1921]). The second genre is made up of ethnographic and auto-ethnographic accounts dating to the early twentieth century. In this vein, the early topology of malevolent spirits offered in A. J. Irwin, "Some Siamese Ghost-Lore and Demonology," *Journal of the Siam Society* 4, no. 2 (1907) has held up remarkably well. The auto-ethnographic work of Phraya Anuman Rajathon offers a more empirical account of Siamese cultural practices and beliefs. Another useful source is Robert B. Textor, *Roster of the Gods: An Ethnography of the Supernatural in a Thai Village*. Finally, recent ethnographic scholarship has tried to come to terms with a revival in aspects of the culture of unnatural death, specifically the idea that the conditions of (post-)modernity have produced a proliferation of the spirits of bad deaths (*phi tai hong*); see, for example, Andrew Alan Johnson, *Ghosts of the New City*, and Rosalind Morris, *In the Place of Origins*.

Perhaps the most important characteristic of the culture of inauspicious death is its heterogeneity and cosmopolitan nature. It was sufficiently indeterminate as to capture and combine elements of different religious traditions, including animism and Buddhism, with different practices from distinct ethnic groups. This flexibility, which has been referred to as "syncretism," has long been among the defining characteristics of Thai religious life. See, for example, Donald Swearer's classic *Buddhist World of Southeast Asia*. For a recent challenge to the "syncretic" paradigm in the study of Thai religious culture, particularly with respect to recent developments, see Pattana Kitiarsa, "Beyond Syncretism: Hybridization of Popular Religion in Contemporary Thailand," *Journal of Southeast Asian Studies* 36, no. 3 (2005).

To this day, trees remain a fixture of local spiritual beliefs, with ordinations held for auspicious trees and offerings made to threatening ones. Contemporary ethnographic accounts of beliefs about tree-inhabiting spirits in Thailand include "Supernatural Objects That Dwell in Trees" in Textor, *Roster of the Gods*, 552–64; and Andrew Alan Johnson, "Naming Chaos: Accident, Precariousness, and the Spirits of Wildness in Urban Thai Spirit Cults," *American Ethnologist* 39, no. 4 (2012). Ethnographic evidence from contemporary northern Thailand reveals that trees—and the spirits believed to inhabit them— still play a role in discourses about causality for misfortune; see Engel, "Globalization and the Decline," 481; Engel, "Discourses of Causation," 259; and Engel & Engel, *Tort, Custom, and Karma*, 21–32. Finally, trees are also at the center of Buddhist-informed conservation efforts; see Susan M. Darlington, "The Ordination of a Tree: The Buddhist Ecology Movement in Thailand," *Ethnology* 37, no. 1 (1998).

"Funerary payments" (*ngoen tham khwan*) and other terms used to describe the kinds of culturally expected social action taken in the aftermath of sudden and unexpected losses of human life help to contextualize how people made sense of loss in late nineteenth-century Siam. The vocabulary of loss and remediation hints at the broader habits of mind that reveal the nature of personal loss as a spiritual problem rooted in a metaphysical belief system with broad ramifications for both this-worldly social life and transcendent soteriological concerns. Government documents dealing with the subject of unnatural or inauspicious death from the late nineteenth century, including those in the "Death by various causes" files compiled by the Ministry of the Capital, suggest that many of the terms were used in an essentially interchangeable manner. Despite the close semantic connections between the ideas, the most common terms can be grouped into broad categories based on their reference to the spiritual and bodily elements of the victim of sudden or unnatural death.

It is appropriate to begin with a term for compensatory action that contains within itself an explicit reference to the spiritual component of the human being, namely, *kan-tham khwan*. This term, a nominalized form of the verb (*tham khwan*), refers to a broad range of ritual and compensatory actions aimed at restoring the spirit of an injured party that had become disembodied through the trauma of injury or sudden death. *Kan-tham khwan* signifies efforts to make the victim of unexpected trauma or loss whole again; it is best understood as a restorative action aimed at returning the victim to his or her rightful situation.[1] In the late nineteenth century, the term *tham khwan* was often appended to the word for money, *ngoen*, making a compound that signified a compensatory payment for an injury or death (*ngoen tham khwan*).

Another subset of terms associated with compensation for the accidental or unnatural loss of life includes a range of words signifying fees (*bia* or *kha*) paid to cover the cost of funerary expenses. The associated ritual expenses include the cost of cremation rites, which are referred to as the *bia* or *kha phao tua* (the fee or cost of cremating the body), and the cost of the wake or vigil for the deceased known as the *bia* or *kha pluk tua*.[2] Documents from this period suggest that the Thai term *phi*, which is today commonly rendered as "ghost," was also frequently used with both of these expressions, that is, *phao phi* and *pluk phi*. Although the literal translation would suggest (the cost of) cremating or waking the ghost, in actuality the terms signify something closer to the idea of feting the spirit of the deceased, and especially of performing religious rites to secure merit for the deceased in the interests of helping him or her acquire a more auspicious rebirth. The Thai terms *kan-thot thaen* and (*kha*) *chot choie*, meaning to compensate and compensation, respectively, constitute another group of terms used to describe appropriate actions in the aftermath of an accidental injury or death.

Historicizing the Khwan

The notion of bad or inauspicious death in late nineteenth century Siam implied a complex metaphysical system for explaining the causes and implications of such tragedies, which was predicated on the fate of the spiritual
component of the person, the *khwan*. The *khwan* has been subject to extensive anthropological and philosophical analysis by scholars of Thai religion and
culture. See, for example, Grant A. Olson, "Filling the Void: Thai Khwan and
Burmese Leip-pya, the Stuff of Which Souls Are Made," in *Socially Engaged
Spirituality: Essays in Honor of Sulak Sivaraksa on his 70th Birthday*, ed. David W.
Chappell (Bangkok: Sathirakoses-Nagapradipa Foundation, 2003); Ruth-Inge
Heinze, *Tham Khwan: How to Contain the Essence of Life: A Socio-Psychological
Comparison of a Thai Custom* (Singapore: Singapore University Press, [1982]);
Shigeharu Tanabe, "The Person in Transformation: Body, Mind, and Cultural
Appropriation," in *Cultural Crisis and Social Memory: Modernity and Identity in
Thailand and Laos*, ed. Shigeharu Tanabe and Charles F. Keyes (Honolulu: Uni-
versity of Hawai'i Press, 2002), 44–49; and Phraya Anuman Rajathon, "The
Khwan and Its Ceremonies," *Journal of the Siam Society* 50 (1962). In general,
these studies have tended to regard the *khwan* synchronically as part of an eth-
nographic present, or ahistorically as a constituent of a timeless and enduring
Thai Buddhist worldview.

One of the central aims of this study has been an effort to historicize the
khwan: that is, to step back from the level of ahistorical generalization and examine the invocation of the *khwan* at a particular historical moment. Among
the crucial findings of my research is that the use of the *khwan* in turn-of-the-
twentieth-century Siam does not conform to contemporary and general accounts of its meaning and usage in Thai culture. Studies including Engel and
Engel's *Tort, Custom, and Karma*, and Grant Olson's "Filling the Void" outline
a stark distinction between the *khwan* and the *winyan*, which they see as at-
tributes of human identity that are associated with states of (nonfatal) injury
and death, respectively. This distinction is not evidenced in the archival documents that I worked with. In matters relating to compensatory payments for
accidental or wrongful death, the *khwan* was often invoked to name the spirit
of the deceased as the party to whom compensatory payments were offered.
Even the limited scholarship that has attempted to consider the *khwan* dia-
chronically has overlooked its usage as part of the sociolegal actions surrounding the aftermath of unnatural death; see Wilaiwan Kanittanan and
James Placzek, "Historical and Contemporary Meanings of Thai *Khwan*: The
Use of Lexical Meaning as an Indicator of Cultural Change," in *Religion, Val-*

ues, and Development in Southeast Asia, ed. Bruce Matthews and Judith Nagata (Singapore: Institute of Southeast Asian Studies, 1986).

There are several possible explanations for this discrepancy between the specific historical invocations of the *khwan* in turn-of-the century Bangkok and the widespread conventions surrounding its use in traditional philosophical and contemporary legal discourse. It is quite possible, for example, that bureaucratic and legalistic discourses and forms of action were inattentive to the particularities of religiocultural beliefs and instead viewed metaphysical principles like the *khwan* as mere vehicles for pragmatic sociolegal forms of interaction and exchange. As was argued in chapter 3, the concerned parties—especially when they were cultural outsiders like the foreign managers of the Bangkok Tramway Company—engaged with these traditional notions of injury, death, and compensation in order to bring about efficient and expeditious outcomes for the injurer and were not especially concerned with or committed to the underlying social and cultural logic of the practices and associated discourses. The same might equally be said of Siamese social elites, who seemed to participate in these transactions in a more or less unilateral way. Other potential explanations include the sheer cosmopolitan nature of the Siamese capital city, where Siamese metaphysical ideas would have existed in more or less constant conversation and competition with other cultural worlds. It was in all likelihood a combination of these factors that helped to constitute the *khwan* as a viable facet of the legal identity of the subaltern subject, as life (and death) was transformed under conditions of constrained sovereignty in the transimperial environment of a colonial port city.

Of Tramways and Transitions

The Bangkok Tramway Company was founded in 1887, when the government of the kingdom of Siam granted a concession to build a tramway system to two foreign entrepreneurs who were longtime residents of the city ("Tramway Concession, Bangkok, 5th May 1887"; NA Microfilm R5 N/128). To date, the (admittedly limited) historiography of the Bangkok Tramway Company and urban transportation in Siam/Thailand has tended to focus either on matters of infrastructure and operations or the experience of elite travelers. On the former, see Ichiro Kakizaki, *Trams, Buses, and Rails: The History of Urban Transport in Bangkok*, 19–50. On the latter, see Chali Iamkrasin, *Mueang thai samai kon* [Thailand in the past], 107–12, which offers an account of King Chulalongkorn's inaugural journey on the electric tramway in 1893. In a

welcome departure, Lawrence Chua, "The City and the City: Race, Nationalism, and Architecture in Early Twentieth-Century Bangkok," *Journal of Urban
History* 40, no. 5 (2014) attends to the intersections of race and space in Bangkok through an examination of tramway lines operated by the Siam Electricity Company.

The accidents, injuries, dismemberment, and death that are foregrounded
in this book have not, to my knowledge, previously been discussed in historical scholarship or popular history. Given this oversight, it is not surprising that
scholars have similarly failed to register the efforts of the tramway company,
its managers, and investors to deal with the repercussions of these tragedies
in the plural legal arena of turn-of-the-century Bangkok. Beyond the legal
machinations, much remains to be said about the tramways from the perspective of social history, the history of technology, and mobility studies. The
technological history, for example, might focus on actions taken by the managers of the tramway company to prevent such accidents by introducing innovations such as cowcatchers, handbrakes, and later a "self-acting wicket"
designed to prevent pedestrians from traversing portions of the city's bridges
designated for use by the tramway cars. Details of these and other developments can be found in my dissertation, *Bodies Politic: Civil Law and Forensic Medicine in Colonial-Era Bangkok* (PhD diss., Cornell University, 2014).

Yet we should not be content with narrating the actions of foreign entrepreneurs and engineers; there is more work to be done on the question of how
subaltern Siamese perceived and experienced the arrival of new forms of mobility. In correspondence related to the death of Jin Kim Hok, for example, the
electric tramway cars are consistently referred to as "steam-powered trains"
(*ai rot fai fa*), which suggests something of the chasm between the agents of
the company and the residents of the capital city who lived among the trains
(NA R5 N 23/23). By the time of Jin Kim Hok's death in May 1895, the tramway cars were in fact powered by overhead electrical lines (see figure 3); before that, they were drawn by horses. The cars had never been powered by
steam engines.

Archival research also reveals efforts by Bangkok residents to sabotage the
tramcars, perhaps in an effort to reclaim the public thoroughfares or to reas-
sert manual and vernacular modes of mobility. From the outset of tramway
service, young men emboldened by the cover of night would lodge rocks into
the metal tracks in hopes of derailing an approaching tramcar (NA R5 N 21/4;
BT 20 June 1894). As the Bangkok Tramway Company transitioned to electric
power, would-be saboteurs turned their attention to the overhead lines that
powered the tramcars. The press tended to dismiss these acts of apparent sabotage, which often resulted in fatal electrocution, as misguided curiosity for

the wonders of electrical power. In February 1893, the *Bangkok Times* reported the electrocution of a man who tried to conduct his own unauthorized experiments in electricity and conduction outside of the Bangkok Tramway Company's newly built electrical plant (*BT* 25 February 1893). Rickshaw and hackney drivers would seem to have had the clearest motive for sabotaging the tramway, but newspaper reports never suggest this explanation, preferring to count the disaffected as luddites and idiots. Such matters of perception and conception, as well as acts of outright resistance, beg further exploration.

A final note on the subject of tramways and transitions pertains to the relations between technological and legal change. As discussed in chapters 2 through 4, passenger rail travel was associated with important developments in law and society in metropolitan legal jurisdictions in the middle to late nineteenth century. These developments have long attracted the attention of scholars of legal history. Interested readers will be rewarded by consulting such works as Morton J. Horwitz, *The Transformation of American Law: 1870–1960: The Crisis of Legal Orthodoxy*; Randolph Bergstrom, *Courting Danger: Injury and Law in New York City, 1870–1910*; William G. Thomas, *Lawyering for the Railroad: Business, Law, and Power in the New South*; Lawrence M. Friedman, "Civil Wrongs: Personal Injury Law in the Late Nineteenth Century," *American Bar Foundation Research Journal* 12, no. 2/3 (1987): 351–78; Friedman, *A History of American Law*; Joyce Sterling and Nancy Reichman, "The Cultural Agenda of Tort Litigation: Constructing Responsibility in the Rocky Mountain Frontier," in *Fault Lines: Tort Law as Cultural Practice*, ed. David M. Engel and Michael McCann (Stanford, CA: Stanford University Press, 2009); and Barbara Young Welke, *Recasting American Liberty: Gender, Race, Law, and the Railroad Revolution*.

It is my sincere hope that this book might prompt further comparative analysis of these developments in metropolitan versus (semi-)colonial jurisdictions. For the purposes of this study, however, my intention has been to render the Siamese narrative as an autonomous process of historical change—albeit one that is informed by imperial and transimperial dynamics—and not as merely a local iteration of metropolitan historical precedents. My focus has therefore been on the local, peculiar, and pragmatic history, rather than the universal and modular. The latter history remains to be written.

Notes

Introduction

1. *"Tae boranakan nai nai ma manut tai pai duai het dai het nueng sueng mi chai tai doi prokati chen kap thuk fa pha tai nai phloeng tok nam tai thuk ying sad fan thaeng mai wa phra in phra phrom arai pen phu tham hai tai tha nai krung pen nathi khong krasuang mueang ja tong nam khwam khuen krap bang khom thun phra karuna doi than thi"* (NA R5 S.Th. 99/17). I am immensely grateful to Arwut (Meng) Teeraeak for this reference.

2. A. B. Griswold and Prasert na Nagara, "The Inscription of King Rama Gam Hen [Ramkhamhaeng] of Sukhodaya (1292 AD): Epigraphic and Historical Studies 9," *Journal of the Siam Society* 59, no. 2 (1971): 205, 208. The authenticity of the monument has long been debated; see James F. Chamberlain, ed., *The Ramkhamhaeng Controversy: Collected Papers* (Bangkok: Siam Society, 1991).

3. The population figure of half a million at 1900 relies on Larry Sternstein's revision of the 1909 census in his "Bangkok at the Turn of the Century: Mongkut and Chulalongkorn Entertain the West," *Journal of the Siam Society* 54, no. 1 (1966): 70. For a detailed analysis of the wildly disparate available data, see Porphant Ouyyanont, "Bangkok's Population & The Ministry of the Capital in Early 20th Century Thai History," *Southeast Asian Studies* 35, no. 2 (1997): 240–43.

4. Anya Bernstein, *Religious Bodies Politic: Rituals of Sovereignty in Buryat Buddhism* (Chicago: University of Chicago Press, 2013); Zoë Crossland, *Ancestral Encounters in Highland Madagascar: Material Signs and Traces of the Dead* (Cambridge: Cambridge University Press, 2014); Heonik Kwon, *Ghosts of War in Vietnam* (Cambridge: Cambridge University Press, 2008); Jean Langford, *Consoling Ghosts: Stories of Medicine and Mourning from Southeast Asians in Exile* (Minneapolis: University of Minnesota Press, 2013); Katherine Verdery, *The Political Lives of Dead Bodies: Reburial and Postsocialist Change* (New York: Columbia University Press, 1999).

5. Michael Herzfeld, *Siege of the Spirits: Community and Polity in Bangkok* (Chicago: University of Chicago Press, 2016); Andrew Alan Johnson, *Ghosts of the New City: Spirits, Urbanity, and the Ruins of Progress in Chiang Mai* (Honolulu: University of Hawai'i Press, 2014); Andrew Alan Johnson, "Naming Chaos: Accident, Precariousness, and the Spirits of Wildness in Urban Thai Spirit Cults," *American Ethnologist* 39, no. 4 (2012); Alan Klima, *The Funeral Casino: Meditation, Massacre, and Exchange with the Dead in Thailand* (Princeton, NJ: Princeton University Press, 2002); Rosalind C. Morris, *In the Place of Origins: Modernity and Its Mediums in Northern Thailand* (Durham, NC: Duke University Press, 2010); Rosalind Morris, "Giving Up Ghosts: Notes on Trauma and the Possibility of the Political from Southeast Asia," *Positions* 16, no. 1 (2008); and Rosalind C. Morris, "Surviving Pleasure at the Periphery: Chiang Mai and

the Photographies of Political Trauma in Thailand, 1976–1992," *Public Culture* 10, no. 2 (1998). Justin McDaniel highlights the prominence of the dead in liturgical and ritual practice as well in *The Lovelorn Ghost and the Magical Monk: Practicing Buddhism in Modern Thailand* (New York: Columbia University Press, 2011).

6. Philippe Ariès, *The Hour of Our Death* (New York: Knopf, 1981); Stanley Brandes, "The Cremated Catholic: The Ends of a Deceased Guatemalan," *Body & Society* 7, no. 2–3 (2001); Thomas Laqueur, *The Work of the Dead: A Cultural History of Mortal Remains* (Princeton, NJ: Princeton University Press, 2015); Stefan Timmermans, *Postmortem: How Medical Examiners Explain Suspicious Death* (Chicago: University of Chicago Press, 2006); Alexei Yurchak, "Bodies of Lenin: The Hidden Science of Communist Sovereignty," *Representations* 129, no. 1 (2015): 116–57.

7. Samson Lim, *Siam's New Detectives: Visualizing Crime and Conspiracy in Modern Thailand* (Honolulu: University of Hawai'i Press, 2016) likewise offers compelling evidence of how material practices surrounding death shape the cultural realm.

8. Michael T. Taussig, "Culture of Terror—Space of Death," in *Colonialism and Culture*, ed. Nicholas B. Dirks (Ann Arbor: University of Michigan Press, 1992).

9. Claudio Lomnitz, *Death and the Idea of Mexico* (New York: Zone Books, 2005), 18.

10. Tony Ballantyne, *Entanglements of Empire: Missionaries, Moari, and the Question of the Body* (Durham, NC: Duke University Press, 2014), 175.

11. Erik Seeman, *Death in the New World: Cross-Cultural Encounters, 1492–1800* (Philadelphia: University of Pennsylvania Press, 2010), 291; Vincent Brown, *The Reaper's Garden: Death and Power in the World of Atlantic Slavery* (Cambridge, MA: Harvard University Press, 2008). See also, Greg Dening, *Islands and Beaches: Discourse on a Silent Land, Marquesas 1774–1880* (Chicago: Dorsey Press, 1980), chap.7, "Violent Death."

12. *A Week in Siam: January 1867* (Bangkok: The Siam Society, 1986 [1870]), 50. *See also Jacob T. Child, The Pearl of Asia* (Chicago: Donohue, Henneberry & Co., 1892), 136–41; *and Lucien Fournereau, Bangkok in 1892, ed. Walter E. J. Tips* (Bangkok: While Lotus Press, 1998), 147–56.

13. The account, which was first published as a news item in the *Bangkok Times* (a local English-language newspaper), would have an unexpected afterlife as a long-standing appendix in annual issues of an English-language almanac for foreign residents; see "A Siamese Execution," *Bangkok Times* (hereafter *BT*), 4 September 1889, and *The Directory for Bangkok and Siam for 1891: A Handy and Perfectly Reliable Book of Reference for All Classes* (Bangkok: Bangkok Times, [1891]).

14. On the former, see Akin Rabibhadana, *The Organization of Thai Society in the Early Bangkok Period 1782–1873* (Bangkok: Amarin, 1996); on the latter, see Hong Lysa, *Thailand in the Nineteenth Century: Evolution of the Economy and Society* (Singapore: Institute of Southeast Asian Studies, 1984), chap. 4.

15. Anya Bernstein, "The Post-Soviet Treasure Hunt: Time, Space, and Necropolitics in Siberian Buddhism," *Comparative Studies in Society and History* 53, no. 3 (2011): 624.

16. Charnvit Kasetsiri, "Thai Historiography from Ancient Times to the Modern Period," in *Perceptions of the Past in Southeast Asia*, ed. Anthony Reid and David Marr (Singapore: Asian Studies Association of Australia, 1979).

17. Thongchai Winichakul, "Prawatisat thai baeb rachachat niyom" ["Thai History in the Royal-Nationalist Mode"], *Sinlapa watthanatham* [*Art & Culture*] 23, no. 1 (2001).

The idea that the Siamese elite possessed a unique ability to selectively adapt Western ideas continues to appear in scholarship on Thai intellectual history; see, for example, Thanet Aphornsuvan, "The West and Siam's Quest for Modernity: Siamese Responses to Nineteenth Century American Missionaries," *South East Asia Research* 17, no. 3 (2009).

18. On the former, see Hong Lysa, *Thailand*; and Pasuk Phongpaichit and Chris Baker, *Thailand: Economy and Politics*, 2nd ed. (New York: Oxford, 2002). On the latter, see Tamara Loos, *Subject Siam: Family, Law, and Colonial Modernity in Thailand* (Ithaca, NY: Cornell University Press, 2006), 40–43.

19. Akin Rabibhadana, *The Organization of Thai Society*; Hong Lysa, *Thailand*, chap. 4.

20. Jit Phumisak's *Chomna khong sakdina thai nai patchuban* [*The real face of Thai feudalism today*] (1957) is the best-known work; see Craig Reynolds, trans., *Thai Radical Discourse: The Real Face of Thai Feudalism Today* (Ithaca, NY: Southeast Asia Program, Cornell University, 1987). See also Craig J. Reynolds and Hong Lysa, "Marxism in Thai Historical Studies," *Journal of Asian Studies* 43, no. 1 (1983) and Craig J. Reynolds, "Feudalism as a Trope for the Past," *Seditious Histories: Contesting Thai and Southeast Asian Pasts* (Seattle: University of Washington Press, 2006).

21. See Thongchai Winichakul, *Siam Mapped: History of the Geo-Body of a Nation* (Honolulu: University of Hawai'i Press, 1997); Shane Strate, *The Lost Territories: Thailand's History of National Humiliation* (Honolulu: University of Hawai'i Press, 2015); Loos, *Subject Siam*; David Streckfuss, *Truth on Trial in Thailand: Defamation, Treason, and Lèse-majesté* (London: Routledge, 2011); Davisakd Puaksom, *Chua rok rang kai lae rat wetchakam: prawatisat kan-phaet samai mai nai sangkhom thai* [*Disease, the body, and the medicalizing state: The history of modern medicine in Thai society*] (Bangkok: Chulalongkorn University Press, 2007); Davisakd Puaksom, "Of Germs, Public Hygiene and the Healthy Body: The Making of the Medicalizing State in Thailand," *Journal of Asian Studies* 66, no. 2 (2007); and Claudia Merli, *Bodily Practices and Medical Identities in Southern Thailand* (Uppsala: Uppsala University Press, 2008).

22. Michael Herzfeld has made the case that these conditions were not, in fact, as unique as the Thai exceptionalist narrative would claim. He identifies a distinctive brand of denial as the fixed pillar around which cultural life has evolved in "crypto-colonial" states; see his "The Absent Presence: Discourses of Crypto-Colonialism," *South Atlantic Quarterly* 101, no. 4 (2002).

23. See, respectively, Danilyn Rutherford, *Laughing at Leviathan: Sovereignty and Audience in West Papua* (Chicago: University of Chicago Press, 2012), 13; and Giorgio Agamben, *Homo Sacer: Sovereign Power and Bare Life* (Stanford, CA: Stanford University Press, 1998).

24. The clearest statement of this Hobbesian tradition can be found in Max Weber, "Politics as Vocation," in *Weber's Rationalism and Modern Society*, ed. Tony Waters and Dagmar Waters (New York: Palgrave Macmillan Books, 2015), 129–98, esp. 136.

25. Thomas Blom Hansen and Finn Stepputat, *Sovereign Bodies: Citizens, Migrants, and States in the Postcolonial World* (Princeton, NJ: Princeton University Press, 2005).

26. Samera Esmeir, *Juridical Humanity: A Colonial History* (Stanford, CA: Stanford University Press, 2012).

27. J. A. Mbembe, "Necropolitics," *Public Culture* 15, no. 1 (2003): 25–26.

28. Michel Foucault, *Birth of Biopolitics* (New York: Picador, 2008). For an insightful elaboration of Foucault's ideas, see Matthew Coleman and Kevin Grove, "Biopolitics,

Biopower, and the Return of Sovereignty," *Environment and Planning D: Society and Space* 27, no. 3 (2009).

29. Murray, "Thanatopolitics," 193; William Pietz, "The Fetish of Civilization: Sacrificial Blood and Monetary Debt," in *Colonial Subjects: Essays on the Practical History of Anthropology*, ed. Peter Pels and Oscar Salemink (Ann Arbor: University of Michigan Press, 1999), 53–81.

30. Mbembe, "Necropolitics," 11. Mbembe's understanding is formulated in response to major works on violence and sovereignty, including Agamben, *Homo Sacer*, and Michel Foucault, *"Society Must Be Defended": Lectures at the Collège de France, 1975–76* (New York: Picador, 2003).

31. Agamben, *Homo Sacer*; Murray, "Thanatopolitics"; and Roberto Esposito, *Bíos: Biopolitics and Philosophy*, trans. Timothy C. Campbell (Minneapolis: University of Minnesota Press, 2008).

32. Mark Driscoll, *Absolute Erotic, Absolute Grotesque: The Living and the Dead in Japan's Imperialism, 1895–1945* (Durham, NC: Duke University Press, 2010); Sherene H. Razack, *Dying from Improvement: Inquests and Inquiries into Indigenous Deaths in Custody* (Toronto: University of Toronto Press 2015); Mark Munsterhjelm, *Living Dead in the Pacific: Contested Sovereignty and Racism in Genetic Research on Taiwan Aborigines* (Vancouver: University of British Columbia Press, 2014).

33. Benedict R. O'G. Anderson, "Studies of the Thai State: The State of Thai Studies," in *The Study of Thailand: Analyses of Knowledge, Approaches, and Prospects in Anthropology, Art History, Economics, History and Political Science*, ed. Eliezer B. Ayal (Athens: Center for International Studies, Ohio University, 1978); Hong Lysa, *Thailand*, 127.

34. Dararat Mettarikanond, *"Kotmai sopheni 'ti-tabian' khrang raek nai prathet thai"* ["The first law of the registration of prostitutes in Thailand"], *Sinlapa Watthanatham* 5, no. 8 (1984).

35. David K. Wyatt, *Thailand: A Short History* (New Haven, CT: Yale University Press, 1982), 217.

36. National Archives of Thailand (NA), Documents from the Fifth Reign (R5), Records of the Ministry of the Capital (N), Division 23.

37. The king's letter reports that after investigation by police, the accident was found to be unintentional and that "the queen had bestowed money to cover the funerary expenses [of the deceased], which is appropriate" (*somdet phra borom osathirat prathan ngoen hai tham sop jin khien ko pen kan-somkhuan*), NA R5 S.Th. 99/17.

38. They fall under Roberto Mangabeira Unger's classical definition of customary law as "patterns of interactions to which moral obligations attach"; from his *Knowledge and Politics* (New York: The Free Press, 1975), cited in Lauren Benton, *Law and Colonial Cultures: Legal Regimes in World History, 1400–1900* (Cambridge: Cambridge University Press, 2002), 8.

39. Benton, *Law and Colonial Cultures*, 10.

40. Daniel Asen, *Death in Beijing: Murder and Forensic Science in Republican China* (Cambridge: Cambridge University Press, 2016), 7.

41. These conditions constituted what Christopher Hamlin has called the "arch anxieties" that determine the nature of historically distinct forensic regimes; see his "Forensic Cultures in Historical Perspective: Technologies of Witness, Testimony, Judgment (and Justice?)," *Studies in History and Philosophy of Biological and Biomedical Sciences* 44 (2013): 4–15.

42. Elizabeth Kolsky, *Colonial Justice in British India* (Cambridge: Cambridge University Press, 2010).

43. Susan Leigh Star and James R. Griesemer, "Institutional Ecology, 'Translation,' and Boundary Objects: Amateurs and Professionals in Berkeley's Museum of Vertebrate Zoology, 1907–39," *Social Studies of Science* 19, no. 3 (1989).

1. Bad Death

1. Ann Laura Stoler, *Along the Archival Grain: Epistemic Anxieties and Colonial Common Sense* (Princeton, NJ: Princeton University Press, 2009), 26.

2. NA R5 N 23 / 1.

3. Naret would likely also have learned about inquests when he visited Singapore along with King Chulalongkorn in 1890 in order to study British municipal governance and policing; see Samson W. Lim, "The Aesthetics of Evidence: Crime and Conspiracy in Thailand's Popular Press" (PhD diss., Cornell University, 2012), 84–87. For more on Naret's early career, travels, and his position within the royal hierarchy, see Tamara Loos, *Bones Around My Neck: The Life and Exile of a Prince Provocateur* (Ithaca, NY: Cornell University Press, 2016), 26–49.

4. NA R5 N 23 / 11.

5. *"Ratsadon phu tai duai het song sai"* (NA R5 N 23 / 151).

6. Walter F. Vella, *The Impact of the West on Government in Thailand* (Berkeley: University of California Press, 1955), 328–31.

7. Pasuk Phongpaichit and Chris Baker, *Thailand: Economy and Politics*, 2nd ed. (New York: Oxford University Press, 2002), 24–26.

8. Akin Rabibhadana, *The Organization of Thai Society in the Early Bangkok Period 1782–1873* (Bangkok: Amarin, 1996). For newly arrived Chinese laborers, Jin Pao perhaps among them, whose ranks had been growing rapidly since the mid-nineteenth century, there was an obligatory triennial "head tax," which was justified as a tax levied on those who were exempted from the obligation to provide corvée labor service to the state; see G. William Skinner, *Chinese Society in Thailand: An Analytical History* (Ithaca, NY: Cornell University Press, 1957), 128.

9. Andrew Turton, "Thai Institutions of Slavery," in *Asian and African Systems of Slavery*, ed. James L. Watson (Berkeley: University of California Press, 1980), 262–72.

10. By the late nineteenth century, the Ministry of the Capital kept tabs on such debt contracts; official records can be found in NA R5 N 26, *Chabab nangsue samkhan* (Records of contracts).

11. These changes represent part of a concomitant decline of one regime of property rights (rights in man) and the rise of another (rights in land); see David Feeny, "The Decline of Property Rights in Man in Thailand, 1800–1913," *Journal of Economic History* 49, no. 2 (1989).

12. See the appendix for a more detailed discussion of relevant literature.

13. Janet Hoskins attests to a similar sense of unanticipated death in Kodi culture; see her *Biographical Objects: How Things Tell the Stories of People's Lives* (New York: Routledge, 1998), 161–81.

14. Stanley J. Tambiah, *Buddhism and the Spirit Cults in North-East Thailand* (Cambridge: Cambridge University Press, 1970), 189.

15. Tambiah, *Buddhism and the Spirit Cults*.

16. Tambiah, *Buddhism and the Spirit Cults,*193.

17. Aage Westenholz, "Street Railways in Siam, and Siamese Customs," *The Street Railway Journal* 7 (August 1891): 414.

18. *BT*, May 23, 1895.

19. See, for example, *BT*, August 10, 1895.

20. Shigeharu Tanabe, "The Person in Transformation: Body, Mind and Cultural Appropriation," in *Cultural Crisis and Social Memory: Modernity and Identity in Thailand and Laos*, ed. S. Tanabe and C. F. Keyes (Honolulu: University of Hawai'i Press, 2002), 43–67; cited in David M. Engel, "Landscapes of the Law: Injury, Remedy, and Social Change in Thailand," in *Law & Society Review* 43, no. 1 (2009): 67. Engel's own ethnographic work on personal injury, law, and justice suggests that these beliefs surrounding the communal implications of individual injury persisted in Northern Thailand well into the late twentieth century; see "Globalization and the Decline of Legal Consciousness: Torts, Ghosts, and Karma in Thailand," *Law & Social Inquiry* 30, no. 3 (2005): 482–83.

21. NA R5 N 23 / 6. As described in the introduction, Wat Saket was infamous among Western travelers to Bangkok in the late nineteenth century.

22. *"Hai jat jaeng ao asop thi klao ma ni khuen sia hai phon nai lam khlong nai kham wan ni"* (NA R5 N 23 / 6).

23. *"Mai pen kan-somkhuan loei"* (NA R5 N 23 / 6).

24. The *Bangkok Times* would often report corpses lying in the street for days before police would intervene (see, for example, *BT*, October 12, 1898). There were also jurisdictional disputes over cases of unnatural death, whereby Siamese police would engage in arguments with local officials, including the tax farmers who owned the gambling dens where cases of sudden and unnatural death often occurred (see, for example, NA R5 N 23 / 151).

25. This was no less true of jurisdictions outside of the capital, where forensic investigations likewise fell to district- and provincial-level officials (*hua mueang*) without any special expertise. Records of criminal cases forwarded from outside regions to the Ministry of the Justice corroborate this; see, for example, NA R5 N 45.7 / 4, which discusses the case of a fatal stabbing in Prachinburi.

26. The "Death by various causes" files show an almost endless variation in the spelling of the terms *"sop"* and *"asop"* (corpse), the latter spelling being an archaic form closer to its Pali-Sanskrit roots.

27. See, for example, NA R5 N 23 / 9.

28. See NA R5 N 23 / 7 for an account of a particularly crowded postmortem examination on temple grounds. That crowds gathered on the occasion of police inquests is in some respects counterintuitive to the logic of inauspicious death. It seems plausible, however, that the presence of police somehow had the effect of defusing or deactivating the menace posed by the corpse; perhaps villagers understood that through their willful interference with the corpse police had taken the risk upon themselves.

29. When the British Police Inspector A. J. A. Jardine arrived in Bangkok (see chapter 4), he noted with frustration that most of the local police stations in the western districts of the city were "either broke down bamboo sheds or 'Salas' [temple pavilions] etc. lent by the Priests" to the local police officers (A. J. A. Jardine, *Report on the Police Administration of Bangkok, Suburbs, and Railway Divisions for 1898–1899*, 68; NA R5 N/96, box 6). Even as late as March 1899, Mr. E. W. Grove, a foreigner serving as

assistant divisional superintendent of police for the western districts of the city (Thonburi) was using a temple *sala* to oversee police business for the eleven stations under his charge (*BT*, March 8, 1899).

30. Open-air examinations at temples also had the added advantage of ventilation: corpses that had languished in the city's waterways for several days were likely well on their way to putrefaction.

31. While cremation was the most common mode of disposing of the dead at the time, corpses were often buried soon after death to allow for decomposition, only to be disinterred at a later date—when only bones remained—in preparation for (often mass-) cremation rites.

32. *Lucien Fournereau, Bangkok in 1892, ed. Walter E. J. Tips (Bangkok: While Lotus Press, 1998),* 151.

33. NA R5 Y 13.4/6.

34. NA R5 Y 13.4/8.

35. Cases showing evidence of police awareness of the tendency of corpses to drift downstream are numerous; see, for example, the cases of Nai Pao discussed earlier, as well as the case of a criminal who jumped into the river in order to evade police (NA R5 N 23/72).

36. NA R5 Y 13.4/2.

37. *Rai ngan kan-prachum senabodi sapha ro. so. 111* [*Minutes of the meetings of the government ministers for the year 1893*], vol. 1 (Krungthep: Amarin, 2550 [2007]), 210.

38. Naret alone was in charge of municipal governance beginning in 1889; see David K. Wyatt, "Family Politics in Nineteenth Century Thailand," *Journal of Southeast Asian History* 9, no. 2 (1968): 226.

39. On taxes: see James A. Warren, *Gambling, the State, and Society in Thailand c. 1800–1945* (New York: Routledge, 2013), chaps. 3 and 5. On policing: Naret's own efforts to reform the municipal police force date back to 1889 (see NA R5 N 8.1/1 and N 11.3/1). On medicine: early documents from the hospital department (*krom phayaban*) pertaining to cholera and vaccination, for example, can be found at NA R5 N 49.3.

40. Porphant Ouyyanont, "Bangkok's Population & The Ministry of the Capital in Early 20th Century Thai History," *Southeast Asian Studies* 35, no. 2 (1997): 256.

41. On the former, see, for example, NA R5 N 5.2/6–7; N 5.2/14; NA R5 N 5.7/1–2; N 5.7/5; N 5.7/8; N 5.7/11; N 5.7/13ff. On the latter, see NA 5 R N 8.1/151, which contains a monthly registry of burials and cremations at city temples; NA R5 N 8.1/165, which deals with efforts to prohibit the burial of cholera victims; and NA R5 N 8.11/1–34, which contains records of requests to move corpses in and out of the city for the purpose of burial.

42. The microfilm reels for the "Death by various causes" files are labeled "NA R5 N," and they span reel numbers 328–34.

43. NA R5 N 23/7. The death of Jin Bua in May 1891 is another interesting case for considering the role of executive authority over unnatural death (NA R5 N 23/3). In responding to police documents concerning the (rather complicated) case, Naret teases out the distinctions between murder and manslaughter (unintentional homicide) and their respective penal or civil repercussions.

44. *"Nai rai ngan khong than ha dai khwam krajat chad khwam talot mai"* (NA R5 N 23/7, letter dated January 5, 1892).

45. *"Nam het thi mi het plaek palat ni khun"* (NA R5 N 23/7).

46. The case file contains the minutes of the inquest held at the Police Court on the morning of January 6, 1892 (NA R5 N 23/7).

47. "*Kae tam kham jaeng ni doem khwam long mai laeo nam rang thawai*" (NA R5 N 23/7).

48. "*Sia jarit khum di [khum] rai ha prokati mai*" (NA R5 N 23/7).

49. On the office of the coroner, see Ian A. Burney, *Bodies of Evidence: Medicine and the Politics of the English Inquest, 1830–1926* (Baltimore: Johns Hopkins University Press, 2000).

50. NA R5 N 23/9.

51. NA R5 N 23/11.

52. "*Bang thi ja pen chu det khrai kan phro amdaeng muan phuk kho tai laeo jin to than ko kin ya phit tai nai wan rung khuen dang ni*" (NA R5 N 23/11).

53. In these cases, it is tempting to imagine Naret, who had served as Siam's ambassador to Britain for several years in the 1880s, as channeling his inner Sherlock Holmes. The latter had made his literary debut in 1887, and Naret was very likely acquainted with the work of Arthur Conan Doyle's fictional detective by this time.

54. "*Kan-rueang ni phikhro tam nai rueang khwam ko du pen na ja thuk ya bua mao jing* [. . .] *hen wa khwam rueang ni pen khwam tai doi phit prokati thamada*" (NA R5 23/10).

55. NA R5 N 23/16.

56. For an overview of these changes, see William J. Siffin, *The Thai Bureaucracy: Institutional Change and Development* (Honolulu: East-West Center Press, 1966), 51–90.

57. Siffin, *The Thai Bureaucracy*, 110. Siffin suggests that in time status within the bureaucracy did take on some meritocratic characteristics, but while "the old hierarchical status system was rationalized and adapted . . . it was never transcended" (111).

58. This disparity between vernacular and legalistic modes of thought can be found in contemporary Thai civil law as well, where discourses about causality can differ wildly between colloquial contexts and state legal institutions; see David M. Engel, "Discourses of Causation in Injury Cases: Exploring Thai and American Legal Cultures," in *Fault Lines: Tort Law as Cultural Practice*, ed. David M. Engel and Michael McCann (Stanford, CA: Stanford University Press, 2009).

59. "*Tai ton malako*" (NA R5 N 23/7).

60. "*Hen nai won phuk kho tai yu thi king mamuang suan nai nak*," NA R5 N 23/55, letter dated May 2, 115 [1897].

61. NA R5 N 23/221.

62. For a demonstration of how this process operates in contemporary civil proceedings, see Engel, "Discourses of Causation," 251.

63. See also, NA R5 N 23/127; NA R5 N 23/207; NA R5 N 23/208; NA R5 N 23/214; NA R5 N 23/221; NA R5 N 23/224; NA R5 N 23/227; NA R5 N 23/236; NA R5 N 23/244; NA R5 N 23/260; NA R5 N 23/266; NA R5 N 23/284; NA R5 N 23/321; NA R5 N 23/325; NA R5 N 23/341; NA R5 N 23/347; NA R5 N 23/390; NA R5 N 23/400; NA R5 N 23/432; NA R5 N 23/445; NA R5 N 23/448; NA R5 N 23/551; NA R5 N 23/572; NA R5 N 23/619; NA R5 N 23/627; NA R5 N 23/632.

64. Several of the trees mentioned above, including *sok* and *phikun*, are among those listed by Anuman Rajathon in his catalog of inauspicious trees that are not to be grown within the grounds of a private dwelling; see Anuman Rajathon, "Some Siamese Superstitions about Trees and Plants," *Journal of the Siam Society* 49, no. 1 (1961): 57–59.

65. See, respectively, NA R5 N 23/207 and NA R5 N 23/208.

66. Such haunting spirits have found a home in the sociological study of place; see Michael Mayerfeld Bell, "The Ghosts of Place," *Theory and Society* 26, no. 6 (1997).

67. "The Mysterious Disappearance," *BT*, September 5, 1894, 3.

68. "The Mysterious Disappearance," *BT*, September 5, 1894, 3.

69. See, for example, *BT*, May 18, 1895; *BT*, June 20, 1899.

70. *BT*, December 23, 1901.

71. *BT*, December 7, 1889.

72. "WANTED[:] A CORPSE," *BT*, August 10, 1898.

73. *BT*, June 5, 1900.

74. *BT*, June 29, 1900.

75. *BT*, June 29, 1900.

76. *BT*, August 10, 1895.

77. *BT*, August 10, 1895.

78. *BT*, August 10, 1895.

79. NA R5 N 23/151, for instance, relates a dispute between police and the Chinese owner of a gambling den over who was responsible for removing a corpse from the street in front of that establishment.

80. See, for example, Khaled Fahmy, "The Anatomy of Justice: Forensic Medicine and Criminal Law in Nineteenth Century Egypt," *Islamic Law & Society* 6, no. 2 (1999); David Arnold, *Colonizing the Body: State Medicine and Epidemic Disease in Nineteenth-Century India* (Berkeley: University of California Press, 1993), 211; Florence Bernault, "Body, Power, and Sacrifice in Equatorial Africa," *Journal of African History* 47, no. 2 (2006): 217–18; Elisa M. Becker, *Medicine, Law and the State in Imperial Russia* (Budapest: Central European University Press, 2011); and Warwick Anderson, "Objectivity and Its Discontents," *Social Studies of Science* 43, no. 4 (2012).

2. Indemnity and Identity

1. *BT*, August 10, 1889.

2. Events such as this do not figure in the (admittedly limited) historiography of the Bangkok Tramway Company; see the appendix.

3. Cited in Paul Virilio, *The Original Accident*, trans. Julie Rose (Malden, MA: Polity Press, 2007), 3.

4. Virilio, *The Original Accident*, 3.

5. Virilio, *The Original Accident*, 9, 5.

6. Virilio, *The Original Accident*, 10 (original emphasis).

7. Paul Virilio, *Politics of the Very Worst* (New York: Semiotext(e), 1999), 12, 89.

8. See Loos, *Subject Siam*; M. B. Hooker, "The 'Europeanization' of Siam's Law 1855–1908," in *The Laws of South-East Asia*, vol. 2, *European Laws in South-East Asia*, ed. M. B. Hooker (St. Paul, MN: Butterworths, 1988), 531–607; and Andrew J. Harding, "The Eclipse of the Astrologers: King Mongkut, His Successors, and the Reformation of Law in Thailand," in *Examining Practice, Interrogating Theory: Comparative Legal Studies in Asia*, ed. Penelope Nicholson and Sarah Biddulph (Leiden: Martinus Nijhoff, 2008), 307–41.

9. See, for example, Thanet Aphornsuvan, "Slavery and Modernity: Freedom in the Making of Modern Siam," in *Asian Freedoms: The Idea of Freedom in South and Southeast Asia*, ed. David Kelly and Anthony Reid (Cambridge: Cambridge University Press,

1998), 163–64; and Tamara Loos, "Issaraphap: Limits of Individual Liberty in Thai Jurisprudence," *Crossroads: An Interdisciplinary Journal of Southeast Asian Studies* 12 (1998). In addition to positive law, scholars have also traced ideological and institutional aspects of this project: elite discourses concerning the opposition of slavery and freedom were devoid of any sense of freedom as a "positive social value for the common people" (Thanet, "Slavery and Modernity," 182), and the national justice system employed a traditional hierarchical vision of access to truth based on Theravada Buddhism, which favored those possessed of high social status (David Streckfuss, *Truth on Trial in Thailand: Defamation, Treason, and Lèse-majesté* [London: Routledge, 2011], 22, 36).

10. Loos, *Subject Siam*, 29–71; Streckfuss, *Truth on Trial*, 36, 81.

11. As Dipesh Chakrabarty has argued, "The universal concepts of political modernity encounter preexisting concepts, categories, institutions, and practices through which they get translated and configured differently" (*Provincializing Europe: Postcolonial Thought and Historical Difference* [Princeton, NJ: Princeton University Press, 2008], xii). Attending to these precedents can help us to avoid the inclination toward "primitivism" and paternalism in the study of traditional forms of legal life; see Uday Chandra, "Liberalism and Its Other: The Politics of Primitivism in Colonial and Postcolonial Law," *Law & Society Review* 47 (2013): 135–68.

12. See, for example, Samera Esmeir, *Juridical Humanity: A Colonial History* (Stanford, CA: Stanford University Press, 2012); Baudouin Dupret, ed., *Standing Trial: Law and the Person in the Modern Middle East* (London: I.B. Tauris, 2004); and Talal Asad, "Conscripts of Western Civilization," in *Dialectical Anthropology: Essays in Honor of Stanley Diamond*, vol. 1, ed. Christine Ward Gailey (Tallahassee: University Press of Florida, 1992).

13. Aage Westenholz, "Street Railways in Siam, and Siamese Customs," *The Street Railway Journal* 7 (August 1891): 414. The management of the Bangkok Tramway Company realized soon after the introduction of the service that horse bells alone were insufficient to alert people of the oncoming cars, so bugles were introduced with different tunes to announce inbound and outbound tramcars.

14. *BT*, November 2, 1889.

15. "Tramway Concession, Bangkok, 5th May 1887" (NA Microfilm R5 N/128), 1. The signatories to the concession also included a British attorney named Edward Blair Michell (serving as notary); Michell's professional career in Siam would continue to intersect with the tramway company in a number of different ways as described in the following chapters.

16. "Tramway Concession," 12.

17. "Tramway Concession," 6.

18. Westenholz, "Street Railways in Siam," 414.

19. NA R5 N 8.1/21.

20. "The Bangkok Tramways Company," *Street Railway Journal* 9, no. 8 (1893): 510.

21. "Electric Railways," *Western Electrician* 10–11 (April 30, 1892): 169; "The Bangkok Tramways Company," 510.

22. "Short Electric Railway Notes," *Street Railway Journal* 8 (May 1892): 317.

23. "The Bangkok Tramways Company," 510.

24. "Industrial and Trade Notes," *Electrical World* 19 (April 30, 1893): 305.

25. Westenholz, "Street Railways," 415.

26. Westenholz, "Street Railways," 414. Westenholz's comments seem to suggest that accidents and injury law alike may not have been as emphatically gendered as Barbara Young Welke has shown they were in the American context; see her "Unreasonable Women: Gender and the Law of Accidental Injury, 1870–1920," *Law and Social Inquiry* 19 (1994).

27. *BT*, April 4, 1895.

28. *BT*, November 2, 1889.

29. *BT*, November 2, 1889.

30. *BT*, February 17, 1892.

31. Dr. Hays's somewhat compromised position as both a shareholder in the Bangkok Tramway Company and the physician of first resort for those injured by the tramcars—not to mention his role as an expert medical witness in civil cases involving the company—is discussed in chapter 3. Hays also reappears in the discussion of the introduction of forensic medicine in Siam (chapter 5).

32. The dismal state of the roads in Bangkok was a common complaint in the press. The *Bangkok Times* proposed "Holes, ruts, sloughs, puddles and occasional dry spots (very treacherous ones though)," as the "special vocabulary" needed to describe them (*BT*, October 19, 1889). The condition of the roads was one reason why (foreign) residents called for the extension of tramway service provided by the Bangkok Tramway Company, which was solely responsible for maintaining the roadbeds wherever its tracks had been laid down.

33. NA R5 N 23/8.

34. Wat Sam Jin, or "the temple of the three Chinese [men]," is today known as Wat Traimit ("the temple of three friends"); it is a large and opulent temple compound at the southeastern gateway to the city's Chinatown.

35. "*Kampani rot traem we kho ao ngoen tham khwan hai amdaeng jan phi nong nai ao*" (NA R5 N 23/8, 2).

36. "*Rueang ni kampani sia bia pluk tua phu tai hai kae yat ko khuan laeo*" (NA R5 N 23/8, 3–4).

37. For an introduction to these ideas and practices, see Tambiah, *Buddhism and the Spirit Cults*, 189–94 and 312–26.

38. While the *khwan* was consistently used to refer to the spirit of the *deceased* in documents pertaining to accidental death from the late nineteenth century, this use does not conform to contemporary usage; see the appendix for more on this discrepancy and for references to relevant historical and ethnographic literature.

39. M. B. Hooker, *Legal Pluralism: An Introduction to Colonial and Neo-Colonial Laws* (Oxford: Clarendon Press, 1975), 372.

40. Hooker, *Legal Pluralism*, 372.

41. Hooker, *Legal Pluralism*, 373. Richard A. O'Connor offers some specific illustrations of how traditional law related to the system of feudal social ordering in "Law as Indigenous Social Theory: A Siamese Thai Case," *American Ethnologist* 8 (1981): 228–29.

42. "*Kampani dai tham khwan hai kae yat phu tai laeo mai tong sang an dai to pai*" (NA R5 N 23/8, 6).

43. NA R5 N 23/8, 6.

44. "*Phu khap [rot traem we] mi khwam phit doi khwam loen loe*" (NA R5 N 23/8, 8).

45. David M. Engel, *Law and Kingship in Thailand during the Reign of King Chulalongkorn* (Ann Arbor: University of Michigan [Center for South and Southeast Asian

Studies], 1975), 61–62; Tamara Loos, "Gender Adjudicated: Translating Modern Legal Subjects in Siam" (PhD diss., Cornell University, 1999), 80–89.

46. See Luang Wisut's final report (NA R5 N 23/8, 8).

47. "The idiom of ex gratia payments is of unilateral action, absence of obligation, ability to pay rather than fault, and need rather than entitlement"; see Marc Galanter, "India's Tort Deficit: Sketch for a Historical Portrait," in *Fault Lines: Tort Law as Cultural Practice*, ed. David M. Engel and Michael McCann (Stanford, CA: Stanford University Press, 2009), 64.

48. Engel, *Law and Kingship*, 59–93.

49. See R. Lingat, "Note sur la Revision des Lois Siamoises en 1805," *Journal of the Siam Society* 23 (1929): 19–27. It was been reproduced as a five-volume set in *Kotmai tra sam duang* [*Law of the Three Seals*] (Osaka, Japan: National Museum of Ethnography, 1981). See also Chris Baker and Pasuk Phongpaichit, eds., *The Palace Law of Ayutthaya and the Thammasat: Law and Kingship in Siam* (Ithaca, NY: Southeast Asia Program Publications, 2016).

50. This discussion refers to Siamese law pertaining to laypeople; religious life in Buddhist temples was governed by the *vinaya*, the laws for Buddhist renunciants (both male and female) that was part of the Pali canonical tradition.

51. R. Lingat, "Evolution of the Concept of Law in Burma and Siam" *Journal of the Siam Society* 38 (1950): 23.

52. For a review of Thai-language scholarship on this question in the northeastern region of Isan, see Nitilak Kaewchandee, "*Kotmai boran isan: sathanaphap ong khwam ru lae kho khit hen bang prakan*" ["Isan ancient law: State of knowledge and some reflections"], *Proceedings of the 16th Annual Meeting of Sociology and Anthropology Branches, Princess Maha Chakri Sirindhorn Anthropology Centre and Naresuan University* 2559 (2016): 79–99, 90–91; and for evidence attesting to the diffusion of law to the southern periphery, see *Prachum phongsawadan phak thi 2* [*Collected Chronicles, No. 2*] (Bangkok: Rongphim Thai, 1914), 44–49. Thanks to Davisakd Puaksom and Krijakara Kokpuak for these references.

53. Loos, *Subject Siam*, 33–34.

54. Streckfuss, *Truth on Trial*, 71.

55. Streckfuss, *Truth on Trial*, 71. See also Thanapol Limapichart, "The Emergence of the Siamese Public Sphere: Colonial Modernity, Print Culture, and the Practice of Criticism (1860s–1910s)," *South-East Asia Research* 17, no. 3 (2009): 371.

56. Loos, *Subject Siam*, 40.

57. Loos, *Subject Siam*, 40.

58. William J. Archer, *Siamese Law on Disputes and Assault* (Bangkok: S. J. Smith's Office, 1886); and Archer, "*The Siamese Laws on Debts* (Bangkok: S. J. Smith's Office, Bangk'olem Point, 1885).

59. NA R5 N 23/23.

60. Kim Hok's injuries are described in a police report (NA R5 N 23/23, 6).

61. See the appendix for a discussion of related terminology for such compensatory payments.

62. "*Kan-tai chen ni tham nangsue sanya prajam to hai mai dai klua ja mi khwam phit*" (NA R5 N 23/23, 2).

63. "*Hai jin pin thao jin hok huai amdaeng phring tham hai pen samkhan*" (NA R5 N 23/23, 2).

64. *"Jin kim hok doen phit thang lat khuen pai bon taphan rot ai fai fa thi chong khaep khaep"* (NA R5 N 23/23, 4). Note the description of the tramway as "steam-powered"; see the appendix for further comment on this.

65. *"Hen phrom kan wa . . . [Jin Kim Hok] mi khwam phit doen khao nai thang ai rot fai fa"* (NA R5 N 23/23, 4). The letter refers only obliquely to the legal rights granted to the tramway company by its concession, which was signed in 1887, through an abbreviated allusion [*"sueng dai rap anuyat to lae oen oen"*].

66. *"Mai tit jai fong rong kampani traem we"* (NA R5 N 23/23, 4).

67. *"Mi khwam metta kap jin kim hok phu tai ok ngoen sam chang hai pen kha phao phi kae jin kim hok phu tai"* (NA R5 N 23/23, 4).

68. See, for example, the note concerning the actions *pluk tua* and *pluk phi* in Archer, *Siamese Law on Disputes*, 2, which likewise emphasizes the payments as an attempt to "do merit for the deceased."

69. *"Tem jai mi khwam yin di rap ngoen sam chang to nai hang kampani traem we pai"* (NA R5 N 23/23, 4).

70. On the planned institutional reforms and King Chulalongkorn's speech on the subject, see Loos, *Subject Siam*, 44.

71. See Engel, *Law and Kingship*, 66–67.

72. An official code of civil procedure would not be promulgated until 1908 (Engel, *Law and Kingship*, 74).

73. Westenholz, "Street Railways in Siam," 414–15.

74. Westenholz, "Street Railways in Siam," 414–15.

75. NA R5 N 23/30.

76. NA R5 N 23/30, 4.

77. NA R5 N 23/30, 5.

78. The letter reads: *"Tae thi khang nai na ok nan ja pen prakan dai luea thi ja phikro"* (NA R5 N 23/30, 5).

79. *BT* 31 August 1892.

80. NA R5 N 23/30, 8. The diagnosis of "bad blood" (*lueat rai*) in the lungs is likely a description of a collapsed or punctured lung.

81. *"Phikhro du na ja pen antarai [thueng chiwit] ko ja pen dai"* (NA R5 N 23/30, 11).

82. *"Prathan ngoen tham khwan rue rap pai jat kan-raksa phayaban ko ja pen kan-di"* (NA R5 N 23/30, 11).

83. *"Phon kho khwam sueng ja mi phu ti tiem nai phra ong than phro dai uea fuea karuna kae ratsadon thi jep buai nan tam somkhuan laeo mom chan hen khwam dang ni"* (NA R5 N 23/30, 11).

84. The ministry was formed on March 25, 1892, with another of King Chulalongkorn's brothers at the helm (Prince Svasti Sobhon); Prince Phichit was appointed in October 1894 (Loos, *Subject Siam*, 49).

85. Engel, *Law and Kingship*, 9. Phichit's literary works also shed some light on what might be called his "traditional" mindset; see Thanet, "Slavery and Modernity," 180 and n. 51.

86. Akiko Iijima, "The 'International Court' System in the Colonial History of Siam," *Taiwan Journal of Southeast Asian Studies* 5, no. 1 (2008): 53–54.

87. *BT*, October 17, 1898.

88. *BT*, November 7, 1898; the child died soon after the accident (*BT*, November 8, 1898).

89. *BT*, April 4, 1894.

90. Karuna Mantena, *Alibis of Empire: Henry Maine and the Ends of Liberal Imperialism* (Princeton, NJ: Princeton University Press, 2010), 2, 6–7.

91. John McCracken, "Customary Law in Colonial Africa," *Journal of African History* 28, no. 1 (1987): 169. See Martin Chanock, *Law, Custom, and Social Order: The Colonial Experience in Malawi and Zambia* (Cambridge: Cambridge University Press, 1985); and Sally Falk Moore, *Social Facts and Fabrications: "Customary" Law on Kilimanjaro, 1880–1908* (Cambridge: Cambridge University Press, 1986).

92. cf. Harding, "The Eclipse of the Astrologers."

93. Sally Engle Merry, *Colonizing Hawai'i: The Cultural Power of Law* (Princeton, NJ: Princeton University Press, 2000), 13.

94. Merry, *Colonizing Hawai'i*, 16.

95. Samera Esmeir, "At Once Human & Not Human: Law, Gender, and Historical Becoming in Colonial Egypt," *Gender & History* 23, no. 2 (2011): 236.

96. Here I mean to suggest a status analogous to Mbembe's conception of a "third zone between subjecthood and objecthood" ("Necropolitics," 25–26).

97. Loos, "Issaraphap"; Thanet, "Slavery and Modernity."

98. From Michel Foucault's "What Is Enlightenment?," in *The Foucault Reader*, ed. Paul Rabinow (New York: Pantheon, 1984), cited in Ian Hacking, *Historical Ontology* (Cambridge, MA: Harvard University Press, 2002), 2.

3. Treaty Port and Tort

1. *BT*, January 27, 1892.

2. Although the *Bangkok Times* refers to the award in "dollars," the award was most likely in the amount of six thousand *ticals* or *baht*.

3. Sheila Jasanoff, *Science at the Bar: Law, Science, and Technology in America* (Cambridge, MA: Harvard University Press, 1995), 19.

4. Jasanoff, *Science at the Bar*, 20.

5. Lauren Benton, *Law and Colonial Cultures: Legal Regimes in World History, 1400–1900* (Cambridge: Cambridge University Press, 2002), 10.

6. Lauren Benton, "Law and Empire in Global Perspective: Introduction," *American Historical Review* 117, no. 4 (2012): 1093.

7. Teresa Sutton, "The Deodand and Responsibility for Death," *The Journal of Legal History* 18, no. 3 (1997): 44.

8. Jacob J. Finkelstein, "The Goring Ox: Some Historical Perspectives on Deodands, Forfeitures, Wrongful Death and the Western Notion of Sovereignty," *Temple Law Quarterly* 46, no. 2 (1973): 197.

9. Finkelstein, "The Goring Ox," 183.

10. Elisabeth Cawthon, "New Life for the Deodand: Coroner's Inquests and Occupational Deaths in England, 1830–46," *American Journal of Legal History* 33 (1989): 137.

11. Harry Smith, "From Deodand to Dependency," *American Journal of Legal History* 11, no. 4 (1967): 390.

12. Smith, "From Deodand to Dependency," 389.

13. While the value of the deodands awarded by coroner's juries had become nominal by the middle of the eighteenth century (Smith, "From Deodand to

Dependency," 394), there were important exceptions to this rule, which might be suggestive of an emerging trend in the use of the legal instrument (Sutton, "The Deodand," 49).

14. Smith, "From Deodand to Dependency," 395.

15. Sutton, "The Deodand and Responsibility for Death," 46–47.

16. Smith, "From Deodand to Dependency," 395; Sutton, "The Deodand," 46.

17. Roger Cooter, "The Moment of the Accident: Culture, Militarism and Modernity in Late-Victorian Britain," in *Accidents in History: Injuries, Fatalities, and Social Relations*, ed. Roger Cooter and Bill Luckin (Atlanta: Editions Rodopi, 1997), 112.

18. Sutton, "The Deodand," 46.

19. Finkelstein, "The Goring Ox," 170–80.

20. Lawrence M. Friedman, *A History of American Law*, 3rd ed. (New York: Touchstone, 2005), 351.

21. See, for example, Robert A. Silverman, *Law and Urban Growth: Civil Litigation in the Boston Trial Courts, 1880–1900* (Princeton, NJ: Princeton University Press, 1981), 99–121; Randolph Bergstrom, *Courting Danger: Injury and Law in New York City, 1870–1910* (Ithaca, NY: Cornell University Press, 1992).

22. "The Law and the Profits," *BT*, January 27, 1892.

23. "The Law and the Profits."

24. Cf. Mitra Sharafi, *Law and Identity in Colonial South Asia: Parsi Legal Culture, 1772–1947* (Cambridge: Cambridge University Press, 2014), 193; see also, Kalyani Ramnath, "The Colonial Difference between Law and Fact: Notes on the Criminal Jury in India," *Indian Economic Social History Review* 50, no. 3 (2013).

25. Robert Bickers, "Legal Fiction: Extraterritoriality as an Instrument of British Power in China in the 'Long Nineteenth Century,'" in *Empire in Asia: A New Global History*, vol. 2, *The Long Nineteenth Century*, ed. Donna Brunero and Brian P. Farrell (New York: Bloomsbury Academic, 2018), 59.

26. Bickers, "Legal Fiction," 59.

27. Bickers, "Legal Fiction," 62.

28. Both claims/verdicts are in stark contrast to the compensatory payments offered by the Bangkok Tramway Company in cases involving the death of Siamese subjects, which were commonly limited to eighty baht (see chapter 2).

29. "The Law and the Profits," *BT*, January 27, 1892.

30. "The Law and the Profits," *BT*, January 27, 1892. The "Grand Panjandrum" is a somewhat obscure literary or theatrical reference to a grandiose character.

31. *BT*, September 19,1892. Maclachlan was also a shareholder in the Bangkok Tramway Company; his stake in the company would come back to haunt him just a year later in an entirely different way, when he was the first shareholder to be sued by a lawyer attempting to test the limits of foreign incorporation (see below).

32. Barbara Young Welke, *Recasting American Liberty: Gender, Race, Law, and the Railroad Revolution* (New York: Cambridge University Press, 2001), 81, 93.

33. John G. Burke, "Bursting Boilers and the Federal Power," *Technology and Culture* 7, no. 1 (1966); Peter W. J. Bartrip, "The State and the Steam-Boiler in Nineteenth Century Britain," *International Review of Social History* 25, no. 1 (1980).

34. "Liability for Criminal Negligence," *BT*, May 30, 1895.

35. King Chulalongkorn (King Rama V) was also a major shareholder in the Bangkok Tramway Company, which might help to explain its peculiar inviolability when it

came to discussions of negligence and liability. Edward Blair Michell, a British lawyer and sometime legal adviser to the Siamese state, served as notary on the occasion. Michell's role in legal change is discussed further below and in chapter 4.

36. "Tramway Concession, Bangkok, 5th May 1887" (NA R5 N/128).

37. The metaphysical nature of such legal notions and the process of their negotiation in Siam are discussed at length in chapter 4.

38. James W. Ely Jr., *Railroads and American Law, 1780–1860* (Lawrence: University Press of Kansas, 2001); see the appendix for further reading on this subject.

39. *BT*, May 30, 1895.

40. *BT*, May 30, 1895; Loos, *Subject Siam*, 103. Imperial rivalries often played out in the pages of the foreign-language newspapers; see Hong Lysa, "'Stranger within the Gates': Knowing Semi-Colonial Siam as Extraterritorials," *Modern Asian Studies* 38, no. 2 (2004): 337.

41. Jasanoff, *Science at the Bar*, 19.

42. Aage Westenholz, "Street Railways in Siam, and Siamese Customs," *The Street Railway Journal* 7 (August 1891): 414–15.

43. "The Bangkok Tramway Company," *Straits Times*, March 14, 1892.

44. "The Bangkok Tramway Company," *Straits Times*, March 14, 1892; "The Tramway Company's Troubles," *BT*, February 21, 1894.

45. "The Bangkok Tramway Company," *Straits Times*, March 14, 1892.

46. Susan M. Martin, *The UP Saga* (Copenhagen: Nordic Institute of Asian Studies, 2003), 20.

47. "The Bangkok Tramway Company," *Straits Times*, March 14, 1892.

48. "The Bangkok Tramway Company," *Straits Times*, March 14, 1892. The dissenter's name appears as "Machlachlan" in the article but is consistently spelled "Maclachlan" elsewhere in the Bangkok press (see below).

49. "A Few Days in Bangkok," *Singapore Free Press and Mercantile Advertiser*, July 17, 893.

50. *BT*, October 25, 1893.

51. *BT*, October 25, 1893.

52. *BT*, November 11, 1893.

53. An entry for "Maclachlan, J." appears in *The Chronicle & Directory for China, Corea [sic], Japan, The Philippines, Indo-China, Straits Settlements, Siam, Bornea, Malay States, &c. for the year 1892* (Hong Kong: The Daily Press, 1892), which lists his profession as "superintendent engineer, Hluang Narison Rice Mill" (587). By 1894, Maclachlan had moved to Wat Takien Rice Mill, where he worked as superintendent engineer for Chesug Teng (*The Chronicle & Directory . . . for the year 1894* [Hong Kong: The Daily Press, 1894], 328).

54. *BT*, November 29, 1893. By this time, Michell had long been at odds with British consular representatives in Siam, and with the consular court in particular; see Catherine Layton, *The Life and Times of Mary, Dowager Duchess of Sutherland: Power Play* (Newcastle upon Tyne: Cambridge Scholars Publishing, 2018), 192–95.

55. *BT*, November 29,1893.

56. *BT*, November 29, 1893.

57. The outcome of Tilleke's suit against Michell, which claimed 750 ticals in damages, is unclear.

58. "The Tramway Company's Troubles," *BT*, February 21, 1894.

59. "The Tramway Company's Troubles" (*BT*, February 21, 1894) identifies the Limited Liabilities Act (1855) as the relevant legislation, but in fact the Companies Act (1862), which applied to corporations consisting of at least seven shareholders, was the relevant law governing companies in Great Britain. British corporate endeavors in Asia, however, were more properly viewed as subject to the Indian Companies Ordinance 1866 (revised in 1882).

60. "The Tramway Company's Position," *BT*, March 10, 1894.

61. "The Tramway Company's Position," *BT*, March 10, 1894.

62. "The Tramway Company's Position," *BT*, March 10, 1894.

63. *BT*, March 31, 1894.

64. Simon Deakin, Angus Johnston, and Basil Markesinis, *Markesinis and Deakin's Tort Law*, 7th ed. (New York: Oxford University Press, 2012), 554; Fleming James Jr., "Vicarious Liability," *Tulane Law Review* 28 (1954).

65. Friedman, *A History of American Law*, 222–25, 350–66; Morton J. Horowitz, *The Transformation of American Law, 1870–1960: The Crisis of Legal Orthodoxy* (New York: Oxford University Press, 1992), 39–45.

66. Strangely, the newspaper failed to highlight the farcical background of cases such as Tilleke *v.* Michell (above), which seem ripe for satire.

67. "Philanthropy," *BT*, April 14, 1894.

68. *BT*, August 16, 892.

69. "Philanthropy," *BT*, April 14, 1894.

70. *BT*, November 16, 1895.

71. *BT*, August 24, 1898.

72. *BT*, November 5, 1897.

73. *BT*, December 29, 1894.

74. *BT*, December 21, 1899.

75. "History," on firm's website, accessed May 29, 2018, http://www.tilleke.com /firm/history.

76. Hays was also Chief Medical Officer to the Royal Siamese Navy, among other government appointments; see Arnold Wright, ed., *Twentieth Century Impressions of Siam* (London: Lloyd's Greater Britain, 1908), 134, 275.

77. See, for example, *BT*, May 9, 1894 and *BT*, June 20, 1898.

78. John Barrett, "Street and Other Railways in Siam," *Street Railway Journal* 13, no. 7 (1897): 400. This designation may be apocryphal—or was perhaps an interim appointment—as the position was most likely occupied by Admiral de Richelieu, the founder and holder of the concession.

79. "Supreme Court," *Straits Times Weekly Issue*, July 5, 1892, 3.

80. "Supreme Court," *Straits Times Weekly Issue*, July 5, 1892, 3.

81. "Supreme Court," *Straits Times Weekly Issue*, July 5, 1892, 3.

82. On Gowan's service to the king, see NA R5 S 24/2.

83. *BT*, February 16, 1899; *BT*, April 28, 1899.

84. *BT*, June 20, 1895.

85. *BT*, June 20, 1895.

86. *BT*, June 20, 1895.

87. Benton, *Law and Colonial Cultures*, 29.

88. See, for example, Sheila Jasanoff, "Bhopal's Trials of Knowledge and Ignorance," *Isis* 98, no. 2 (2007): 346.

89. Harding, "The Eclipse," 307.

90. Bruno Latour, "Postmodern? No, Simply Amodern. Steps Towards an Anthropology of Science: An Essay Review," *Studies in History and Philosophy of Science* 21, no. 1 (1990): 147.

91. Will Hanley, *Identifying with Nationality: Europeans, Ottomans, and Egyptians in Alexandria* (New York: Columbia University Press, 2017), 31.

92. Bruno Latour, "Morality and Technology: The End of the Means," trans. Couze Venn, *Theory, Culture & Society* 19, no. 5–6 (2002).

93. Matthew P. Fitzpatrick, ed., *Liberal Imperialism in Europe* (New York: Palgrave Macmillan, 2012).

94. On the former, see Jennifer Pitts, *A Turn to Empire: The Rise of Imperial Liberalism in Britain and France* (Princeton, NJ: Princeton University Press, 2006).

95. Kolsky, *Colonial Justice*; Shannon Lee Dawdy, *Building the Devil's Empire: French Colonial New Orleans* (Chicago: University of Chicago Press, 2008).

96. Darryl E. Flaherty has provided a complementary analysis in *Public Law, Private Practice: Politics, Profit, and the Legal Profession in Nineteenth-Century Japan* (Cambridge, MA: Harvard University Press, 2013), 11–26.

4. Accidental Metaphysics

1. David Delaney, "Making Nature / Marking Humans: Law as a Site of (Cultural) Production," *Annals of the Association of American Geographers* 91, no. 3 (2001).

2. Nancy A. Weston, "The Metaphysics of Modern Tort Theory," *Valparaiso University Law Review* 28, no. 3 (1994).

3. Bruno Latour, *We Have Never Been Modern* (Cambridge, MA: Harvard University Press, 1993).

4. Cooter, "The Moment," 116.

5. Judith Green, "Accidents: The Remnants of a Modern Classificatory System," in *Accidents in History*, ed. Roger Cooter and Bill Luckin (Atlanta: Editions Rodopi, 1997), 49.

6. Green, "Accidents."

7. John C. Burnham, *Accident Prone: A History of Technology, Psychology, and Misfits of the Machine Age* (Chicago: University of Chicago Press, 2009).

8. François Ewald, *L'Etat Providence* (Paris: B. Grasset, 1986); François Ewald, "The Return of Descartes' Malicious Demon: An Outline of a Philosophy of Precaution," in *Embracing Risk: The Changing Culture of Insurance and Responsibility*, ed. Tom Baker and Jonathan Simon (Chicago: University of Chicago Press, 2002).

9. David Wade Chambers and Richard Gillespie, "Locality in the History of Science: Colonial Science, Technoscience, and Indigenous Knowledge," *Osiris* 15, no. 1 (2000): 229.

10. Carol Gluck, "Words in Motion," in *Words in Motion: Toward a Global Lexicon*, ed. Carol Gluck and Anna Lowenhaupt Tsing (Durham, NC: Duke University Press, 2009), 5.

11. E. B. Michell, *A Siamese-English Dictionary for the Use of Students in Both Languages* (Freeport, NY: Books for Libraries Press, 1973 [1892]).

12. Further evidence of Michell's practical struggle to mediate Western law in the Siamese context can be found the marginalia of his personal copy of *The Directory for*

Bangkok and Siam Directory for the Year 1892 (Bangkok: Bangkok Times, [1892]), where he scribbled notes about specific aspects of Siamese civil and penal law (see the first page of the "Advertisements" section after the final appendix). The volume, which is part of Cornell's Kroch collection, bears the initials "E.B.M." in the inside front cover.

13. Michell, *A Siamese-English Dictionary*, 36.

14. Michell, *A Siamese-English Dictionary*.

15. Michell, *A Siamese-English Dictionary*, 151.

16. Michell, *A Siamese-English Dictionary*, xviii.

17. Michell, *A Siamese-English Dictionary*, xviii.

18. Henry Alabaster, *The Wheel of Law: Buddhism Illustrated from Siamese Sources* (London: Trübner & Co., 1871).

19. Thiphakorawong, *Nangsue sadaeng kitchanukit* [*A book explaining various things*] (Bangkok: Khuru Sapha, 1971 [1867]).

20. Craig J. Reynolds, "Buddhist Cosmography in Thai History, with Special Reference to Nineteenth-Century Culture Change," *Journal of Asian Studies* 35, no. 2 (1976): 214–18.

21. Alabaster, *The Wheel of Law*, 223, 236.

22. Gregory Schopen, "Archaeology and Protestant Presuppositions in the Study of Indian Buddhism," *History of Religions* 31, no. 1 (1991).

23. Samuel J. Smith, *A Comprehensive Anglo-Siamese Dictionary* (Bangkok: Bangkolem Press, 1899 [1899–1908]); see vol. 3, 89 and vol. 4, 132.

24. "*Phu rue sing thi tham khwan khrueang chai hai kae phit khlat*" (Smith, *A Comprehensive Anglo-Siamese Dictionary*, vol. 1, 775). It should be noted, however, that in some ways Smith's dictionary offers a divergent view of the subject of civil legal actions in his translation of the civil wrong of "libel." In Smith's work, libel is no longer an action against the *khwan*, but is instead against the person ("*than phu uen*," 357).

25. Samuel Gamble McFarland and George B. McFarland, *An English-Siamese Dictionary Containing 14,000 Words and Idiomatic Expressions* (Bangkok: American Presbyterian Mission Press, 1903) draws on Samuel Gamble McFarland, *An English-Siamese Dictionary* (Bangkok: American Presbyterian Mission Press, 1865). George McFarland later published an expanded version in Bangkok in 1941, which was republished in the United States beginning in 1944; see George Bradley McFarland, *Thai-English Dictionary* (Stanford, CA: Stanford University Press, 1960); especially Mary R. Haas, "Foreword to the Second Printing."

26. McFarland, *Thai-English Dictionary*, 144–45; Mary R. Haas's review, "*Thai-English Dictionary* by George Bradley McFarland," *Journal of the American Oriental Society* 65 (1945): 270–73, esp. 270.

27. Mary R. Haas's reivew, "*Thai-English Dictionary* by George Bradley McFarland," 270.

28. George B. McFarland, *Thai-English Dictionary*, 489.

29. For modern Thai law codes on tort and compensation, see *Thailand Civil and Commercial Code, Title V: Wrongful Acts*. See also David M. Engel and Jaruwan S. Engel, *Tort, Custom, and Karma: Globalization and Legal Consciousness in Thailand* (Stanford, CA: Stanford University Press, 2010), 53–54; and Isara Lovanich, "Personal Injury and Damages for Non-Pecuniary Loss in the Law of Torts and the Product Liability Law" (MA thesis, Thammasat University, 2011).

30. "Tramway Concession, Bangkok, 5th May 1887" (NA Microfilm R5 N/128).

31. NA R5 N 21/1, 27ff.; clause 6, which mentions "Acts of God," appears on p. 40.

32. "*Het thi koed khuen, het kan thi koed*"; Prayut Payutto, *Photjanukrom phutthasasanam chabab pramuan sap* [*Dictionary of the Buddhist religion, collected terms*] (Bangkok: Maha Chulalongkorn University, 2527 [1984]), 433.

33. Margaret Cone, *A Dictionary of Pāli, Part I* (Oxford: Pali Text Society, 2001), 493–94.

34. T. W. Rhys Davis and William Stede, *The Pali-English Dictionary* (London: Luzac, 1959 [1921]), 151, 733.

35. Steven Collins, *A Pali Grammar for Students* (Chiang Mai, Thailand: Silkworm, 2005), 131–32.

36. "*Khuan thetsana hai mo kae upattihetu khue sadaeng tham hai khao kap rueang thi koet khuen*"; Payutto, *Photjanukrom*, 433 (my emphasis).

37. *Pali-English Dictionary*, 733, 384. The *Visuddhimagga* seems to confirm this early conflation of the terms; see George D. Bond, *The Word of the Buddha: The Tipiṭaka and Its Interpretation in Theravada Buddhism* (Colombo: Gunasena, 1982), 130.

38. Edmund Hardy, ed., *The Netti-Pakaraṇa, with Extracts from Dhammpāla's Commentary* (London: Pali Text Society, 1961 [1902]), 78. For an English translation, see *The Guide (Netti-Pakaraṇaṁ) according to Kaccāna Thera*, trans. Bhikkhu Ñāṇamoli (London: Pali Text Society, 1977 [1962]), 109–10.

39. See *The Guide (Netti-Pakaraṇaṁ)*, 111, n. 456/2; and Rhys Davids and Stede, *Pali-English Dictionary*, 733, which cites evidence from the *Abhidhamma* as confirmation of *hetu* as a kind of "moral condition."

40. In the early twentieth century, efforts to localize new concepts through translation, transliteration, and neologisms would be centralized in state institutions like The Royal Institute (Ratchabanditaya sathan). See Prince Wan Waithayakon, "Thai Word Coining," *Journal of the Siam Society* 89 (2001): 90–93 and Nitaya Kanchanawan, "Changing to the New World: High-tech Verbalization in Thai," in *Papers from the Fourth Annual Meeting of the Southeast Asian Linguistics Society*, ed. Udom Warotamasikkhadit and Thanyarat Panakul (Phoenix: Arizona State University, Program for Southeast Asian Studies, 1998), 143–56.

41. Prayut, *Photjanukrom*, 433.

42. Another Pali-Thai dictionary ignores the mismatch between the original Pali meaning of the word and its connotations in contemporary Thai; see Prince Kitiyakara Krommaphra Chandaburinarunath, *Pathanukrom bali thai angkrit sansakrit* [Pali-Thai-English-Sanskrit dictionary] (Bangkok: King Mahamakut's Academy, 1977).

43. Wolfgang Schivelbusch, *The Railway Journey: The Industrialization of Time and Space in the 19th Century* (Berkeley: University of California Press, 1987), 127.

44. "*Kan-sueng koet thi mai mai ru kon*," *English and Siamese Vocabulary* (Bangkok: American Presbyterian Mission Press, 1865), 5.

45. McFarland and McFarland, *An English-Siamese Dictionary*. Samuel compiled the dictionary in the 1860s and his son, George, who worked as a physician and professor at the Royal Medical College in Bangkok, later expanded on it; see George Bradley McFarland, *Thai-English Dictionary* (Stanford, CA: Stanford University Press, 1960 [1941]). By the mid-twentieth century, there was greater consistency concerning the translation of "accident"; the younger McFarland's edition of the dictionary contains a subentry for "*ubatihet*," which he defines as "an accident; a causal incident; an accidental event" (*Thai-English Dictionary*, 1006).

46. Michell, *A Siamese-English Dictionary*, xvii, 310.

47. Jean Baptiste Pallegoix, *Sapha phajana phasa thai: Dictionarium Linguae Thai* (Paris, 1854), 842. The title itself seems ahistorical in its reference to the language as "Thai." Along with the subtitle of the dictionary, "Sive Siamensis" [without Siamese], this seems to suggest that Pallegoix compiled his dictionary with a view to excluding certain (antiquated or colloquial?) aspects of the language.

48. Jean Baptiste Pallegoix, *Siphot phasa thai: Siamese-French-English Dictionary*, ed. J. L. Vey (Bangkok: Printing Office of the Catholic Mission, 1896), 1085.

49. *"Nan khue wa antarai tam bali"*; J. Caswell and J. H. Chandler, *A Dictionary of the Siamese Language* (Bangkok: Chulalongkorn University Press, 2544 [2001] [1846]), 960.

50. Luang Ratanayatti (Sangop), *Dikchanari phasa angkrit plae pen thai: English-Siamese Dictionary* (Krungthep: *Rong phim luang, Ro. So.* 120 [1901]), 6. Ratanyatti uses the same term to define the word "casualty" (75).

51. King Chulalongkorn, *"Wa duai het haeng khwam tai nai tham klang ayu"* ["Concerning the causes of death in middle age"], *Wachirayan wiset* (2431 [1888]).

52. Which is not to say, however, that elites did not suffer accidental deaths. In one well-known incident, one of King Chulalongkorn's consorts, Queen Sunantha, a younger sister of Queen Saowapha, lost her life in a boating mishap while traveling by river barge to the retreat palace at Bang Pa-In in 1880. See Prayut Sithiphan, *"Khadi phra nang rua lom"* ["The case of the capsized princess"], in *San thai nai adit* [Thai courts in the past], 2nd ed. (Bangkok: Sang san buk: 2551 [2008]), 227–36; and Nonthaphorn Yumangmi, *"Wipayok klang sai nam kap ruang lao 'Sadet mae Sunantha"* ["Tragedy in Mid-Stream and the Story of 'Royal Mother Sunantha'"], *Sinlapa watthanantham* 31, no. 1 (2009): 76–101.

53. Bernard S. Cohn, *Colonialism and Its Forms of Knowledge: The British in India* (Princeton, NJ: Princeton University Press, 1996), 5.

54. "Mr. A. J. A. Jardine: Officer Who Reorganised Siam Police," *Straits Times*, October 2, 1914, 2.

55. A. J. A. Jardine, *Report on the Police Administration of Bangkok, Suburbs, and Railway Divisions for 1898–1899* (NA R5 N/96, box 6), 4.

56. The numbers in the suburban and railway divisions of the metropolitan police force were far worse according to Jardine (*Report . . . for 1898–1899*, 16).

57. See the Thai-language translation of Jardine's *Report . . . for 1898–1899* at NA R5 N 8.6/3, 29–30.

58. Heather Streets-Salter, *Martial Races: The Military, Race, and Masculinity in British Imperial Culture, 1857–1914* (Manchester: Manchester University Press, 2004).

59. Jardine, *Report . . . for 1898–1899*, 86.

60. Hong Lysa, "Indian Police Subalterns in King Chulalongkorn's Kingdom: Turn of the Twentieth Century Bangkok Pantomime," in *Khu khwam phumjai* [With pride], ed. Sirilak Sampatchalit and Siriporn Yodkamolsat (Bangkok: Sansan, 2545 [2002]). French observers took this as an affront; they considered the Siamese police force to be a de facto standing British army in the Mekhong Valley, which was in direct conflict with treaty provisions concerning Siam's independence ("The French Authorities and the Police," *BT*, December 20, 1898).

61. Jardine, *Report . . . for 1898–1899*, 89.

62. Jardine, *Report . . . for 1898–1899*, 89. On police manuals of the sort envisioned by Jardine, see Lim, *Siam's New Detectives*.

63. Jardine, *Report . . . for 1898–1899*, 40.

64. Jardine had evidently been successful at getting a legal measure called the "Secret Societies Act" passed to address this issue, but he noted with frustration that little had been done in the way of enforcement (Jardine, *Report . . . for 1898–1899*, 40, 49).

65. Kim A. Wagner, *Stranglers and Bandits: A Historical Anthology of Thuggee* (New York: Oxford University Press, 2009).

66. Jardine, *Report . . . for 1898–1899*, 88.

67. Jardine, *Report . . . for 1898–1899*, 89.

68. Jardine, *Report . . . for 1898–1899*, 89.

69. Engel, *Law and Kingship*, 23.

70. Jardine, *Report . . . for 1898–1899*, 1.

71. See, for example, Ian Hacking, *The Taming of Chance* (Cambridge: Cambridge University Press, 1990); Mary Poovey, *A History of the Modern Fact: Problems of Knowledge in the Science of Wealth and Society* (Chicago: University of Chicago Press, 1998); and Tong Lam, *A Passion for Facts: Social Surveys and the Construction of the Chinese Nation-State, 1900–1949* (Berkeley: University of California Press, 2011).

72. Burney, *Bodies of Evidence*, 3, 65.

73. Jardine, *Report . . . for 1898–1899*, 77.

74. Jardine, *Report . . . for 1898–1899*, 77. Inquest records for the Ministry of the Capital confirm Jardine's description of opium-eater's dysentery: "habitual opium eaters become poor, are unable to purchase the drug, and from the want of it get dysentry [*sic*] and die very suddenly" (77). Habitual opium users suffered from chronic constipation, but when they lost access to the drug the opposite condition set in, often with fatal consequences.

75. A. J. A. Jardine, *Report on the Police Administration of Bangkok, Suburbs, and Railway Divisions for 1899–1900* (N R5 N/6–97, 90, 94).

76. Jardine, *Report on the Police Administration, 1899–1900*, 94.

77. Jardine, *Report on the Police Administration, 1899–1900*, 94.

78. *BT*, May 11, 1899.

79. "*Banchi khon thi tai doi 'aek si den' nai pi 118*" (NA R5 N 8.6/5, 105).

80. Michel Foucault, "Governmentality," in *Power: Essential Works of Foucault, 1954–1984*, vol. 3, ed. James D. Faubion (London: Penguin, 2001).

81. On Farr's contributions to "British vital statistics," see Hacking, *The Taming of Chance*, 53. On John Snow's work in epidemiology, see Steven Johnson, *The Ghost Map: The Story of London's Most Terrifying Epidemic and How it Changed Science, Cities, and the Modern World* (New York: Riverhead Books, 2007).

82. Green, "Accidents: The Remnants," 49. See also Geoffrey C. Bowker and Susan Leigh Star, *Sorting Things Out: Classification and Its Consequences* (Cambridge, MA: MIT Press, 1999).

83. Michel Foucault's ideas from *The History of Sexuality, Volume 1: An Introduction* (New York: Vintage, 1990 [1978]), quoted in Brain C. J. Singer and Lorna Weir, "Politics and Sovereign Power: Considerations on Foucault," *European Journal of Social Theory* 9, no. 4 (2006): 450.

84. Jardine, *Report . . . for 1898–1899*, 89.

85. *BT*, April 18, 1900.

86. *BT*, August 21, 1901.

87. *BT*, August 21, 1901.

88. The suggestion that a particular driver might have been more prone to accidents than another is likewise an idea with its own peculiar cultural histories; see Burnham, *Accident Prone*.

89. *BT*, September 18, 1901.

90. *BT*, September 18, 1901.

91. *BT*, September 18, 1901.

92. "Shocking Accident," *BT*, February 8, 1899.

93. "A New Danger in Klong Kut Mai," *BT*, February 8, 1899; *BT*, February 9, 1899.

94. "Shocking Accident," *BT*, February 8, 1899.

95. "Shocking Accident," *BT*, February 8, 1899.

96. *BT*, February 15, 1899.

97. See, respectively, Pallegoix, *Sapha phajana*, 130, 405, 769, 775.

98. Pallegoix, *Sapha phajana*, passim (e.g., 181, 188, 195, 222, 397, 477, 576, 837, 877, 884).

99. Pallegoix, *Siphot phasa thai*, 768. Prayut Payutto notes that the Thai term *pramat* comes from the Pali *pamâda*, meaning heedlessness, carelessness, negligence, indolence, remissness (*Potjanukrom putthasat chabab pramuan tham* [Bangkok: Mahachulalongkorn University, 2528 (1985)], 389). He defines this original Pali sense of the term as equivalent to the contemporary Thai terms: *khwam loen loe, khwam phloe, khwam khat sati, khwam ploi pla la loei* (149).

100. Pallegoix, *Siphot phasa thai*, 768.

101. Michell, *A Siamese-English Dictionary*, 150.

102. Ratanayatti, *Dikchanari phasa angkrit*, 332. There is the possibility, however, that the association of *pramat* with (*khwam*) *loen loe* in legalistic terminology was a later development, and that at the turn of the twentieth century *khwam loen loe* retained a fundamentally colloquial sense. The early dictionary of the Presbyterian Mission in Siam (1865), for example, defines "negligence" as *khwam loen loe* (*English and Siamese Vocabulary*, 193).

103. "Negligence" appears in volume 3 of Smith's five-volume dictionary, which was published in 1905 (*A Comprehensive Dictionary Vol. III*, 682). "Negligence" remains ill-defined in the modern Thai Civil and Commercial Code, leaving legal scholars to work with a comparable definition from the Penal Code; see Engel and Engel, *Tort, Custom, Karma*, 53. See also Engel, "Landscapes of the Law," 75.

104. *BT* 5 March 1900, 2.

105. Engel, *Law and Kingship*, 68–69. For more detailed information on the establishment and jurisdiction of these courts, see *Prachum kotmai prajam sok* (Collected laws, arranged chronologically), ed. Sathian Wichailak (Bangkok: Niti Wet, 1935–1953), vols. 14–15.

106. *BT*, March 5, 1900.

107. *BT*, March 13, 1900.

108. *BT*, March 13, 1900.

109. "Tramway Concession" (NA R5 N 21/1).

110. *BT*, March 13, 1900, 2.

111. *BT*, March 13, 1900, 2.

112. *BT*, November 13, 1901.

113. *BT*, February 15, 1899.

114. Evans-Pritchard, *Witchcraft, Oracles and Magic among the Azande* (Oxford: Clarendon Press, 1937) is the locus classicus. See also Jean Comaroff and John

Comaroff, eds., *Modernity and Its Malcontents: Ritual and Power in Postcolonial Africa* (Chicago: University of Chicago Press, 1993); Peter Geschiere, "Witchcraft and the Limits of the Law: Cameroon and South Africa," in *Law and Disorder in the Postcolony*, ed. Jean Comaroff and John Comaroff (Chicago: University of Chicago Press, 2006). See also, Nile Green's exploration of moral competition in a cosmopolitan colonial port in *Bombay Islam: The Religious Economy of the West Indian Ocean, 1840–1915* (Cambridge: Cambridge University Press, 2011), esp. introduction and chap. 2.

115. Engel and Engel, *Tort, Custom, Karma*, passim.

116. Latour, *We Have Never Been Modern*, passim.

117. Cohn, *Colonialism and Its Forms*, 4.

118. Cohn, *Colonialism and Its Forms*, 4.

119. Chakrabarty, *Provincializing Europe*, xii.

5. Morbid Subjects

1. Nigel Brailey, ed., *The Satow Siam Papers: The Private Diaries and Correspondence of Ernest Satow, Vol. 1, 1884–1885* (Bangkok: The Historical Society under the Patronage of H.R.H. Princess Maha Chakri Sirindhorn, 1997), 15. Thanks to Chalong Soontravanich for suggesting this source.

2. Burney, *Bodies of Evidence*, 23–28.

3. Burney, *Bodies of Evidence*, 16–51.

4. Warwick Anderson, *Colonial Pathologies: American Tropical Medicine, Race, and Hygiene in the Philippines* (Durham, NC: Duke University Press, 2006), 74–103; David Arnold, *Colonizing the Body: State Medicine and Epidemic Disease in Nineteenth-Century India* (Berkeley: University of California Press, 1993), 42.

5. Meghan Vaughan, *Curing Their Ills: Colonial Power and African Illness* (Stanford, CA: Stanford University Press, 1991).

6. Kolsky, *Colonial Justice*, 135; Jordanna Bailkin, "The Boot and the Spleen: When Was Murder Possible in British India?," *Comparative Studies in Society and History* 48 (2006). While citing cases that seem to corroborate the sense of injustice associated with colonial consular courts, Will Hanley also challenges that narrative in *Identifying with Nationality: Europeans, Ottomans, and Egyptians in Alexandria* (New York: Columbia University Press, 2017), 155–72.

7. Loos, *Subject Siam*, 42–44; Hong Lysa, "Extraterritoriality in Bangkok in the Reign of King Chulalongkorn, 1868–1910: The Cacophonies of Semi-Colonial Cosmopolitanism," *Itinerario: European Journal of Overseas History* 27 (2003).

8. Bernstein, "The Post-Soviet Treasure Hunt," 624.

9. Mbembe, "Necropolitics," 11. Mbembe's theory is formulated in response to major works on violence and sovereignty, including Giorgio Agamben, *Homo Sacer: Sovereign Power and Bare Life* (Stanford, CA: Stanford University Press, 1998); and Michel Foucault, *"Society Must Be Defended": Lectures at the Collège de France, 1975–76* (New York: Picador, 2003).

10. Jeshuran Chandran, "British Foreign Policy and the Extraterritorial Question in Siam, 1891–1900," *Journal of the Malaysian Branch of the Royal Asiatic Society* 38 (1965): 290.

11. *BT*, August 6, 1892.

12. Trial by jury was itself a facet of the British legal system without precedent in a Siamese legal context.

13. *BT*, August 6, 1892.

14. Norman Chevers, *A Manual of Medical Jurisprudence for Bengal and the North-Western Provinces* (Calcutta: F. Carbery, 1856), 358–59.

15. Pasuk Phongpaichit and Chris Baker, *Thailand: Economy and Politics*, 2nd ed. (Oxford: Oxford University Press, 2002), 95–107.

16. William G. Skinner, *Chinese Society in Thailand: An Analytical History* (Ithaca, NY: Cornell University Press, 1957); Vikrom Koompirocana, "Siam in British Foreign Policy, 1855–1938: The Acquisition and the Relinquishment of British Extra-territorial Rights" (PhD diss., Michigan State University, 1972), 109–24.

17. *BT*, August 28, 1896 (original emphasis). Not long after, one particular case of false registration would provoke the ire of the English-language press in Bangkok: a man named Kadir (alias "Nai Day"), the son of a Siamese official, was able to register himself as a (Cambodian) French protégé while working as captain of a French vessel (*BT*, September 11, 1896).

18. Chandran, "British Foreign Policy," 300.

19. Hong Lysa, "Stranger within the Gates," 333. These figures also hint at the paucity of the available pool of British-born jurors in Siam.

20. Chandran, "British Foreign Policy," 303; Strate, *The Lost Territories*, 32–33. This seems to have been true in other jurisdictions as well; see David Todd, "Beneath Sovereignty: Extraterritoriality and Imperial Internationalism in Nineteenth-Century Egypt," *Law & History Review* 36, no. 1 (2018): 119–21.

21. Chandran, "British Foreign Policy," 295.

22. Strate, *The Lost Territories*, 32.

23. Brailey, *The Satow Siam Papers*, 106–10. Chandran argues that this softening of the imperial stance was in part due to the perceived threat of German imperial designs on the Malay Peninsula ("British Foreign Policy," 294).

24. Chandran, "British Foreign Policy," 297.

25. Chandran, "British Foreign Policy," 292.

26. Akiko Iijima, "The 'International Court.'"

27. Hong, "Extraterritoriality in Bangkok," 126. A telegram (# 10565) dated 17 December 1896 and sent from London to the Siamese Ministry of Foreign Affairs further confirms this was a pressing issue for the state (NA R5 M.5.1ป/6).

28. Bailkin, "The Boot and the Spleen," 473.

29. *BT*, May 16, 1898.

30. See, for example, *BT*, August 23, 1893; *BT*, May 18, 1895; *BT*, June 9, 1898; *BT*, February 3, 1899.

31. Ann Laura Stoler, *Carnal Knowledge and Imperial Power: Race the Intimate in Colonial Rule* (Berkeley: University of California Press, 2002), 24 (emphasis in original). The title of the next section is a play on Stoler's seminal work *Carnal Knowledge and Imperial Power*.

32. "*Duai thuk wan ni mak ja mi khadi khwam thi khon nai bang khap tang prathet kha khon fai sayam tai boi boi khon fai sayam tong pen jot fong khwam yang san kong sun hai phijarana tam nangsue sanya*" (NA R5 S.Th. 8.2.ฉ/1).

33. Loos, *Subject Siam*, 43–45, 107. For a near-contemporaneous articulation of this logic by a sympathetic observer, see P. W. Thornely, *The History of a Transition* (Bangkok: Siam Observer Press, 1923), 119.

34. *"Fai kong sun tat sin khadi doi kotmai nana prathet mai fang ao kham chanasut phlik sop khong phanak ngan amphoe pen lakthan phro wa mai sap akan chat wa tai duai het prakan dai"* (NA R5 S.Th. 8.2.ฌ/1).

35. *"Tha khwam rueang dai fai sayam mai dai hai phaet truat chanasut pha sop jaeng akan thi tai nan laeo kong sun ko yok khwam sia"* (NA R5 S.Th. 8.2.ฌ/1).

36. *"Pen kan-thi khon fai sayam sia priap khon tang prathet yu"* (NA R5 S.Th. 8.2.ฌ/1).

37. The terms recur, sometimes with slight variation, including references to Thai people (*khon thai*, as opposed to *khon* or *fai sayam*), in the correspondence as evidenced below.

38. *"kho phra ratchathan phra borom ratchanuyat hai kong trawaen riak phaet pai pha sop thi mi antarai duai khon sapyek tang prathet kratham rai nan phrom duai amphoe"* (NA R5 S.Th. 8.2.ฌ/1, letter dated December 7, 1892).

39. Fred W. Riggs, *Thailand: The Modernization of a Bureaucratic Polity* (Honolulu: East-West Center, 1966), 117.

40. In the coming years, the oversight of ecclesiastical matters would take a secondary role to education, and in 1902 the Ministry of Religious Affairs (*krasuang thammakan*) would become the Ministry of Education/Public Instruction (*krasuang sueksathikan*); see David K. Wyatt, *The Politics of Reform in Thailand: Education in the Reign of King Chulalongkorn* (New Haven, CT: Yale University Press, 1969), 234.

41. *BT*, April 1, 1893.

42. *"Mo he [Hays] dai rap ngoen duean pen mo nai krom phayaban khuan pen na thi chanasut sop tam het thi krom phayaban pen na thi samrap raksa khai jep khong mahachon nan"* (NA R5 S.Th. 8.2.ฌ/1, letter dated December 7, 1892).

43. NA R5 S.Th. 8.2.ฌ/1, letter dated December 16, 1892.

44. *"Nakrian rongrian phaetyakon thi mi khwam-ru phuea ja tham kan dai ko mi yu lai khon khuan ja hai nak rian pai truat pha sop tam thi krasuang mueang kho ma"* (NA R5 S. Th. 8.2.ฌ/1, letter dated December 16, 1892).

45. Although traditional Siamese legal codes such as the Law of the Three Seals contained elaborate discussions of evidence, including the rules pertaining to potential witnesses, the first formal law of evidence composed according to Western models was not promulgated until February 1895 (*BT*, February 14, 1895).

46. *"Tha pen kan-yai kan-samkhan ja hai mo he [Hays] rue phaet yurop khon nueng khon dai pai chuai truat"* (NA R5 S.Th. 8.2.ฌ/1, letter dated December 17, 1892).

47. *"Mai jam pho tae khon tang prathet kha khon thai yang diao thueng phrai fa pra ratchakon duai kan"* (NA R5 S.Th. 8.2.ฌ/1, letter dated December 17, 1892).

48. Nai Chum, among the inaugural students at the Royal Medical College, cited (and reproduced) his contract when he attempted to appeal his first civil service assignment after graduation in March 1893 (NA R5 S.Th. 8/1).

49. Tony Day and Craig J. Reynolds, "Cosmologies, Truth Regimes, and the State in Southeast Asia," *Modern Asian Studies* 34 (2000); see also Quentin (Trais) Pearson, "'DNA Evidence Cannot Lie': Forensic Science, Truth Regimes, and Civic Epistemology in Thai History," in *Global Forensic Cultures: Making Fact and Justice in the Modern Era*, ed. Ian Burney and Christopher Hamlin (Baltimore: Johns Hopkins University Press, 2019).

50. Jurgen Habermas, *The Structural Transformation of the Public Sphere: An Inquiry into a Category of Bourgeois Society*, trans. Thomas Burger with Frederick Lawrence (Cambridge, MA: MIT Press, 1989), 27–56; Thanapol Limaphichart, "The Emergence

of the Siamese Public Sphere: Colonial Modernity, Print Culture, and the Practice of Criticism (1860s–1910s)," *South East Asia Research* 17 (2009).

51. Burney, *Bodies of Evidence*, 16–51.

52. Cf. Bruno Latour, "When Things Strike Back: A Possible Contribution of 'Science Studies' to the Social Sciences," *British Journal of Sociology* 51 (2000): 115.

53. *"Phu thi pha truat sop ja pen phaet thai rue phaet yurop ko dai khap pha jao mai mi khwam-rang kiat sing dai loei tae phaet phu thi ja truat pha nan tong pen phaet thi mi khwam-ru pho thi ja bok het haeng akan tai hai san kong sun tang prathet chuea thao nan"* (NA R5 S.Th. 8.2.ฎ/1, letter dated January 14, 1893).

54. *"Phuea mi hai kong sun yok het khuen tad sin khwam haeng akan tai dang chen thi khoei tat sin hai yok khwam sia"* (NA R5 S.Th. 8.2.ฎ/1, letter dated January 14, 1893).

55. Naret refers to such documents as "a report of the findings of the autopsy" (*"nangsue rai ngan jaeng khwam tam het thi truat dai"*). The notion of a formal medicolegal document recording the cause of death, a death certificate, had apparently not yet entered the lexicon of Siamese officials. It would soon appear (in transliteration) in the "Death by various causes" archives once formal autopsies began in May 1896 (chap. 6).

56. *"Hai tham rai ngan jaeng khwam tam het thi truat dai"* (NA R5 S.Th. 8.2.ฎ/1, letter dated December 7, 1892).

57. NA R5 S.Th. 8/9.

58. NA R5 S.Th. 8/9, letter dated June 4, 1893.

59. *"Khran ja jang hai mo he [Hays] pha sop ko pen ngoen mak nak hen wa prayot thi ja dai sap mai thao kan thi ja sia ngoen"* (NA R5 S.Th. 8/9, letter dated June 4, 1893).

60. *"Jam tong rip jad kan rueang phaet truat sop hai pen thi man khong sia jueng ja di tha mai rip jad mi het to pai na ja sia kan"* (NA R5 S.Th. 8/9, letter dated June 4, 1893).

61. NA R5 S.Th. 8/9, 1. Damrong Phaetyakhun (Chuen Phuthaphaet, 1881–1953), was later elevated in rank to *phraya* (1923) and served as the first dean of the Faculty of Medicine at Chulalongkorn University (1947–1950).

62. NA R5 S.Th. 8/9, 4; letter dated two days later, on June 6, 1893.

63. *"Hen duai klao wa luang damrong thueng rian phaet dai nangsue samkhan ko jing tae pen kha thun la ong thuli phrabat pen khon thai"* (NA R5 S.Th. 8/9, 4; letter dated two days later, on June 6, 1893).

64. Pauline Kusiak, "Instrumentalized Rationality, Cross-Cultural Mediators, and Civil Epistemologies of Late Colonialism," *Social Studies of Science* 40, no. 6 (2010): 873.

65. Note that these circumstances were not as unique as they might seem. As Will Hanley has recently argued, different gradations of political belonging and their attendant rights and privileges tended to collapse when applied to the "international sphere . . . outside the home state"; see his *Identifying with Nationality*, 59.

66. Vincanne Adams and Warwick Anderson, "Pramoedya's Chickens: Postcolonial Studies of Technoscience," in *The Handbook of Science and Technology Studies*, 3rd ed., ed. Edward J. Hackett et al. (Cambridge, MA: MIT Press, 2008), 188.

67. On the former, see B. J. Terwiel, *Through Traveller's Eyes: An Approach to Early Nineteenth-Century Thai History* (Bangkok: Duang Kamol, 1989). On the latter, see Charles F. Keyes, "Presidential Address: 'The Peoples of Asia'—Science and Politics in the Classification of Ethnic Groups in Thailand, China, and Vietnam," *Journal of Asian Studies* 61, no. 4 (2002): 1177–81; David Streckfuss, "The Mixed Colonial Legacy in

Siam: Origins of Thai Racialist Thought, 1890–1910," in *Autonomous Histories, Particular Truths: Essays in the Honor of John R. W. Smail*, ed. Laurie Sears (Madison, WI: Centre for Southeast Asian Studies, 1993); and Thongchai Winichakul, "The Others Within: Travel and Ethno-Spatial Differentiation of Siamese Subjects, 1883–1910," in *Civility and Savagery: Social Identity in Tai States*, ed. Andrew Turton (Richmond, Surrey: Curzon, 2000).

68. Please consult the discussion of these trends in chapter 1 for sources.

69. Wyatt, *Thailand*, 217.

70. Mbembe, "Necropolitics," 25–26.

71. Weber, "Politics as Vocation."

6. Incisions and Inscriptions

1. NA R5 N 23/64.

2. NA R5 N 23/64.

3. NA R5 N 23/64, 4.

4. Documents concerning the death of Amdaeng Si appear at both NA R5 N 23/64 and NA R5 N 23/67.

5. "*Muea pha laeo ko dai phop akan rok khong khao [khao] dai tai doi pen rok nai pod lae pen rok nai hua jai*" (NA R5 N 23/67).

6. "*Mo nai tin gen* [Nightingale] *pha sop truat do ko ha dai khwam wa pen arai tai mai mo dai ao krapho ahan pai truat ik*" (NA R5 N 23/64, 3). It would not be the last time that Nightingale would remove the stomach from a cadaver in the wake of an (apparently inconclusive) autopsy at the police hospital; see NA R5 N 23/124 and NA R5 N 23/135.

7. "Autopsy," from the original Greek roots, had the etymological sense of seeing (*optos*) for one's self (*autos*).

8. Tony Walter, "Mediator Deathworks," *Death Studies* 29, no. 5 (2005).

9. *BT*, August 31, 1892.

10. *BT*, August 31, 1892.

11. See Naret's original proposal concerning the position of the Chief Physician (*phaet yai*) (NA R5 N 8.1/1).

12. *BT*, September 9, 1898.

13. Charles Mosley, ed., *Burke's Peerage, Baronetage & Knightage*, 107th ed. (Wilmington, DE: Genealogical Books, 2003), vol. 2, 2897–98.

14. *BT*, May 30, 1894.

15. *BT*, May 30, 1894. Dr. W. Willis was the medical attendant of record in 1894, but due to his extended absence from Siam, the American doctor T. Heyward Hays had served as "acting medical attendant" to the legation prior to Nightingale's appointment (*The Directory for Bangkok and Siam for 1894*).

16. *BT*, July 28, 1894.

17. See the listing "Physicians and Surgeons" in *The Directory for Bangkok and Siam for 1895*.

18. *BT*, September 1, 1894. The meanderings of Grant's corpse were discussed briefly in chapter 1.

19. "The Drowning Case," *BT*, September 5, 1894.

20. Anonymous, "The Press," in *Twentieth Century Impressions of Siam*, 295.

21. "The Drowning Case," *BT*, September 5, 1894. Newspaper holdings at the Thai National Archives for this period are limited to the *Bangkok Times*, so my account must rely on one side of the debate.

22. Hong Lysa, "Indian Police Subalterns," 461, 464.

23. *BT*, December 20, 1898.

24. The *Free Press*, quoted in "The Drowning Case," *BT*, September 5, 1894.

25. The *Free Press*, quoted in "The Drowning Case," *BT*, September 5, 1894.

26. *BT*, September 5, 1894.

27. Burney, *Bodies of Evidence*, 109.

28. *BT*, February 2, 1895.

29. *BT*, December 8, 1894.

30. Foreign residents demanded better oversight of the meat sold for consumption at city markets, but regulation was complicated by the fact that butchers—many of whom were foreign residents who enjoyed extraterritorial protection—enjoyed the right of refusal to pay taxes or submit to searches by Siamese authorities.

31. *BT*, March 21, 1896.

32. *BT*, December 6, 1901.

33. NA R5 N 23 / 151, 3.

34. NA R5 N 23 / 95, 7.

35. This is true even in cases where the autopsy was postponed to a later date or time; see, for example, NA R5 N 23 / 106.

36. Jonathan Saha, "'Uncivilized Practitioners': Medical Subordinates, Medico-Legal Evidence and Misconduct in Colonial Burma, 1875–1907," *South East Asia Research* 20, no. 3 (2012): 423.

37. In most cases, Meng Yim's autopsy reports were addressed to Phra Ananno-pharak, an administrative official with the police (*jao krom kong trawaen fai kong raksa*) in the Ministry of the Capital.

38. NA R5 N 23 / 135.

39. NA R5 N 23 / 135, 10.

40. NA R5 N 23 / 135, 10.

41. *"Khap pha jao mi khwam hen wa akan sueng dai tai nan tai duai fai that phikan pen phit duai bang sing thueng kranan ko di khap pha jao ja wa yang yuen hai pen nae thi diao tam thamada yang mai dai"* (NA R5 N 23 / 135, 11).

42. Jean Mulholland, "Thai Traditional Medicine: Ancient Thought and Practice in a Thai Context," *Journal of the Siam Society* 67, no. 2 (1979).

43. NA R5 N 23 / 150, 5.

44. NA R5 N 23 / 150, 5.

45. See, for example, Anderson, *Colonial Pathologies*, 74–103; Arnold, *Colonizing the Body*, 42; Vaughan, *Curing Their Ills*.

46. *"Khon phu ni hen akan pen jing dai wa* [illegible] *pen khon sup ya fin"* (NA R5 N 23 / 150, 6).

47. Susan Leigh Star and James R. Griesemer, "Institutional Ecology, 'Translation,' and Boundary Objects: Amateurs and Professionals in Berkeley's Museum of Vertebrate Zoology, 1907–39," *Social Studies of Science* 19, no. 3 (1989).

48. In the period between May 1896 and September 1898, forensic medical examinations were performed in 17 cases out of a total of 144 inquests included in the "Death by various causes" files; see NA R5 N 23 / 64 (and 67, which contains documents

pertaining to the same case); 95; 106; 121; 124; 125; 135; 150; 151; 153 (missing autopsy report); 157 (medical examination, but no autopsy); 164 (missing autopsy report); 171; 178; 183 (missing autopsy report); 193 (missing autopsy report); 198. Autopsy reports from the same period also appear in other files, including the records of the Ministry of Justice; see, for example, NA R5 Y 13.4/6, 8.

49. *"Sing an sueng boriphok ko ja mi prakot yu nai krapho ahan rue kratham hai krapho ahan lae lam sai pen antarai"* (NA R5 N 23/135, 12).

50. *"Het tai thi pen kho songsai yang ni khuan tong tai suan kho khwam doi la iad phro khwam tai pen khadi mi thot luang yu"* (NA R5 N 23/135, 12).

51. *BT*, January 31, 1898.

52. *BT*, October 3, 1899. See also Nightingale's account of the dispute in his report on the work of the Department of Local Sanitation for the year 1897 (report dated January 21, 1898; NA R5 N 5.6/2, 2–13).

53. NA R5 N 5.6/4, letter dated December 18, 117 (1898).

54. *BT*, September 9, 1898.

55. NA R5 N 5.6/4, letter dated December 18, 117 (1898).

56. *"Khat khong mai yu nai amnat,"* NA R5 N 5.6/4, letter dated December 18, 117 (1898).

57. During this time, in cases where Highet was called away on other duties, Meng Yim assisted other Western physicians in conducting autopsies at the police hospital, including a Dr. J. Ferguson Lis (NA R5 N 23/178); he also appears to have conducted autopsies by himself in at least one case (NA R5 N 23/193).

58. NA R5 N 5.6/4, letter dated July 27, 118 (1899). The event precipitating this new request seems to have been the autopsy of a thirty-one-year-old Chinese woman who died of an apparent opium overdose on 22 July 1899; see NA R5 N 23/198.

59. NA R5 N 5.6/4, letter dated July 27, 118 (1899).

60. NA R5 N 5.6/4, letter dated August 3, 1899.

61. NA R5 N 5.6/4, letter dated August 3, 1899. It should be noted, however, that this would not be the only instance of friction between Dr. Highet and his direct reports. See NA R5 N 5.3/11, regarding an incident from April 1905.

62. NA R5 N 5.6/4, letter dated August 3, 1899.

63. NA R5 N 23/210.

64. NA R5 N 23/210, 2.

65. NA R5 N 23/210, 6 (letter dated September 7, 117 [1898]).

66. *"Kan-thi ja pha sop nan lae truat sop nan ko yang mai dai rap kham sang anuyat prakan dai nai pen kan-nae non nai rawang wela ni,"* NA R5 N 23/210, 6 (letter dated September 7, 117 [1898]).

67. *"Tae wa tha khun luang mi het koet khuen nai thong thi khong khun luang laeo rap than hai khun luang jat kan tam thang ratchakan khong khun luang thoen,"* NA R5 N 23/210, 6 (letter dated September 7, 117 [1898]).

68. *"Anueng to samrap wang sop lae kan-thi ja chai samrap nai kan-pha sop rue sing khong tang tang nan ko phrom yu thi rong phayaban sala daeng nan laeo,"* NA R5 N 23/210, 6 (letter dated September 7, 117 [1898]).

69. NA R5 N 23/210, 4–5 (see note appended to Luang Wisutborihan's report).

70. *"To samrap pha sop nan dai nam pai wai thi sala daeng laeo tae kham sang doem yang mai dai thon,"* NA R5 N 23/210, 5.

71. Bruno Latour, *Reassembling the Social: An Introduction to Actor-Network-Theory* (Oxford: Oxford University Press, 2007), 68.

72. Latour, *Introduction to Actor-Network-Theory* (my emphasis).

73. See, for example, NA R5 N 23/253 and NA R5 N 23/261.

74. In the few cases where physicians did become involved in death investigations, evidence suggests that they were all too willing to bypass the morgue and the surgical procedures required by an autopsy (see NA R5 N 23/219).

75. Sanjay Subrahmanyam, "Between a Rock and a Hard Place: Some Afterthoughts," in *The Brokered World: Go-Betweens and Global Intelligence, 1770–1820*, ed. Simon Schaffer et al. (Sagamore Beach, MA: Science History Publications, 2009).

76. Steven Shapin, *Never Pure: Historical Studies of Science as if It Was Produced by People with Bodies, Situated in Time, Space, Culture, and Society, and Struggling for Credibility and Authority* (Baltimore: Johns Hopkins University Press, 2010).

77. Schaffer, *The Brokered World*; see also Kapil Raj, "Go-Betweens, Travellers, and Cultural Translators," in *A Companion to the History of Science*, ed. Bernard Lightman (Malden, MA: John Wiley & Sons, 2016).

78. David Turnbull, *Masons, Tricksters, and Cartographers: Comparative Studies in the Sociology of Scientific and Indigenous Knowledge* (Amsterdam: Harwood, 2000), 44.

Conclusion

1. *BT*, December 6, 1901.

2. "Appointments," *Lancet*, June 28, 1902, p. 1867.

3. NA R5 N 5.3/8.

4. *BT*, May 23, 1894.

5. *BT*, June 9, 1894. See also NA R5 N 5.4.

6. "The Alleged Case of Plague," *BT*, May 11, 1898.

7. Highet, "Sixth Annual Report of the Medical Officer of Health . . . for the Year ro. so. 121 [1 April 1902–31 March 1903]," NA R5 N 5.5/11, 10–25.

8. NA R5 N 5.7.

9. *BT*, May 16, 1898. Plague did arrive in Siam in 1904; see Davisakd Puaksom, "Of Germs, Public Hygiene and the Healthy Body: The Making of the Medicalizing State in Thailand," *Journal of Asian Studies* 66 (2007): 324–28. And for evidence of how these reports came to the attention of police, see, for example, NA R5 N 23/565.

10. Highet, "Eighth Annual Report of Medical Officer of Health for the Year 123 [April 1, 1904–March 31, 1905]" (NA R5 N 5.5/14).

11. NA R5 N 5.3/13 (letter dated February 11, 1906).

12. Nightingale would continue to participate in this new mode of state medical concern even after his tenure ended: he served as the Siamese delegate to the International Medical Conference at Brussels in 1903 ("The Annus Medicus," *Lancet*, December 26, 1903, 1823).

13. "Registration of Deaths," *BT*, April 18, 1900, 3.

14. The timing of this proposed transition roughly corresponds to what Davisakd Puaksom has identified as "the birth of public sanitation" in May 1897; see his "Of Germs," 318–19. See also Monruethai Chaiwiset, *Prawatisat sangkhom: wa duai suam lae khrueang sukkhaphan nai prathet thai* [*Social history: Of lavatories and sanitary ware in Thailand*] (Bangkok: Matichon, 2545 [2002]).

15. Ruth Rogaski, *Hygienic Modernity: Meanings of Health and Disease in Treaty-Port China* (Berkeley: University of California Press, 2004).

16. Benton, *Law and Colonial Cultures*; Pär Kristoffer Cassel, *Grounds of Judgment: Extraterritoriality and Imperial Power in Nineteenth-Century China and Japan* (New York: Oxford University Press, 2012); Will Hanley, *Identifying with Nationality*. On the "culture of legalities," see John L. Comaroff, "Colonialism, Culture, and the Law: A Foreword," *Law & Social Inquiry* 26, no. 2 (2001): 311.

17. Sheila Jasanoff, *Science at the Bar: Law, Science, and Technology in America* (Cambridge, MA: Harvard University Press, 1995), 19.

18. Dan Bouk, *How Our Days Became Numbered: Risk and the Rise of the Statistical Individual* (Chicago: University of Chicago Press, 2015), xv.

19. While this study has focused on accidental injury and death on the tracks of the Bangkok Tramway Company in the late nineteenth century, preliminary research suggests that the very same forms of compensatory arrangements carried over into the era of automobility at the start of twentieth century. I intend to explore these continuities in future research.

20. Esmeir, *Juridical Humanity*.

21. On the notion of alternative modernity, an idea that is closely related to Dipesh Chakrabarty's clarion call to "provincialize Europe" by attempting to write histories outside the logic of Eurocentric paradigms, see Loos, *Subject Siam*, 18–24.

22. Wyatt, *Thailand*, 217.

23. Wyatt, *Thailand*, 217.

24. Wyatt, *Thailand*, 217.

25. Adam T. Smith, *The Political Machine: Assembling Sovereignty in the Bronze Age Caucus* (Princeton, NJ: Princeton University Press, 2015); Will Hanley, *Identifying with Nationality*, 19.

Epilogue

1. Kittiphong Maneerit, "'Anna Reese' *sing* [*sic: sueng*] *bens chon rot tamruat dap*" ["Anna Reese," whose Benz struck and killed a police officer], last modified June 25, 2015, https://www.youtube.com/watch?v=XrPZk-t4SD0&noredirect=1.

2. "'Anna Reese' Rejects 6.2M Settlement Sought by Cop's Family," *Khoasod English*, August 10, 2015, http://www.khaosodenglish.com/news/crimecourtscalamity/2015/08/10/1439198419/.

3. Thai Criminal Procedure Code, Title 3: Criminal Prosecutions and Penal Action, chapter 1: Criminal Prosecutions, Sections 38–9, and especially chapter 2: Penal Actions, Section 44/I. See also Prathan Watanavanich, "The Emergence of Victims' Rights in Thailand: Twenty Years After The U.N. Declaration of Basic Principles of Justice for Victims of Crime and Abuse of Power," *United Nations Asia and Far East Institute for the Prevention of Crime and the Treatment of Offenders Resource Material Series* 70 (2006).

4. "Actress Charged with Deadly Car Crash Says Victim's Ghost Forgave Her," *Khoasod English*, July 3, 2015, http://www.khaosodenglish.com/detail.php?newsid=1435918909.

5. "'Anna Reese' Rejects 6.2 Million Settlement," *Khoasod English*, August 10, 2015.

6. "Anna Reese Settles with Family of Dead Policeman," *Khaosod English*, August 24, 2015, http://www.khaosodenglish.com/life/2015/08/24/1440417488/.

7. Zoë Crossland, "The Agency of the Dead," in *Distributed Agency*, ed. N. J. Enfield and Paul Kockelman (Oxford: Oxford University Press, 2017), 182.

8. Crossland, "The Agency of the Dead."

9. Crossland, "The Agency of the Dead."

10. David M. Engel and Jaruwan S. Engel, *Tort, Custom, and Karma: Globalization and Legal Consciousness in Thailand* (Stanford, CA: Stanford University Press, 2010), 56–75.

11. See, respectively, Jonathan Head, "Thailand's Wealthy Untouchables," *BBC News*, April 7, 2008, http://news.bbc.co.uk/2/hi/asia-pacific/7328054.stm; "Teen Crash Driver Gets Suspended Jail," *Bangkok Post*, August 31, 2012, http://www.bangkokpost.com/archive/teenage-driver-praewa-gets-2-yrs-in-jail/310202; Luke Hunt, "Lao Death Sparks Thai Outrage," *The Diplomat*, March 29, 2011, http://thediplomat.com/2011/03/laos-death-sparks-thai-outrage/; "Drink-Driving Killer Given 2 Years, Bailed," *Bangkok Post*, May 31, 2016, http://www.bangkokpost.com/archive/drink-driving-killer-given-2-years-bailed/996313; and Poppy Danby, "Uproar in Thailand after wealthy young driver who killed two students when he rear-ended them in his expensive Mercedes gets away without alcohol or drugs tests," *Daily Mail*, March 23, 2016, http://www.dailymail.co.uk/news/article-3506770/Mercedes-crash-KILLED-two-students-ignites-uproar-Thailand-wealthy-young-driver-refuses-alcohol-drugs-tests.html.

12. "Model-Actress Anna Charged with Drink Driving, Hit and Run," *The Nation*, May 22, 2017, http://www.nationmultimedia.com/news/national/30315915.

13. Kelly McLaughlin, "Red Bull Gives You . . . Immunity," *Daily Mail*, April 3, 2017, http://www.dailymail.co.uk/news/article-4375556/Wanted-Red-Bull-heir-pictured-partying-hit-run.html.

14. In a notable rebuke to this system of ex gratia compensatory payments and indemnification, however, the families of the victims of Janepob Verraporn rejected the efforts of the court to bring them together with the defendant in order to reach a settlement; see Teeranai Charuvastra, "Victims' Families Refuse Cash, Demand Full Prosection of Jenphop [Janepob]," *Khaosod English*, July 12, 2016, http://www.khaosodenglish.com/news/crimecourtscalamity/courts/2016/07/12/victims-families-refuse-cash-demand-full-prosecution-jenphop/.

15. Thomas Fuller, "Hit-and-Run Case Seen as Reflection of Inequality in Thailand," *New York Times*, September 2, 2013, http://www.nytimes.com/2013/09/03/world/asia/wealthy-thai-fails-to-show-for-hearing-over-hit-and-run.html; Pasuk Phongpaichit and Chris Baker, eds., *Unequal Thailand: Aspects of Wealth, Income, and Power* (Singapore: National University of Singapore Press, 2015); and Kevin Hewison, "Considerations on Inequality and Politics in Thailand," *Democratization* 21, no. 5 (2014).

16. Engel and Engel, *Tort, Custom, and Karma*, 21–32, 157.

17. Engel and Engel, *Tort, Custom, and Karma*, 77–94.

18. Engel and Engel, *Tort, Custom, and Karma*, 78–79, 156–58.

Appendix

1. Engel, "Discourses of Causation," 257.

2. While *phao tua* has all but disappeared in contemporary usage, *ngan phao phi* remains a common colloquialism for describing a wake.

Bibliography

Archival Materials

Most of the archival materials cited in this study are from the National Archives of
Thailand (NA). Documents at the National Archives are organized chronologically according to the reign dates; the documents cited date to the Fifth
Chakri Reign (1868–1910; Thai: *ratchakan thi 5*) and are thus labeled "R5." The
documents are then divided according to the government ministry from
which they came (see below for abbreviations), then the division number,
followed by the document number, and in some cases a page number or other
specifying marker (such as a date for letters).

National Archives of Thailand

Documents from the Fifth Reign (1868–1910), by Ministry

M	Ministry of the Interior (*Krasuang Mahatthai*)
	Division 5.1 บ Department of Corrections. Suspects and Prisoners.
N	Ministry of the Capital (*Krasuang Nakhonban*)
	Division 5.3 Department of Sanitation. Civil Servants.
	Division 5.5 Department of Sanitation. Reports.
	Division 5.6 Department of Sanitation. Division of Physicians.
	Division 5.7 Department of Sanitation. Disease Inspection and Prevention.
	Division 8.1 Metropolitan Police.
	Division 8.6 Metropolitan Police. Miscellaneous Reports.
	Division 21 Tramway.
	Division 23 Death by Various Causes.
	Division 26 Records of Contracts.
	Division 49.3 Correspondence with the Ministry of Public Instruction. Hospital Department.
S.	Ministry of Public Instruction (*Krasuang Sueksathikan*)
	Division 24 Hospitals.
S.Th.	Ministry of Public Instruction/Religious Affairs (*Krasuang Sueksathikan/Thammakan*)
	Division 8 Hospital Department. Records.
	Division 8.2.ฌ Hospital Department. Bangrak Hospital.
	Division 99 Miscellaneous Documents.
Y	Ministry of Justice (*Krasuang Yutitham*)
	Division 13.4 Court Cases. Assault and Murder.

Newspapers and Magazines

Bangkok Times (BT), 1889–1905.
Electrical World, 1893.
The Lancet, 1902–3.
The Singapore Free Press and Mercantile Advertiser, 1893.
The Straits Times, 1892.
The Straits Times Weekly Issue, 1892.
The Street Railway Journal, 1892–93.
Wachirayan wiset, 1888.
Western Electrician, 1892.

Printed Primary Sources, Books, and Selected Articles

Alabaster, Henry. *The Wheel of Law: Buddhism Illustrated from Siamese Sources.*
    London: Trübner & Co., 1871.
Archer, William J. *Siamese Law on Disputes and Assault.* Bangkok: S. J. Smith's Office, 1886.
——. *"The Siamese Laws on Debts, translated by W. J. Archer of H.B.M.'s Legation."*
    Bangkok: S. J. Smith's Office, Bangk'olem Point, 1885.
Barrett, John. "Street and Other Railways in Siam." *Street Railway Journal* 13, no. 7
    (July 1897): 400.
Beauvoir, Ludovic, Marquis de. *A Week in Siam: January 1867.* Bangkok: The Siam
    Society, 1986 [1870].
Bradford, E. R. C. *Statements of the Crimes of Dacoity and Poisoning in British Territory
    for the Year 1875.* Simla: Government Central Branch Press, 1877.
Caswell, J., and J. H. Chandler, comps. *A Dictionary of the Siamese Language.* Bangkok:
    Chulalongkorn University Press, 2544 [2001] [1846].
*The Chronicle & Directory for China, Corea [sic], Japan, The Philippines, Indo-China,
    Straits Settlements, Siam, Bornea, Malay States, &c. for the year 1892.* Hong Kong:
    Daily Press, 1892.
Chulalongkorn, King. *"Wa duai het haeng khwam tai nai tham klang ayu"* ["On the
    causes of death in middle age"]. *Wachirayan wiset*, 2431 [1888].
Collins, Steven. *A Pali Grammar for Students.* Chiang Mai, Thailand: Silkworm Books,
    2005.
Cone, Margaret. *A Dictionary of Pāli, Part I.* Oxford: Pali Text Society, 2001.
*The Directory for Bangkok and Siam for 1891: A Handy and Perfectly Reliable Book of
    Reference for All Classes.* Bangkok: Bangkok Times, [1891].
English and Siamese Vocabulary. Bangkok: American Presbyterian Mission Press, 1865.
Fournereau, Lucien. *Bangkok in 1892.* Edited by Walter E. J. Tips. Bangkok: White
    Lotus Press, 1998.
The Guide According to Kaccāna Thera (Netti-Pakaraṇaṁ), translated by Bhikkhu
    Ñāṇamoli. London: Pali Text Society, 1977 [1962].
Hardy, E., ed. *The Netti-Pakaraṇa, with Extracts From Dhammpāla's Commentary.*
    London: Pali Text Society, 1961 [1902].
Kitiyakara Krommaphra Chandaburinarunath, Prince, comp. *Pathanukrom bali thai
    angkrit sansakrit [Pali-Thai-English-Sanskrit dictionary].* Bangkok: King Maha-
    makut's Academy, 1977.

Kotmai tra sam duang [*Law of the Three Seals*], vols. 1–5. Osaka, Japan: National Museum of Ethnography, 1981.

Map of the Kingdom of Siam and Its Dependencies. Edinburgh: W. & A. K. Johnston, [1900?].

McFarland, George B. *Thai-English Dictionary.* Stanford, CA: Stanford University Press, 1960.

McFarland, Samuel Gamble. *An English-Siamese Dictionary.* Bangkok: American Presbyterian Mission Press, 1865.

McFarland, Samuel Gamble, and George B. McFarland. *An English-Siamese Dictionary Containing 14,000 Words and Idiomatic Expressions.* Bangkok: American Presbyterian Mission Press, 1903 [1865].

Michell, E. B. "Boxing." In *Fencing, Boxing, Wrestling,* edited by the Duke of Beaufort. London: Longman, Greene, and Co., 1897.

———. *A Siamese-English Dictionary for the Use of Students in Both Languages.* Freeport, NY: Books for Libraries Press, 1973 [1892].

Oberlies, Thomas. *Pāli: A Grammar of the Language of the Theravāda Tipiṭaka.* Berlin: Walter de Gruyter, 2001.

Pallegoix, Jean Baptiste. *Sapha phajana phasa thai: Dictionarium Linguae Thai.* Paris, 1854.

———. *Siphot phasa thai: Siamese-French-English Dictionary,* edited by J. L. Vey. Bangkok: Printing Office of the Catholic Mission, 1896.

Prachum phongsawadan phak thi 2 [*Collected Chronicles, No. 2*]. Bangkok: Rongphim Thai, 2457 [1914].

Prayut Payutto, Phra. *Photjanukrom phutthasasanam chabab pramuan sap* [*Dictionary of the Buddhist religion, collected terms*]. Bangkok: Maha Chulalongkorn University, 2527 [1984].

———. *Photjanukrom phutthasat chabab pramuan tham* [*Dictionary of Buddhism*]. Bangkok: Mahachulalongkorn University, 2528 [1985].

Rai ngan kan-prachum senabodi sapha ro. so. 111 [*Minutes of the meetings of the government ministers for the year 1893*], vols. 1–3. Krung thep: Amarin, 2550 [2007].

Ratanayatti, Luang (Sangop). *Dikchanari phasa angkrit plae pen thai: English-Siamese Dictionary.* Krungthep: Rong phim luang, Ro. So. 120 [1901].

Rhys Davids, T. W., and Wilhelm Stede. *Pali-English Dictionary.* London: Pali Text Society, 1959 [1921–25].

Sathian Wichailak, comp. *Prachum kotmai prajam sok* [*Collected laws, arranged chronologically*]. Bangkok: Niti Wet, 1935–53.

Si Saowaphang, Prince. *Wa duai amnat phi lae phi lok* [*On the power of spirits*]. Krungthep: Rong phim luang nai phra borom maha ratchawang, 2464 [1921].

Smith, Samuel J. *A Comprehensive Anglo-Siamese Dictionary,* vols. 1–5. Bangkok: Bangkolem Press, 1899–1908.

Straits Settlements. *The Laws of the Straits Settlements 1835–1900: Revised up to and including the 31st Day of December, 1919.* London: Waterlow & Sons, 1920.

Thiphakorawong, Chao Phraya. *Nangsue sadaeng kitchanukit* [*A book explaining various things*]. Bangkok: Khuru Sapha, 1971 [1867].

Westenholz, Aage. "Street Railways in Siam, and Siamese Customs." *Street Railway Journal* 7 (August 1891): 414–15.

Wright, Arnold, and Oliver T. Breakspear, eds. *Twentieth Century Impressions of Siam: Its History, People, Commerce, Industries, and Resources*. London: Lloyd's, 1908.

Secondary Printed Sources, Books, and Articles

Agamben, Giorgio. *Homo Sacer: Sovereign Power and Bare Life*. Stanford, CA: Stanford University Press, 1998.

Akiko Iijima. "The 'International Court' System in the Colonial History of Siam." *Taiwan Journal of Southeast Asian Studies* 5, no. 1 (2008): 31–64.

Akin Rabibhadana. "Clientship and Class Structure in the Early Bangkok Period." In *Change and Persistence in Thai Society: Essays in Honor of Lauriston Sharp*, edited by G. William Skinner and A. Thomas Kirsch, 93–124. Ithaca, NY: Cornell University Press, 1975.

——. *The Organization of Thai Society in the Early Bangkok Period 1782–1873*. Bangkok: Amarin, 1996.

Amster, Ellen J. *Medicine and the Saints: Science, Islam, and the Colonial Encounter in Morocco, 1877–1956*. Austin: University of Texas Press, 2013.

Anderson, Benedict R. O'G. "Studies of the Thai State: The State of Thai Studies." In *The Study of Thailand: Analyses of Knowledge, Approaches, and Prospects in Anthropology, Art History, Economics, History and Political Science*, edited by Eliezer B. Ayal, 193–247. Athens: Center for International Studies, Ohio University, 1978.

Anderson, Warwick. *Colonial Pathologies: American Tropical Medicine, Race, and Hygiene in The Philippines*. Durham, NC: Duke University Press, 2006.

——. "Objectivity & Its Discontents." *Social Studies of Science* 43, no. 4 (2012).

Anuman Rajathon, Phraya. "The Khwan and Its Ceremonies." *Journal of the Siam Society* 50, no. 2 (1962): 119–64.

——. "Some Siamese Superstitions about Trees and Plants." *Journal of the Siam Society* 49, no. 1 (1961): 57–63.

Anusaranasasanakiarti, Phra Khru, and Charles F. Keyes. "Funerary Rites and the Buddhist Meaning of Death: An Interpretive Text from Northern Thailand." *Journal of the Siam Society* 68, no. 1 (1980): 1–28.

Ariès, Philippe. *The Hour of Our Death*. New York: Knopf, 1981.

Arnold, David. *Colonizing the Body: State Medicine and Epidemic Disease in Nineteenth-Century India*. Berkeley: University of California Press, 1993.

Asen, Daniel. *Death in Beijing: Murder and Forensic Science in Republican China*. Cambridge: Cambridge University Press, 2016.

Au, Sokhieng. *Mixed Medicines: Health and Culture in French Colonial Indochina*. Chicago: University of Chicago Press, 2013.

Bailkin, Jordanna. "The Boot and the Spleen: When Was Murder Possible in British India?" *Comparative Studies in Society and History* 48, no. 2 (2005): 462–93.

Baker, Chris, and Pasuk Phongpaichit. *A History of Thailand*. Cambridge: Cambridge University Press, 2005.

——, eds. *The Palace Law of Ayutthaya and the Thammasat: Law and Kingship in Siam*. Ithaca, NY: Cornell University Southeast Asia Program Publications, 2016.

Ballantyne, Tony. *Entanglements of Empire: Missionaries, Moari, and the Question of the Body*. Durham, NC: Duke University Press, 2014.

Becker, Elisa M. *Medicine, Law and the State in Imperial Russia*. Budapest: Central European University Press, 2011.

Bell, Michael Mayerfeld. "The Ghosts of Place." *Theory and Society* 26, no. 6 (1997): 813–36.

Benjamin, Walter. *Selected Writings Volume 4, 1938–1940*. Edited by Howard Eiland and Michael W. Jennings. Cambridge, MA: Belknap Press, 2003.

Benton, Lauren. *Law and Colonial Cultures: Legal Regimes in World History, 1400–1900*. Cambridge: Cambridge University Press, 2002.

——. "Law and Empire in Global Perspective: Introduction." *American Historical Review* 117, no. 4 (2012): 1092–100.

Bergstrom, Randolph. *Courting Danger: Injury and Law in New York City, 1870–1910*. Ithaca, NY: Cornell University Press, 1992.

Bernault, Florence. "Body, Power, and Sacrifice in Equatorial Africa." *Journal of African History* 47, no. 2 (2006): 207–39.

Bernstein, Anya. "The Post-Soviet Treasure Hunt: Time, Space, and Necropolitics in Siberian Buddhism." *Comparative Studies in Society and History* 53, no. 3 (2011): 623–53.

——. *Religious Bodies Politic: Rituals of Sovereignty in Buryat Buddhism*. Chicago: University of Chicago Press, 2013.

Bickers, Robert. "Legal Fiction: Extraterritoriality as an Instrument of British Power in China in the 'Long Nineteenth Century.'" In *Empire in Asia: A New Global History*, vol. 2, edited by Donna Brunero and Brian P. Farrell, 53–80. New York: Bloomsbury Academic, 2018.

Blackburn, Anne M. *Locations of Buddhism: Colonialism & Modernity in Sri Lanka*. Chicago: University of Chicago Press, 2010.

Boem Bangphli. *"Khru samit, pho so 2363–2452"* ["Rev. Smith, 1820–1909"]. *Sinlapa watthanatham [Art & culture]* 28, no. 3 (2007): 130–45.

Bond, George D. *The Word of the Buddha: The Tipiṭaka and Its Interpretation in Theravada Buddhism*. Colombo, Sri Lanka: Gunasena, 1982.

Bowker, Geoffrey C., and Susan Leigh Star. *Sorting Things Out: Classification and Its Consequences*. Cambridge, MA: MIT Press, 1999.

Brailey, Nigel, ed. *The Satow Siam Papers: The Private Diaries and Correspondence of Ernest Satow, Vol. 1, 1884–1885*. Bangkok: The Historical Society under the Patronage of H.R.H. Princess Maha Chakri Sirindhorn, 1997.

Brown, Vincent. *The Reaper's Garden: Death and Power in the World of Atlantic Slavery*. Cambridge, MA: Harvard University Press, 2008.

Burney, Ian A. *Bodies of Evidence: Medicine and the Politics of the English Inquest, 1830–1926*. Baltimore: Johns Hopkins University Press, 2000.

Burnham, John C. *Accident Prone: A History of Technology, Psychology, and Misfits of the Machine Age*. Chicago: University of Chicago Press, 2009.

Callon, Michel. "Some Elements of a Sociology of Translation: Domestication of Scallops and the Fishermen of St. Brieuc Bay." In *Power, Action and Belief: A New Sociology of Knowledge?*, edited by John Law, 196–233. London: Routledge, 1986.

Cassel, Pär Kristoffer. *Grounds of Judgment: Extraterritoriality and Imperial Power in Nineteenth-Century China and Japan.* New York: Oxford University Press, 2012.

Cawthon, Elisabeth. "New Life for the Deodand: Coroner's Inquests and Occupational Deaths in England, 1830–46." *American Journal of Legal History* 33, no. 2 (1989): 137–47.

——. "Thomas Wakley and the Medical Coronership: Occupational Death and the Judicial Process." *Medical History* 30, no. 2 (1986): 191–202.

Chaiyan Rajchagool. *The Rise and Fall of the Thai Absolute Monarchy.* Bangkok: White Lotus, 1994.

Chakrabarty, Dipesh. *Provincializing Europe: Postcolonial Thought and Historical Difference.* Princeton, NJ: Princeton University Press, 2000.

Chali Iamkrasin. *Mueang thai samai kon* [*Thailand in the past*]. Bangkok: Samnak Phim Dok Mali, 1991.

Chamberlain, James F., ed. *The Ramkhamhaeng Controversy: Collected Papers.* Bangkok: Siam Society, 1991.

Chambers, David Wade, and Richard Gillespie. "Locality in the History of Science: Colonial Science, Technoscience, and Indigenous Knowledge." *Osiris* 15, no. 1 (2000): 221–40.

Chandra, Uday. "Liberalism and Its Other: The Politics of Primitivism in Colonial and Postcolonial Law." *Law & Society Review* 47, no. 1 (2013): 135–68.

Chandran, Jeshuran. "British Foreign Policy and the Extraterritorial Question in Siam, 1891–1900." *Journal of the Malaysian Branch of the Royal Asiatic Society* 38, pt. 2 (1965): 290–313.

——. "The Anglo-French Declaration of 1896 and the Independence of Siam." *Journal of the Siam Society* 28, pt. 2 (1970): 105–26.

Chanock, Martin. *Law, Custom, and Social Order: The Colonial Experience in Malawi and Zambia.* Cambridge: Cambridge University Press, 1985.

Charnvit Kasetsiri. "Thai Historiography from Ancient Times to the Modern Period." In *Perceptions of the Past in Southeast Asia*, edited by Anthony Reid and David Marr, 156–70. Singapore: Asian Studies Association of Australia, 1979.

Chatichai Muksong, and Komatra Chuengsatiansup. "Medicine and Public Health in Thai Historiography." In *Global Movements, Local Concerns: Medicine and Health in Southeast Asia*, edited by Laurence Monnais and Harold J. Cook, 226–45. Singapore: NUS Press, 2012.

Chua, Lawrence. "The City and the City: Race, Nationalism, and Architecture in Early Twentieth-Century Bangkok." *Journal of Urban History* 40, no. 5 (2014): 933–58.

Cohn, Bernard. *Colonialism and Its Forms of Knowledge: The British in India.* Princeton, NJ: Princeton University Press, 1996.

Coleman, Matthew, and Kevin Grove. "Biopolitics, Biopower, and the Return of Sovereignty." *Environment and Planning D: Society and Space* 27, no. 3 (2009): 489–507.

Cooter, Roger. "The Moment of the Accident: Culture, Militarism and Modernity in Late-Victorian Britain." In *Accidents in History*, edited by Roger Cooter and Bill Luckin, 107–57. Atlanta, GA: Editions Rodopi, 1997.

Crossland, Zoë. *Ancestral Encounters in Highland Madagascar: Material Signs and Traces of the Dead.* Cambridge: Cambridge University Press, 2014.

——. Epilogue to *Necropolitics: Mass Graves and Exhumations in the Age of Human Rights*, edited by Francisco Ferrándiz and Antonius C. G. M. Robben, 240–52. Philadelphia: University of Pennsylvania Press, 2015.

Dararat Mettarikanond. *"Kotmai sopheni 'ti-tabian' khrang raek nai prathet thai"* ["The First Law of the Registration of Prostitutes in Thailand"]. *Sinlapa watthanatham [Art & culture]* 5, no. 5 (1984): 6–19.

Darlington, Susan M. "The Ordination of a Tree: The Buddhist Ecology Movement in Thailand." *Ethnology* 37, no. 1 (1998): 1–15.

Davies, Paul L., ed. *Gowers and Davies: The Principles of Modern Company Law*, 6th ed. London: Sweet & Maxwell, 1997.

Davisakd Puaksom. *Chua rok rang kai lae rat wetchakam: prawatisat kan-phaet samai mai nai sangkhom thai* [*Disease, the Body, and the Medicalizing State: The History of Modern Medicine in Thai Society*]. Bangkok: Chulalongkorn University Press, 2007.

——. "Of Germs, Public Hygiene, and the Healthy Body: The Making of the Medicalizing State in Thailand." *Journal of Asian Studies* 66, no. 2 (2007): 311–44.

Dawdy, Shannon Lee. *Building the Devil's Empire: French Colonial New Orleans*. Chicago: University of Chicago Press, 2008.

Day, Tony, and Craig J. Reynolds. "Cosmologies, Truth Regimes, and the State in Southeast Asia." *Modern Asian Studies* 34, no. 1 (2000): 1–55.

Deakin, Simon, Angus Johnston, and Basil Markesinis. *Markesinis and Deakin's Tort Law*, 7th ed. New York: Oxford University Press, 2012.

Delaney, David. *Law and Nature*. New York: Cambridge University Press, 2003.

——. "Making Nature/Marking Humans: Law as a Site of (Cultural) Production." *Annals of the Association of American Geographers* 91, no. 3 (2001): 487–503.

Dening, Greg. *Islands and Beaches: Discourse on a Silent Land, Marquesas 1774–1880*. Chicago: Dorsey Press, 1980.

Dirks, Nicholas B. Foreword to *Colonialism and Its Forms of Knowledge: The British in India*, Bernard S. Cohn, ix–xvii. Princeton, NJ: Princeton University Press, 1996.

Driscoll, Mark. *Absolute Erotic, Absolute Grotesque: The Living and the Dead in Japan's Imperialism, 1895–1945*. Durham, NC: Duke University Press, 2010.

Ely, James W. Jr. *Railroads and American Law*. Lawrence: University Press of Kansas, 2001.

Engel, David M. *Code and Custom in a Thai Provincial Court*. Tucson: University of Arizona Press, 1978.

——. "Discourses of Causation in Injury Cases: Exploring Thai and American Legal Cultures." In *Fault Lines: Tort Law as Cultural Practice*, edited by David M. Engel and Michael McCann, 251–68. Stanford, CA: Stanford University Press, 2009.

——. "Globalization and the Decline of Legal Consciousness: Torts, Ghosts, and Karma in Thailand." *Law & Social Inquiry* 30, no. 3 (2005): 469–514.

——. "Landscapes of the Law: Injury, Remedy, and Social Change in Thailand." *Law & Society Review* 43, no. 1 (2009): 61–94.

——. *Law and Kingship in Thailand during the Reign of King Chulalongkorn*. Ann Arbor: Center for South and Southeast Asian Studies, University of Michigan, 1975.

Engel, David M., and Jaruwan S. Engel. *Tort, Custom, and Karma: Globalization and Legal Consciousness in Thailand*. Stanford, CA: Stanford University Press, 2010.

Esmeir, Samera. "At Once Human & Not Human: Law, Gender, and Historical Becoming in Colonial Egypt." *Gender & History* 23, no. 2 (2011): 235–49.

——. *Juridical Humanity: A Colonial History*. Stanford, CA: Stanford University Press, 2012.

Esposito, Roberto. *Bíos: Biopolitics and Philosophy*. Translated by Timothy C. Campbell. Minneapolis: University of Minnesota Press, 2008.

Ewald, François. *L'Etat Providence*. Paris: B. Grasset, 1986.

——. "The Return of Descartes' Malicious Demon: An Outline of a Philosophy of Precaution." In *Embracing Risk: The Changing Culture of Insurance and Responsibility*, edited by Tom Baker and Jonathan Simon, 273–301. Chicago: University of Chicago Press, 2002.

Ezrahi, Yaron. *The Descent of Icarus: Science and the Transformation of Contemporary Democracy*. Cambridge, MA: Harvard University Press, 1990.

Fahmy, Khaled. "The Anatomy of Justice: Forensic Medicine and Criminal Law in Nineteenth Century Egypt." *Islamic Law & Society* 6, no. 2 (1999): 224–71.

Feeny, David. "The Decline of Property Rights in Man in Thailand, 1800–1913." *Journal of Economic History* 49, no. 2 (1989): 285–96.

Figlio, Karl. "What Is an Accident?" In *The Social History of Occupational Health*, edited by Paul Weindling, 180–206. London: Croom Helm, 1985.

Finkelstein, Jacob J. "The Goring Ox: Some Historical Perspectives on Deodands, Forfeitures, Wrongful Death and the Western Notion of Sovereignty." *Temple Law Quarterly* 46, no. 2 (1973): 169–290.

Fischer, Michael M. J. *Emergent Forms of Life and the Anthropological Voice*. Durham, NC: Duke University Press, 2003.

——. "Technoscientific Infrastructures and Emergent Forms of Life: A Commentary." *American Anthropologist* 107, no. 1 (2005): 55–61.

Fitzpatrick, Matthew P., ed. *Liberal Imperialism in Europe*. New York: Palgrave Macmillan, 2012.

Flaherty, Darryl E. *Public Law, Private Practice: Politics, Profit, and the Legal Profession in Nineteenth-Century Japan*. Cambridge, MA: Harvard University Press, 2013.

Forbes, Thomas R. "By What Disease or Casualty: The Changing Face of Death in London." *Journal of the History of Medicine and Allied Sciences* 31 (1976): 395–420.

Foucault, Michel. *Birth of Biopolitics*. New York: Picador, 2008.

——. *The Birth of the Clinic: An Archaeology of Medical Perception*. New York: Vintage Books, 1994 [1973].

——. "Governmentality." In *Power: Essential Works of Foucault, 1954–1984, Vol. III*, edited by James D. Faubion, 201–22. London: Penguin, 2001.

——. *Madness and Civilization: A History of Insanity in the Age of Reason*. New York: Vintage Books, 1973 [1965].

——. *The Order of Things: An Archeology of the Human Sciences*. New York: Vintage Books, 1994 [1970].

——. "Society Must Be Defended": Lectures at the Collège de France, 1975–76. New York: Picador, 2003.

——. "What Is Enlightenment?" In *The Foucault Reader*, edited by Paul Rabinow, 32–50. New York: Pantheon, 1984.

Friedman, Lawrence. *A History of American Law*, 3rd ed. New York: Touchstone, 2005.

Galanter, Marc. "India's Tort Deficit: Sketch for a Historical Portrait." In *Fault Lines: Tort Law as Cultural Practice*, edited by David M. Engel and Michael McCann, 47–65. Stanford, CA: Stanford University Press, 2009.

Gluck, Carol. "Words in Motion." In *Words in Motion: Toward a Global Lexicon*, edited by Carol Gluck and Anna Lowenhaupt Tsing, 3–10. Durham, NC: Duke University Press, 2009.

Gramsci, Antonio. *Selections from the Prison Notebooks*. Edited and translated by Quintin Hoare and Geoffrey Nowell-Smith. London: Lawrence & Wishart, 1971.

Green, Judith. "Accidents: The Remnants of a Modern Classificatory System." In *Accidents in History*, edited by Roger Cooter and Bill Luckin, 35–58. Atlanta, GA: Editions Rodopi, 1997.

——. *Risk and Misfortune: A Social Construction of Accidents*. London: University College London, 1997.

Green, Nile. *Bombay Islam: The Religious Economy of the West Indian Ocean, 1840–1915*. Cambridge: Cambridge University Press, 2011.

——. "Moral Competition and the Thrill of the Spectacular: Recounting Catastrophe in Colonial Bombay." *South Asia Research* 28, no. 3 (2008): 239–51.

Griswold, A. B., and Prasert na Nagara. "The Inscription of King Rama Gam Hen [Ramkhamhaeng] of Sukhodaya (1292 AD): Epigraphic and Historical Studies 9." *Journal of the Siam Society* 59, no. 2 (1971): 179–228.

Habermas, Jurgen. *The Structural Transformation of the Public Sphere: An Inquiry into a Category of Bourgeois Society*. Translated by Thomas Burger with Frederick Lawrence. Cambridge, MA: MIT Press, 1989.

Hacking, Ian. *Historical Ontology*. Cambridge, MA: Harvard University Press, 2002.

——. *The Taming of Chance*. Cambridge: Cambridge University Press, 1990.

Halliday, Simon, and Patrick Schmidt, eds. *Conducting Law and Society Research: Reflections on Methods and Practices*. New York: Cambridge University Press, 2009.

Hamlin, Christopher. "Forensic Cultures in Historical Perspective: Technologies of Witness, Testimony, Judgment (and Justice?)." *Studies in History and Philosophy of Biological and Biomedical Sciences* 44 (2013): 4–15.

Hanley, Will. *Identifying with Nationality: Europeans, Ottomans, and Egyptians in Alexandria*. New York: Columbia University Press, 2017.

Hansen, Thomas Blom, and Finn Stepputat. *Sovereign Bodies: Citizens, Migrants, and States in the Postcolonial World*. Princeton, NJ: Princeton University Press, 2005.

Harding, Andrew J. "The Eclipse of the Astrologers: King Mongkut, His Successors, and the Reformation of Law in Thailand." In *Examining Practice, Interrogating Theory: Comparative Legal Studies in Asia*, edited by Penelope Nicholson and Sarah Biddulph, 307–41. Leiden: Martinus Nijhoff, 2008.

Heinze, Ruth-Inge. *Tham Khwan: How to Contain the Essence of Life: A Socio-Psychological Comparison of a Thai Custom*. Singapore: Singapore University Press, 1982.

Herzfeld, Michael. "The Absent Presence: Discourses of Crypto-Colonialism." *South Atlantic Quarterly* 101, no. 4 (2002): 899–926.

——. "The Conceptual Allure of the West: Dilemmas and Ambiguities of Crypto-Colonialism in Thailand." In *The Ambiguous Allure of the West: Traces of the*

Colonial in Thailand, edited by Rachel V. Harrison and Peter A. Jackson, 173–86. Hong Kong: Hong Kong University Press, 2010.

——. *Siege of the Spirits: Community and Polity in Bangkok*. Chicago: University of Chicago Press, 2016.

Hong Lysa. "Extraterritoriality in Bangkok in the Reign of King Chulalongkorn, 1868–1910: The Cacophonies of Semi-Colonial Cosmopolitanism." *Itinerario: European Journal of Overseas History* 27, no. 1 (2003): 125–46.

——. "Indian Police Subalterns in King Chulalongkorn's Kingdom: Turn of the Twentieth Century Bangkok Pantomime." In *Khu khwam phumjai* [With pride], edited by Sirilak Sampatchalit and Siriporn Yodkamolsat, 453–73. Bangkok: Sansan, 2545 [2002].

——. "'Stranger within the Gates': Knowing Semi-Colonial Siam as Extraterritorials." *Modern Asian Studies* 38, no. 2 (2004): 327–54.

——. *Thailand in the Nineteenth Century: Evolution of the Economy and Society*. Singapore: Institute of Southeast Asian Studies, 1984.

Hooker, M. B. "The 'Europeanization' of Siam's Law 1855–1908." In *The Laws of South-East Asia, Volume II: European Laws in South-East Asia*, edited by M. B. Hooker, 531–607. St. Paul, MN: Butterworths, 1988.

——. *Legal Pluralism: An Introduction to Colonial and Neo-Colonial Laws*. Oxford: Clarendon Press, 1975.

Horwitz, Morton J. *The Transformation of American Law, 1870–1960: The Crisis of Legal Orthodoxy*. New York: Oxford University Press, 1992.

Hoskins, Janet. *Biographical Objects: How Things Tell the Stories of People's Lives*. New York: Routledge, 1998.

Ichiro Kakizaki. *Trams, Buses, and Rails: The History of Urban Transport in Bangkok*. Seattle: University of Washington Press, 2015.

Irwin, A. J. "Some Siamese Ghost-Lore and Demonology." *Journal of the Siam Society* 4, no. 2 (1907): 19–46.

Isara Lovanich. "Personal Injury and Damages for Non-Pecuniary Loss in the Law of Torts and the Product Liability Law." MA thesis, Thammasat University, 2011.

Jackson, Peter. "Autonomy and Subordination on Thai History: The Case for Semicolonial Analysis." *Inter-Asia Cultural Studies* 8, no. 3 (2007): 329–48.

James, Fleming, Jr. "Vicarious Liability." *Tulane Law Review* 28 (1954): 161–215.

Jasanoff, Sheila, ed. "Bhopal's Trials of Knowledge and Ignorance." *Isis* 98, no. 2 (2007): 344–50.

——. *Designs on Nature: Science and Democracy in Europe and the United States*. Princeton, NJ: Princeton University Press, 2005.

——. *Science at the Bar: Law, Science, and Technology in America*. Cambridge, MA: Harvard University Press, 1995.

——. *States of Knowledge: The Co-Production of Science and Social Order*. New York: Routledge, 2004.

Johnson, Andrew Alan. *Ghosts of the New City: Spirits, Urbanity, and the Ruins of Progress in Chiang Mai*. Honolulu: University of Hawai'i Press, 2014.

——. "Naming Chaos: Accident, Precariousness, and the Spirits of Wildness in Urban Thai Spirit Cults." *American Ethnologist* 39, no. 4 (2012): 766–78.

——. "Rebuilding Lanna: Constructing and Consuming the Past in Urban Northern Thailand." PhD diss., Cornell University, 2010.

Johnson, Steven. *The Ghost Map: The Story of London's Most Terrifying Epidemic and How It Changed Science, Cities, and the Modern World*. New York: Riverhead Books, 2007.

Keane, Webb. *Christian Moderns: Freedom & Fetish in the Mission Encounter*. Berkeley: University of California Press, 2006.

Klima, Alan. *The Funeral Casino: Meditation, Massacre, and Exchange with the Dead in Thailand*. Princeton, NJ: Princeton University Press, 2002.

Kolsky, Elizabeth. *Colonial Justice in British India*. Cambridge: Cambridge University Press, 2010.

Kostal, R. W. *Law and English Railway Capitalism, 1825–1875*. Oxford: Clarendon Press, 1994.

Kusiak, Pauline. "Instrumentalized Rationality, Cross-Cultural Mediators, and Civil Epistemologies of Late Colonialism." *Social Studies of Science* 40, no. 6 (2010): 871–902.

Kwon, Heonik. *Ghosts of War in Vietnam*. Cambridge: Cambridge University Press, 2008.

Lam, Tong. *A Passion for Facts: Social Surveys and the Construction of the Chinese Nation-State, 1900–1949*. Berkeley: University of California Press, 2011.

Langford, Jean. *Consoling Ghosts: Stories of Medicine and Mourning from Southeast Asians in Exile*. Minneapolis: University of Minnesota Press, 2013.

Laqueur, Thomas. *The Work of the Dead: A Cultural History of Mortal Remains*. Princeton, NJ: Princeton University Press, 2015.

Latour, Bruno. "Morality and Technology: The End of the Means." Translated by Couze Venn. *Theory, Culture & Society* 19, no. 5–6 (2002): 247–60.

——. *The Pasteurization of France*. Cambridge, MA: Harvard University Press, 1988.

——. "Postmodern? No, Simply Amodern. Steps Towards an Anthropology of Science: An Essay Review." *Studies in History and Philosophy of Science* 21, no. 1 (1990): 145–71.

——. *Reassembling the Social: An Introduction to Actor-Network-Theory*. Oxford: Oxford University Press, 2005.

——. *We Have Never Been Modern*. Cambridge, MA: Harvard University Press, 1993.

Lawan Chotamara. *Moradok thai: ruam rueang rao khong watthanatham na ru thi an sanuk yang mai na chua* [*Thai heritage: A Collection of entertaining and incredible stories about our culture*]. Bangkok: Samnak phim Ratchawadi, 2536 [1993].

Layton, Catherine. *The Life and Times of Mary, Dowager Duchess of Sutherland: Power Play*. Newcastle upon Tyne: Cambridge Scholars Publishing, 2018.

Lesy, Michael. *Wisconsin Death Trip*. New York: Pantheon, 1973.

Lim, Samson. "The Aesthetics of Evidence: Crime and Conspiracy in Thailand's Popular Press." PhD diss., Cornell University, 2012.

——. *Siam's New Detectives: Visualizing Crime and Conspiracy in Modern Thailand*. Honolulu: University of Hawai'i Press, 2016.

Lingat, R. "Evolution of the Concept of Law in Burma and Siam." *Journal of the Siam Society* 38, no. 1 (1950): 9–31.

——. "Note sur la Revision des Lois Siamoises en 1805." *Journal of the Siam Society* 23, no. 1 (1929): 19–27.

Liu, Lydia H. "Injury: Incriminating Words and Imperial Power." In *Words in Motion: Toward a Global Lexicon*, edited by Carol Gluck and Anna Lowenhaupt Tsing, 198–218. Durham, NC: Duke University Press, 2009.

Lomnitz, Claudio. *Death and the Idea of Mexico*. Brooklyn, NY: Zone Books, 2005.

Loos, Tamara. *Bones Around My Neck: The Life and Exile of a Prince Provocateur*. Ithaca, NY: Cornell University Press, 2016.

——. "Gender Adjudicated: Translating Modern Legal Subjects in Siam." PhD diss., Cornell University, 1999.

——. "Issaraphap: Limits of Individual Liberty in Thai Jurisprudence." *Crossroads: An Interdisciplinary Journal of Southeast Asian Studies* 12, no. 1 (1998): 35–75.

——. *Subject Siam: Family, Law, and Colonial Modernity in Thailand*. Ithaca, NY: Cornell University Press, 2006.

Mantena, Karuna. *Alibis of Empire: Henry Maine and the Ends of Liberal Imperialism*. Princeton, NJ: Princeton University Press, 2010.

Martin, Susan M. *The UP Saga*. Copenhagen: Nordic Institute of Asian Studies, 2003.

Marx, Karl. "The Eighteenth Brumaire of Louis Bonaparte." In *The Marx-Engels Reader*, edited by Robert C. Tucker, 594–617. New York: W. W. Norton, 1978.

Masaji Chiba, ed. *Asian Indigenous Law: In Interaction with Received Law*. London: KPI, 1986.

Matics, K. I. "Hell Scenes in Thai Murals." *Journal of the Siam Society* 67, no. 2 (1979): 35–39.

Mbembe, J. A. "Necropolitics." Translated by Libby Meintjes. *Public Culture* 15, no. 1 (2003): 11–40.

McCraken, John. "Customary Law in Colonial Africa." *Journal of African History* 28, no. 1 (1987): 169–70.

McDaniel, Justin. *The Lovelorn Ghost and the Magical Monk: Practicing Buddhism in Modern Thailand*. New York: Columbia University Press, 2011.

Mead, Kullada Kesboonchoo. *The Rise and Decline of Thai Absolutism*. London: RoutledgeCurzon, 2004.

Merli, Claudia. *Bodily Practices and Medical Identities in Southern Thailand*. Uppsala: Uppsala University Press, 2008.

Merry, Sally Engle. *Colonizing Hawai'i: The Cultural Power of Law*. Princeton, NJ: Princeton University Press, 2000.

Monnais, Laurence, and Harold J. Cook, eds. *Global Movements, Local Concerns: Medicine and Health in Southeast Asia*. Singapore: NUS Press, 2012.

Monruethai Chaiwiset. "*Prawattisat sangkhom: suam lae khrueang sukkhaphan nai prathet thai (pho. so. 2440–2540)*" ["A social history: Lavatories and sanitary ware in Thailand, 1897–1997"]. Master's thesis, Thammasat University, 2542 [1999].

——. *Prawattisat sangkhom: wa duai suam lae khrueang sukkhaphan nai prathet thai* [A social history of lavatories and sanitary ware in Thailand]. Bangkok: Matichon, 2545 [2002].

Moore, Sally Falk. *Social Facts and Fabrications: "Customary" Law on Kilimanjaro, 1880–1908*. Cambridge: Cambridge University Press, 1986.

Moosa, Ebrahim. "Interface of Science and Jurisprudence: Dissonant Gazes at the Body in Modern Muslim Ethics." In *God, Life and the Cosmos: Christian and Islamic Perspectives*, edited by Ted Peters, Muzzaffar Iqbal, and Syed Nomanul Haq, 329–56. Aldershot, UK: Ashgate, 2002.

Morris, Rosalind C. "Giving Up Ghosts: Notes on Trauma and the Possibility of the Political from Southeast Asia." *Positions* 16, no. 1 (2008): 229–58.

——. *In the Place of Origins: Modernity and Its Mediums in Northern Thailand*. Durham, NC: Duke University Press, 2000.

——. "Surviving Pleasure at the Periphery: Chiang Mai and the Photographies of Political Trauma in Thailand, 1976–1992." *Public Culture* 10, no. 2 (1998): 341–70.

Mosley, Charles, ed. *Burke's Peerage, Baronetage & Knightage*, 107th ed. Wilmington, DE: Genealogical Books, 2003.

Mulholland, Jean. "Thai Traditional Medicine: Ancient Thought and Practice in a Thai Context." *Journal of the Siam Society* 67, no. 2 (1979): 80–115.

Munsterhjelm, Mark. *Living Dead in the Pacific: Contested Sovereignty and Racism in Genetic Research on Taiwan Aborigines*. Vancouver: University of British Columbia Press, 2014.

Murray, Stuart J. "Thanatopolitics: On the Use of Death for Mobilizing Political Life." *Polygraph* 18 (2006): 191–215.

Nitaya Kanchanawan. "Changing to the New World: High-Tech Verbalization in Thai." In *Papers from the Fourth Annual Meeting of the Southeast Asian Linguistics Society*, edited by Udom Warotamasikkhadit and Thanyarat Panakul, 143–56. Phoenix: Arizona State University, Program for Southeast Asian Studies, 1998.

Nitilak Kaewchandee. *"Kotmai boran isan: sathanaphap ong khwam ru lae kho khit hen bang prakan"* ["Isan ancient law: State of knowledge and some reflections"]. *Proceedings of the 16th Annual Meeting of Sociology and Anthropology Branches, Princess Maha Chakri Sirindhorn Anthropology Centre and Naresuan University* 2559 [2016]: 79–99.

Nonthaphorn Yumangmi. *"Wipayok klang sai nam kap ruang lao 'Sadet mae Sunantha'"* ["Tragedy in mid-stream and the story of 'Royal Mother Sunantha'"]. *Sinlapa watthanantham [Art & culture]* 31, no. 1 (2009): 76–101.

O'Connor, Richard A. "Law as Indigenous Social Theory: A Siamese Thai Case." *American Ethnologist* 8, no. 2 (1981): 223–37.

Olson, Grant A. "Filling the Void: Thai Khwan and Burmese Leip-pya, the Stuff of Which Souls Are Made." In *Socially Engaged Spirituality: Essays in Honor of Sulak Sivaraksa on His 70th Birthday*, edited by David W. Chappell, 271–302. Bangkok: Sathirakoses-Nagapradipa Foundation, 2003.

Pasuk Phongpaichit, and Chris Baker. *Thailand: Economy and Politics*, 2nd ed. New York: Oxford, 2002.

Pattana Kitiarsa. "Beyond Syncretism: Hybridization of Popular Religion in Contemporary Thailand." *Journal of Southeast Asian Studies* 36, no. 3 (2005): 461–87.

Pearson, Quentin A. III. *Bodies Politic: Civil Law & Forensic Medicine in Colonial Era Bangkok*. PhD diss., Cornell University, 2014.

——. "'DNA Evidence Cannot Lie': Forensic Science, Truth Regimes, and Civic Epistemology in Thai History." In *Global Forensic Cultures: Making Fact and Justice in the Modern Era*, edited by Ian A. Burney and Christopher Hamlin, 235–54. Baltimore: Johns Hopkins University Press, 2019.

——. "Morbid Subjects: Forensic Medicine and Sovereignty in Siam." *Modern Asian Studies* 52, no. 2 (2018): 394–420.

Peleggi, Maurizio. *Lords of Things: The Fashioning of the Siamese Monarchy's Modern Image*. Honolulu: University of Hawai'i Press, 2002.

Peller, Gary. "The Metaphysics of American Law." *California Law Review* 73, no. 4 (1985): 1151–290.

Philippe Marchat, ed. *Jeune Diplomate Au Siam (1894–1900): Lettres de mon Grand-père Raphaël Réau*. Issy-les-Moulineaux: Muller, 2009.

Pierce, Steven, and Anupama Rao, eds. *Discipline and the Other Body*. Durham, NC: Duke University Press, 2006.

Pietz, William. "Death of the Deodand: Accursed Objects and the Money Value of Human Life." *RES: Anthropology and Aesthetics* 31 (1997): 97–108.

——. "The Fetish of Civilization: Sacrificial Blood and Monetary Debt." In *Colonial Subjects: Essays on the Practical History of Anthropology*, edited by Peter Pels and Oscar Salemink, 53–81. Ann Arbor: University of Michigan Press, 1999.

——. "Person." In *Critical Terms for the Study of Buddhism*, edited by Donald S. Lopez Jr., 188–210. Chicago: University of Chicago Press, 2005.

Pitts, Jennifer. *A Turn to Empire: The Rise of Imperial Liberalism in Britain and France*. Princeton, NJ: Princeton University Press, 2006.

Poovey, Mary. *A History of the Modern Fact: Problems of Knowledge in the Science of Wealth and Society*. Chicago: University of Chicago Press, 1998.

Porphant Ouyyanont. "Bangkok's Population & The Ministry of the Capital in Early 20th Century Thai History." *Southeast Asian Studies* 35, no. 2 (1997): 240–60.

Prakash, Gyan. *Another Reason: Science and the Imagination of Colonial India*. Princeton, NJ: Princeton University Press, 1999.

Prathan Watanavanich. "The Emergence of Victims' Rights in Thailand: Twenty Years after the U.N. Declaration of Basic Principles of Justice for Victims of Crime and Abuse of Power." *United Nations Asia and Far East Institute for the Prevention of Crime and the Treatment of Offenders Resource Material Series* 70 (2006).

Prayut Sithiphan. "*Khadi phra nang rua lom*" ["The case of the capsized princess"]. In *San thai nai adit* [Thai courts in the past], 2nd ed., 227–36. Bangkok: Sang san buk: 2551 [2008].

Ramnath, Kalyani. "The Colonial Difference between Law and Fact: Notes on the Criminal Jury in India." *Indian Economic Social History Review* 50, no. 3 (2013): 341–63.

Razack, Sherene H. *Dying from Improvement: Inquests and Inquiries into Indigenous Deaths in Custody*. Toronto: University of Toronto Press, 2015.

Reynolds, Craig J. "A Seditious Poem and Its History." In *Seditious Histories: Contesting Thai and Southeast Asian Pasts*, 80–101. Seattle: University of Washington Press, 2006.

———. "Buddhist Cosmography in Thai History, with Special Reference to Nineteenth-Century Culture Change." *Journal of Asian Studies* 35, no. 2 (1976): 203–20.

———. "Feudalism as a Trope for the Past." In *Seditious Histories: Contesting Thai and Southeast Asian Pasts*, 102–21. Seattle: University of Washington Press, 2006.

———. "The Plot of Thai History: Theory and Practice." In *Patterns and Illusions: Thai History and Thought*, edited by Gehan Wijeyewardene and E. C. Chapman, 313–32. Canberra: Australia National University, 1992.

———. *Thai Radical Discourse: The Real Face of Thai Feudalism Today*. Ithaca, NY: Southeast Asia Program, Cornell University, 1987.

Reynolds, Craig J., and Hong Lysa. "Marxism in Thai Historical Studies." *Journal of Asian Studies* 43, no. 1 (1983): 77–104.

Rutherford, Danilyn. *Laughing at Leviathan: Sovereignty and Audience in West Papua*. Chicago: University of Chicago Press, 2012.

Saha, Jonathan. "'Uncivilized Practitioners': Medical Subordinates, Medico-legal Evidence and Misconduct in Colonial Burma, 1875–1907." *South East Asia Research* 20, no. 3 (2012): 423–43.

Sartori, Andrew. "The British Empire and Its Liberal Mission." *Journal of Modern History* 78, no. 3 (2006): 623–42.

Sayre, Francis Bowes. "The Passing of Extraterritoriality in Siam." *American Journal of International Law* 22, no. 1 (1928): 70–88.

Scarry, Elaine. "Consent and the Body: Injury, Departure and Desire." *New Literary History* 21, no. 4 (1990): 867–97.

Schopen, Gregory. "Archaeology and Protestant Presuppositions in the Study of Indian Buddhism." *History of Religions* 31, no. 1 (1991): 1–23.

Seeman, Erik. *Death in the New World: Cross-Cultural Encounters, 1492–1800*. Philadelphia: University of Pennsylvania Press, 2010.

Shapin, Steven. *Never Pure: Historical Studies of Science as if It Was Produced by People with Bodies, Situated in Time, Space, Culture, and Society, and Struggling for Credibility and Authority*. Baltimore: Johns Hopkins University Press, 2010.

Sharafi, Mitra. *Law and Identity in Colonial South Asia: Parsi Legal Culture, 1772–1947*. New York: Cambridge University Press, 2014.

Shigeharu Tanabe. "The Person in Transformation: Body, Mind and Cultural Appropriation." In *Cultural Crisis and Social Memory: Modernity and Identity in Thailand and Laos*, edited by S. Tanabe and C. F. Keyes, 43–67. Honolulu: University of Hawai'i Press, 2002.

Siffin, William J. *The Thai Bureaucracy: Institutional Change and Development*. Honolulu: East-West Center Press, 1966.

Silverman, Robert A. *Law and Urban Growth: Civil Litigation in the Boston Trial Courts, 1880–1900*. Princeton, NJ: Princeton University Press, 1981.

Singer, Brain C. J., and Lorna Weir. "Politics and Sovereign Power: Considerations on Foucault." *European Journal of Social Theory* 9, no. 4 (2006): 443–65.

Skinner, G. William. *Chinese Society in Thailand: An Analytical History*. Ithaca, NY: Cornell University Press, 1957.

Smith, Harry. "From Deodand to Dependency." *American Journal of Legal History* 11, no. 4 (1967): 389–403.

Spieker, Sven. *The Big Archive: Art from Bureaucracy*. Cambridge, MA: MIT Press, 2008.

Star, Susan Leigh, and James R. Griesemer. "Institutional Ecology, 'Translation,' and Boundary Objects: Amateurs and Professionals in Berkeley's Museum of Vertebrate Zoology, 1907–39." *Social Studies of Science* 19, no. 3 (1989): 387–420.

Sterling, Joyce, and Nancy Reichman. "The Cultural Agenda of Tort Litigation: Constructing Responsibility in the Rocky Mountain Frontier." In *Fault Lines: Tort Law as Cultural Practice*, edited by David M. Engel and Michael McCann, 287–306. Stanford, CA: Stanford Law Books, 2009.

Sternstein, Larry. "Bangkok at the Turn of the Century: Mongkut and Chulalongkorn Entertain the West." *Journal of the Siam Society* 54, no. 1 (1966): 55–71.

Stoler, Ann Laura. *Along the Archival Grain: Epistemic Anxieties and Colonial Common Sense*. Princeton, NJ: Princeton University Press, 2009.

Strand, David. *Rickshaw Beijing: City People and Politics in the 1920s*. Berkeley: University of California Press, 1989.

Strate, Shane. *The Lost Territories: Thailand's History of National Humiliation*. Honolulu: University of Hawai'i Press, 2015.

Streckfuss, David. *Truth on Trial in Thailand: Defamation, Treason, and Lèse-majesté*. London: Routledge, 2011.

Streets-Salter, Heather. *Martial Races: The Military, Race, and Masculinity in British Imperial Culture, 1857–1914*. Manchester: Manchester University Press, 2004.

Surapong Jankasamepong. "*Bot bat thang kan-phim lae khun upakan khong mo samit to sangkhom thai*" ["The benefaction of Dr. Smith to Thai society and his role in printing"]. *Sinlapa watthanatham* [*Art & culture*] 27, no. 9 (2006): 78–92.

Sutton, Teresa. "The Deodand and Responsibility for Death." *Journal of Legal History* 18, no. 3 (1997): 44–55.

Swearer, Donald. *Buddhist World of Southeast Asia*, 2nd ed. Albany: SUNY Press, 2010.

Takashi Tomosugi. *Reminiscences of Old Bangkok: Memory and the Identification of a Changing Society*. [Tokyo]: The Institute of Oriental Culture, University of Tokyo, 1993.

Tambiah, Stanley J. *Buddhism and the Spirit Cults in North-East Thailand*. Cambridge: Cambridge University Press, 1970.

Taussig, Michael T. "Culture of Terror—Space of Death." In *Colonialism and Culture*, edited by Nicholas B. Dirks, 135–73. Ann Arbor: University of Michigan Press, 1992.

Tej Bunnag. *The Provincial Administration of Siam from 1892 to 1915: The Ministry of the Interior under Prince Damrong Rachanuphap*. New York: Oxford, 1977.

Textor, Robert B. *Roster of the Gods: An Ethnography of the Supernatural in a Thai Village*, vols. 1–6. New Haven, CT: Human Relations Area Files, 1973.

Thanapol Limapichart. "The Emergence of the Siamese Public Sphere: Colonial Modernity, Print Culture, and the Practice of Criticism (1860s–1910s)." *South-East Asia Research* 17, no. 3 (2009): 361–99.

Thanet Aphornsuvan. "Slavery and Modernity: Freedom in the Making of Modern Siam." In *Asian Freedoms: The Idea of Freedom in South and Southeast Asia*, edited by David Kelly and Anthony Reid, 161–86. Cambridge: Cambridge University Press, 1998.

——. "The West and Siam's Quest for Modernity: Siamese Responses to Nineteenth Century American Missionaries." *South East Asia Research* 17, no. 3 (2009): 401–31.

Thongchai Winichakul. *"Prawatisat thai baeb rachachat niyom"* ["Thai history in the royal-nationalist mode"]. *Sinlapa watthanantham [Art & culture]* 23, no. 1 (2001): 56–65.

——. "The Quest for *Siwilai*: A Geographical Discourse of Civilizational Thinking in Late Nineteenth and Early Twentieth-Century Siam." *Journal of Asian Studies* 59, no. 3 (2000): 528–49.

——. *Siam Mapped: History of the Geo-body of a Nation*. Honolulu: University of Hawai'i Press, 1994.

Thornely, P. W. *The History of a Transition*. Bangkok: Siam Observer Press, 1923.

Timmermans, Stefan. *Postmortem: How Medical Examiners Explain Suspicious Death*. Chicago: University of Chicago Press, 2006.

Todd, David. "Beneath Sovereignty: Extraterritoriality and Imperial Internationalism in Nineteenth-Century Egypt." *Law & History Review* 36, no. 1 (2018): 105–37.

Turnbull, David. *Masons, Tricksters, and Cartographers: Comparative Studies in the Sociology of Scientific and Indigenous Knowledge*. Amsterdam: Harwood, 2000.

Turton, Andrew. "Introduction to *Civility and Savagery*." In *Civility and Savagery: Social Identity in Tai States*, edited by Andrew Turton, 3–32. Richmond, Surrey: Curzon, 2000.

——. "Thai Institutions of Slavery." In *Asian and African Systems of Slavery*, edited by James L. Watson, 251–92. Berkeley: University of California Press, 1980.

Unger, Mangabeira. *Knowledge and Politics*. New York: The Free Press, 1975.

Vella, Walter F. *The Impact of the West on Government in Thailand*. Berkeley: University of California Press, 1955.

Verdery, Katherine. *The Political Lives of Dead Bodies: Reburial and Postsocialist Change*. New York: Columbia University Press, 1999.

Virilio, Paul. *The Original Accident*. Malden, MA: Polity Press, 2007.

Wagner, Kim A. *Stranglers and Bandits: A Historical Anthology of Thuggee*. New York: Oxford University Press, 2009.

——. *Thuggee: Banditry and the British in Early Nineteenth-Century India*. New York: Palgrave Macmillan, 2007.

Walter, Tony. "Mediator Deathworks." *Death Studies* 29, no. 5 (2005): 383–412.

Wan Waithayakon, Prince. "Thai Word Coining." *Journal of the Siam Society* 89 (2001): 90–93.

Warren, James A. *Gambling, the State, and Society in Thailand c. 1800–1945*. New York: Routledge, 2013.

Weber, Max. "Politics as Vocation." In *Weber's Rationalism and Modern Society*, edited by Tony Waters and Dagmar Waters, 129–98. New York: Palgrave Macmillan Books, 2015.

Welke, Barbara Young. *Recasting American Liberty: Gender, Race, Law, and the Railroad Revolution*. New York: Cambridge University Press, 2001.

——. "Unreasonable Women: Gender and the Law of Accidental Injury, 1870–1920." *Law and Social Inquiry* 19 (1994): 369–403.

Weston, Nancy A. "The Metaphysics of Modern Tort Theory." *Valparaiso University Law Review* 28, no. 3 (1994): 919–1006.

Wiener, Martin J. *An Empire on Trial: Race, Murder, and Justice under British Rule, 1870–1935.* Cambridge: Cambridge University Press, 2009.

Wilaiwan Kanittanan, and James Placzek. "Historical and Contemporary Meanings of Thai *Khwan*: The Use of Lexical Meaning Change as an Indicator of Cultural Change." In *Religion, Values, and Development in Southeast Asia*, edited by Bruce Matthews and Judith Nagata, 146–67. Singapore: Institute of Southeast Asian Studies, 1986.

Wyatt, David K. "Family Politics in Nineteenth Century Thailand." *Journal of Southeast Asian History* 9, no. 2 (1968): 208–28.

——. *Thailand: A Short History.* New Haven, CT: Yale University Press, 1982.

Yurchak, Alexei. "Bodies of Lenin: The Hidden Science of Communist Sovereignty." *Representations* 129, no. 1 (2015): 116–57.

Zelizer, Viviana A. *Pricing the Priceless Child: The Changing Social Value of Children.* New York: Basic Books, 1985.

Index

Lightning Source UK Ltd.
Milton Keynes UK
UKHW010326140220
358721UK00002B/380/J

9 781501 740152